KETO
comfort foods

family favorite recipes made low-carb and healthy

Maria Emmerich

First Published in 2017 by Victory Belt Publishing Inc.

ISBN-13: 978-1-628602-57-9

The author is not a licensed practitioner, physician, or medical professional and offers no medical diagnoses, treatments, suggestions, or counseling. The information presented herein has not been evaluated by the U.S. Food and Drug Administration, and it is not intended to diagnose, treat, cure, or prevent any disease. Full medical clearance from a licensed physician should be obtained before beginning or modifying any diet, exercise, or lifestyle program, and physicians should be informed of all nutritional changes.

The author/owner claims no responsibility to any person or entity for any liability, loss, or damage caused or alleged to be caused directly or indirectly as a result of the use, application, or interpretation of the information presented herein.

Front and Back Cover Photography by Hayley Mason and Bill Staley

Interior Design by Yordan Terziev and Boryana Yordanova

Printed in Canada

TC 0518

Table of Contents

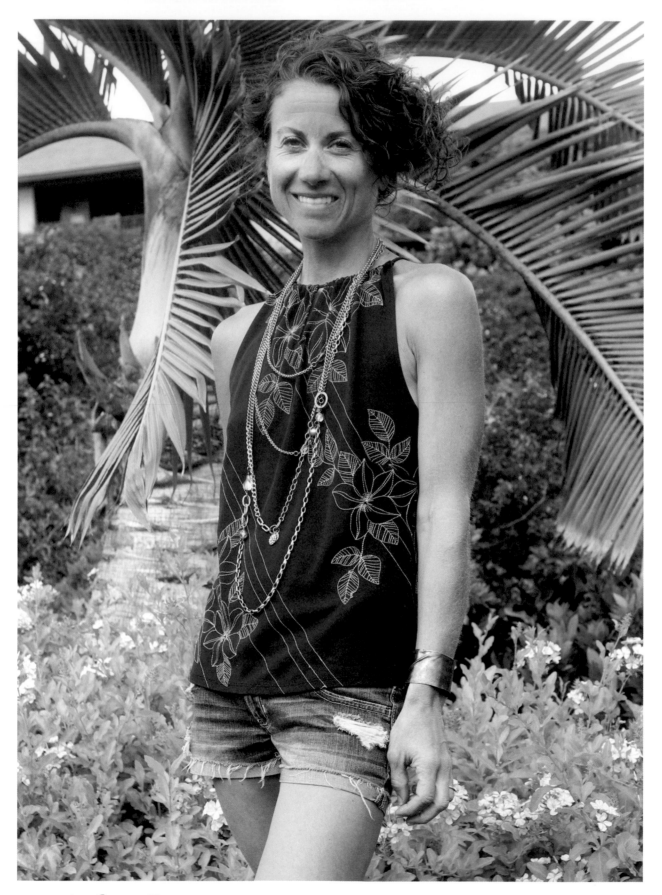

Introduction

food *is celebratory,*
food *triggers memories,*
food *stirs emotions.*

I had the great pleasure to travel to New Orleans for business in 2011 and was taken to eat at an amazing restaurant on Bourbon Street called Muriel's. Our group was seated not in the main dining area, but in a haunted private dining room! I had the étouffée, on which my Crawfish Étouffée recipe (page 246) is based. The kitchen staff also prepared special Swerve-sweetened sugar-free desserts for our table.

A lot of the people I was dining with were locals. They asked me how I stay keto and said that it is extremely difficult to do in New Orleans because the local motto is "live to eat," not "eat to live," which I found quite interesting.

We're often told to regard food as fuel and nothing else, but food is more than that. Even at the young age of two and a half, my son demonstrated how food is more than just nourishment. He would jump into his booster chair, buckle in, and start to sing. It wasn't because he was getting chicken nuggets, boxed macaroni and cheese, or a bowl of ice cream. In one video I have of him, I was making my Meatballs with Brown Gravy (page 216), and he was singing at the top of his lungs simply because it was mealtime. Food is pleasure, food is love. Food should also be nourishing, and that's why I was so excited to write this book. It is filled with pleasure, love, and nourishing foods.

It isn't a bad thing to enjoy food. My goal is for you to fall in love with ketogenic foods so that you can nourish your soul *and* your body.

I have had the pleasure of writing numerous cookbooks, and I will never be able to pick a favorite; however, I think this book was the most fun to write. I really enjoyed reminiscing about my favorite foods from my former unhealthy diet and pondering how to recreate such favorites as Bomba Burgers and Death by Chocolate Cheesecake as keto dishes. What I find extraordinary is that I enjoy the taste of these recipes even more than the traditional carb- and sugar-filled versions!

As I continue to grow with my cooking, I am finding techniques that are fantastic at adding that special "umami" flavor profile. Umami is a savory flavor that is sometimes described as the fifth taste, along with sweet, sour, salty, and bitter. This book is filled with amazing recipes that will make you feel satisfied on your ketogenic journey.

Keto isn't a diet to me or my family; it is a way of life. We enjoy feeling this amazing, so we never want to veer away from ketogenic foods. We aren't tempted by traditional mashed potatoes or wheat-filled breads. I think the main reason we are never enticed is that I'm always on the hunt for new ways to make ketogenic foods even more comforting and delicious.

Food is tradition!

I'm guessing you and your family have a few traditions that are food-related. When I was a child, we always had lasagna on my birthday. I love lasagna, especially BBQ chicken lasagna, and I always made it for my siblings' birthdays. My brothers and sister and I would gather at our parents' house, and we would celebrate with my lasagna and then play a fun game of volleyball outside.

Food is memory!

Many years ago I worked at a restaurant called High View that specialized in fried fish. Whenever I ride my bicycle past the lovely Tin Fish restaurant on Lake Calhoun in Minneapolis, I am immediately transported back to my time working at High View, which also happened to be when I fell in love with my now-husband, Craig. I'm not a huge fan of fried fish, but I adore that smell because of the amazing time in my life that it conjures.

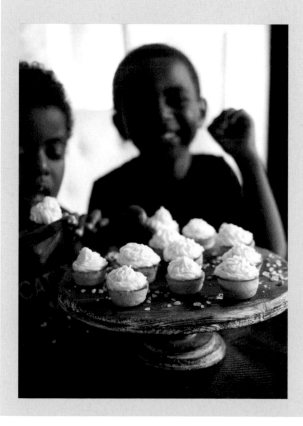

Food is love!

Food is a great way to show love and affection. I often give food-related gifts for the holidays and friends' birthdays. Even when I was a poor college student, I would make homemade food gifts for my friends and family. It was usually caramel apple pie (not healthified!), unbaked and frozen, with a label on it explaining how to bake it so that the recipients could enjoy a fresh-baked pie whenever they desired.

I still love to give food gifts, but I choose healthified gifts now. This past year I made gift baskets filled with a bag of Swerve sweetener, chocolates from ChocoPerfection, and Primal Kitchen Greek salad dressing, as well as my homemade taco seasoning. The reason I love to include this taco seasoning mix is that it also helps educate people. I had a family member tell me that he hadn't been feeling well for quite some time, so he decided to cut out gluten, but it hadn't helped. I asked him if he had cut out smoked meats, beef jerky, spice mixes, and a few other products, all of which contain gluten. He hadn't. Once he started following the rules on my avoid-hidden-gluten plan, he finally began to feel amazing.

Food is celebratory!

When I ran my first marathon, my parents took me out to eat afterward. When I graduated from college, we celebrated at a fun German restaurant filled with traditional German food and accordion music.

We often celebrate major life events with food. Weddings, funerals, and other rites of passage all include food. This isn't a bad thing; food helps bring us together to celebrate someone's life, a couple's commitment to each other, or someone's hard work and achievements. The trick is to learn to celebrate with foods that your body will celebrate, too!

my first food memories

I had a great childhood. I remember going to visit my Grandma Betty and Grandpa Jerry way out in the country. They didn't have much, but going to see them was always fun. Both of my grandparents were amazing musicians, so there was always music. And there were always brownies with more frosting than brownie. You could smell the sweet aroma of chocolate wafting from their mobile home before the door even opened. Grandma Betty always made a pan without crushed walnuts on top because she knew that my brother and I didn't like them with nuts. Grandpa would sing "How Much Is That Doggie in the Window?" while they both played guitar, and my brother and I would dance around with chocolate-coated fingers.

I had a few amazing jobs that centered around food when I was in high school. I worked at the cutest coffee shop called Uncommon Ground, where I learned to make scones (page 48), pumpkin muffins (page 52), mochas (page 36), and Italian sodas (page 298). I adored working there. I loved the morning rush of businesspeople coming in for coffee and a muffin and the fun musicians who played there in the evenings. I still dream of opening up a ketogenic coffee shop where I would serve delicious and nourishing comfort foods, with a variety of musicians playing to accompany the tasty food.

My other job in high school was as a hostess and waitress at High View, the "fancy" steak and seafood restaurant in town. It had a beautiful view of a small quaint lake. I grew up eating at this restaurant. When I was little, my parents would take us there every Friday night. My brother and I would bring our fishing poles, and we would fish until my mother called us in to eat. When I was sixteen, I started to waitress there. High View was known for surf and turf (page 245) and on rare occasions would serve lobster (which inspired my Butter-Poached Lobster on page 254). I still miss the hustle and bustle of the busy restaurant kitchen.

I could go on and on about my memories of food, but my point is that food is a huge part of everyday life. Even the simple smell of fried fish can bring back memories! I love comfort food, and I continue to celebrate holidays by baking special keto treats with my boys so that they will have special memories of time in the kitchen with loved ones just like I do.

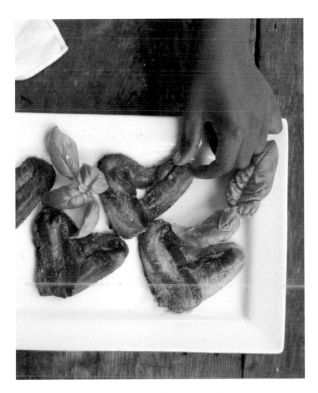

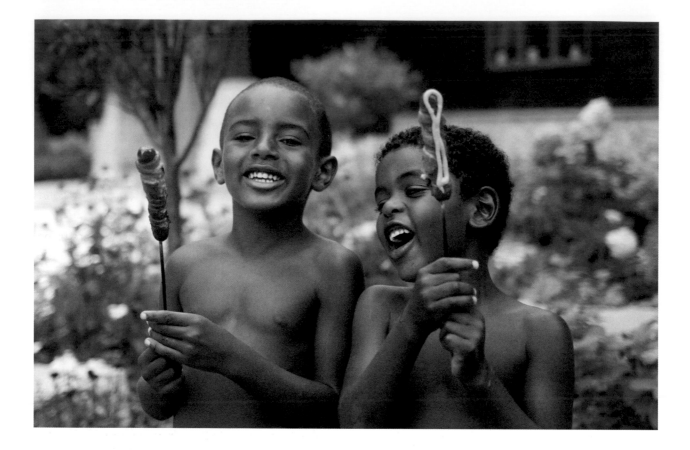

why I wrote a book focused on comfort foods

In 2013, I had the opportunity to speak on a low-carb cruise hosted by my friend and coauthor Jimmy Moore. (Check out our book *The Ketogenic Cookbook.*) While I was on the cruise, one of the ketogenic doctors who spoke asked why I allow sweet treats even if they are made with stevia or Swerve (a natural sweetener like stevia). I proudly stood up, found my most confident voice, and explained that I have two young children who are bombarded with images of cupcakes, candy, juice boxes, and sugary cereals, all in fake bright colors to capture their attention. So to keep my kids from rebelling and pleading for that junk, I offer them safe treats at home. My son Micah even asks if certain foods contain sugar or gluten and

would cause his belly to hurt, and I say yes. Then he asks if we have cupcakes at home that are healthy, and I either say yes or suggest that we bake some together. He gladly chooses the safe treat. He doesn't have celiac disease, but sugar and grains make him feel ill, which often happens to my clients when they consume sugar or starch after months of avoiding them.

I also love to entertain, and that includes serving desserts that we all can enjoy. I even love to throw parties for dolls! Micah has a doll that he named Libby, and he loves her very much. He recently told me that Libby's birthday was in three days. So we had keto cake and keto ice cream to celebrate!

there are a few reasons why i love to make ketogenic comfort foods:

Food marketing to my kids

I'm competing against a multitrillion-dollar food industry that markets products filled with dyes, chemicals, and sugar to children. Providing cute keto treats keeps my kids happy. I also teach them how certain foods will make them feel good, be super-smart, and run fast!

We live in a society that celebrates with food.

What's the first thing that comes to mind when I say . . .

Thanksgiving: I think of pumpkin pie.

Christmas: I think of Christmas cookies and eggnog.

Valentine's Day: Do you think chocolate?

Birthdays: Do you think of cake and ice cream?

State Fair: This annual event is synonymous with deep-fried cheese curds, corn dogs, and deep-fried Twinkies!

They all bring up images of food!

Even when our children learn to go on the potty as toddlers, we reward them with food. Micah always asked for kale chips, but still, food was his reward. I hear all the time from parents who are frustrated when their kids' Little League team goes out for ice cream after every game. One of my clients sent me a picture of the giant bag of Skittles that her type 1 diabetic second grader was given for scoring 100 percent on her math test!

Cooking and baking are my therapy.

I love to create beautiful food. I enjoy being in the kitchen on a rainy day. (If it's nice out, I prefer to be outside on my bicycle or kayak!) I'm not one to meditate on a mat with my eyes closed. I like to think of my cooking and baking time as mindful meditation.

Some healthcare clinics and counselors are using cooking or baking as a therapy tool for people suffering from depression, anxiety, and other mental health problems. Sounds crazy, right? But cooking soothes stress, builds self-esteem, and helps curb negative self-talk by focusing the mind on following a recipe.

It has helped me stick to this lifestyle for over a decade!

If it were up to Craig, I would make meatloaf cake instead of my Death by Chocolate Cheesecake (page 310) for birthdays, but I love dessert. Having keto treats at home helps me say no to a slice of cake at a party. If I never let myself have a treat like keto ice cream (I always have some on hand), I wouldn't be able to say no to sugar-filled treats. Allowing myself keto indulgences ensures that I never feel deprived.

And with the recipes in this book, *you* will never feel deprived, either! Whether your old favorite comfort foods were sugary desserts or carb-laden bowls of pasta, I've got you covered. Enjoy!

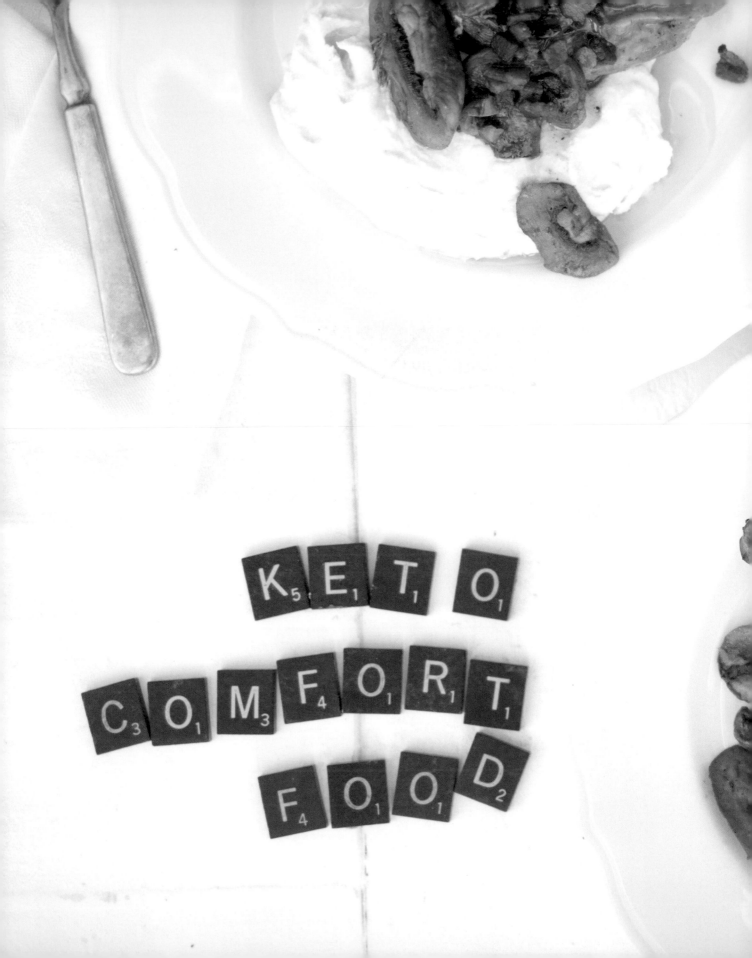

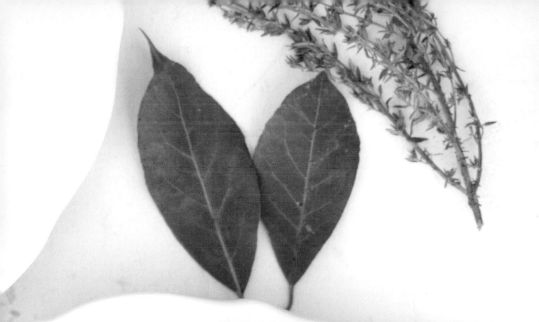

part 1
THE KETOGENIC KITCHEN

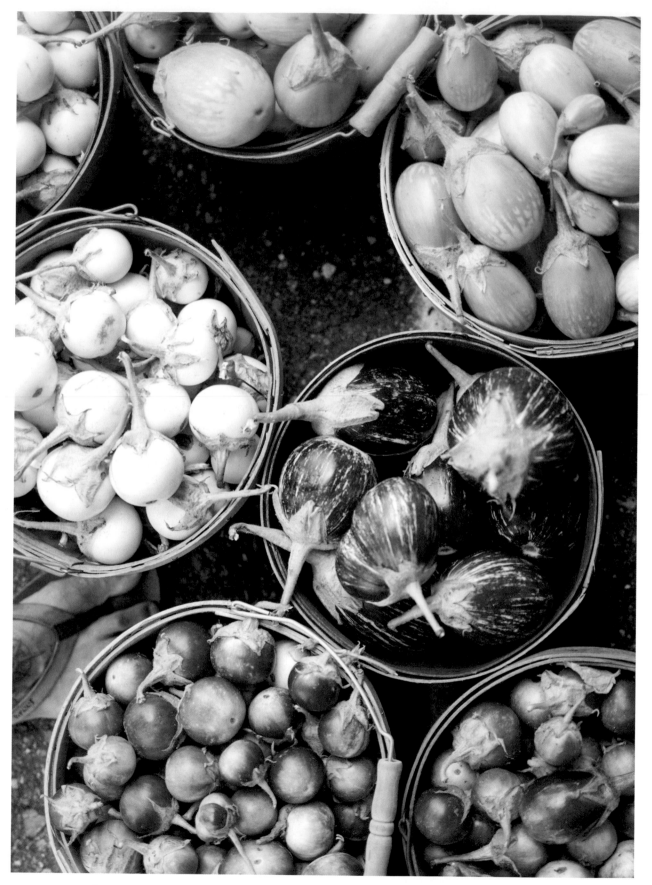

Keto Comfort Foods

Ingredients

The key to any healthy diet is eating real, whole foods. When following a ketogenic diet, you'll want to seek out keto-friendly ingredients and avoid those that aren't.

fats

On a keto diet, you need lots of healthy fat to burn as fuel. But as important as it is to seek out healthy fats, it's just as critical to avoid unhealthy fats.

healthy fats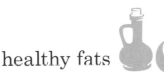

Fats with high amounts of saturated fatty acids (SFAs)—such as MCT oil, coconut oil, butter, ghee, tallow, and lard—are best: they are stable and anti-inflammatory, protect against oxidation, and have many other important health benefits. Organic and grass-fed or pastured sources are always best.

On page 14 is a list of the best fats and oils to use, with their SFA and PUFA content (see page 15 for more on PUFAs). When you see "keto fat" mentioned in a recipe in this book, know that it's fine to use any of these fats—just make sure to take into account whether you need it for a hot or a cold use.

If you're not dairy-sensitive, the following are great healthy, keto-friendly dairy fats to include in your diet:

- **Butter:** 50% SFA, 3.4% PUFA
- **Ghee*:** 48% SFA, 4% PUFA
- **Heavy cream:** 62% SFA, 4% PUFA
- **Cheddar cheese:** 64% SFA, 3% PUFA
- **Cream cheese:** 56% SFA, 4% PUFA
- **Sour cream:** 58% SFA, 4% PUFA
- **Crème fraîche:** 64% SFA, 3% PUFA

You may be able to tolerate ghee even if you're dairy-sensitive because the milk proteins have been removed.

Many of the recipes in this book also use Parmesan cheese. I call for either grated or powdered Parmesan. Powdered Parmesan is simply Parmesan cheese that has been grated to the point of being light, fluffy, and powdery. Fresh pregrated Parmesan cheese available at supermarket cheese counters usually has a powdery texture and can be a convenient option in recipes that call for powdered Parmesan. To make powdered Parmesan at home, place grated Parmesan in a food processor or spice grinder and pulse until it is fluffy and powdery.

MCT OIL

MCT stands for medium-chain triglycerides, which are chains of fatty acids. MCTs are found naturally in coconut oil, palm oil, and dairy, and they're particularly helpful on a keto diet because the body uses them quickly and any MCTs not immediately utilized are converted to ketones.

MCT oil is extracted from coconut or palm oil and contains higher, concentrated levels of MCTs, so it's great for adding ketones to your diet. Whenever MCT oil appears in a recipe in this book, it's always my first choice, but to make the recipes as accessible as possible, I've provided alternative oil choices as well.

Fat	SFA	PUFA	Notes
Almond oil	8.2%	17%	• Has a mild, neutral flavor • Works great for sweet dishes and Thai dishes • Use in nonheat applications, such as salad dressings • Can also be used on the skin
Avocado oil	11%	10%	• Has a mild, neutral flavor • Works great for savory and sweet dishes • Can be heated
Beef tallow	49.8%	3.1%	• Has a mild beef flavor • Works great for savory dishes • Can be heated
Cocoa butter	60%	3%	• Has a mild coconut flavor • Works great for sweet and savory dishes • Can be heated
Coconut oil	92%	1.9%	• Has a strong coconut flavor • Works great for sweet dishes and Thai dishes • Can be heated • Can also be used on the skin
Duck fat	25%	13%	• Has a rich duck flavor • Works great for frying savory foods • Can be heated
Extra-virgin olive oil*	14%	9.9%	• Has a strong olive flavor • Works great for Italian salad dressings • Use in nonheat applications, such as salad dressings
Hazelnut oil	10%	14%	• Has a mild hazelnut flavor • Works great for sweet dishes and Thai dishes • Use in nonheat applications, such as salad dressings
High oleic sunflower oil	8%	9%	• Has a mild sunflower seed flavor • Works great for sweet dishes and Thai dishes • Use in nonheat applications, such as salad dressings
Lard	41%	12%	• Has a mild flavor • Works great for frying sweet or savory foods • Can be heated
Macadamia nut oil	15%	10%	• Has a mild nutty flavor • Works great for salad dressings • Use in nonheat applications, such as salad dressings
MCT oil**	97%	less than 1%	• Has a neutral flavor • Works great for savory dishes and baked goods • Can be heated using low to moderate heat (no higher than 320°F)
Palm kernel oil***	82%	2%	• Has a neutral flavor • Works great for baking • Can be heated

*Extra-virgin olive oil is great for cold applications, such as salad dressings, but should not be used for cooking; heat causes the oil to oxidize, which is harmful to your health.

**MCT oil can be found at most health food stores, but if you have trouble finding it, you can use avocado oil, macadamia nut oil, or extra-virgin olive oil instead, keeping in mind that avocado oil is the most neutral-flavored of the three.

***Be sure to purchase sustainably sourced and processed palm kernel oil. There are ecological concerns associated with some palm oils.

bad fats

Two kinds of fats should be avoided on a ketogenic diet: trans fats and polyunsaturated fatty acids (PUFAs).

Trans fats are the most inflammatory fats; in fact, they are among the worst substances for our health that we can consume. Many studies have shown that eating foods that contain trans fats increases the risk of heart disease and cancer.

Here is a list of trans fats to avoid at all costs:

· Hydrogenated or partially hydrogenated oils (check ingredient labels for these sneaky fats)

· Margarine

· Vegetable shortening

PUFAs should also be limited, as they are prone to oxidation. Many cooking oils are high in PUFAs. Here is a list of the most common ones:

Fat	PUFA
Grapeseed oil	70.6%
Sunflower oil	68%
Flax oil	66%
Safflower oil	65%
Soybean oil	58%
Corn oil	54.6%
Walnut oil	53.9%
Cottonseed oil	52.4%
Vegetable oil	51.4%
Sesame oil	42%
Peanut oil	33.4%
Canola oil	19%

PURCHASING KETO-FRIENDLY INGREDIENTS

You can purchase keto-friendly pantry products on my website, MariaMindBodyHealth.com/store. They're also available in most grocery stores.

To save money, I recommend buying ingredients in bulk—including perishables like meat and fresh veggies. They can be frozen (a chest freezer is a great investment) and thawed later.

Remember, choosing top-quality organic foods is always best.

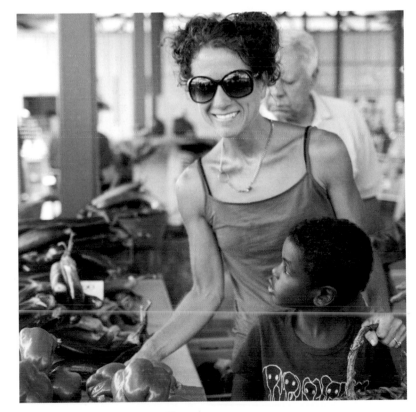

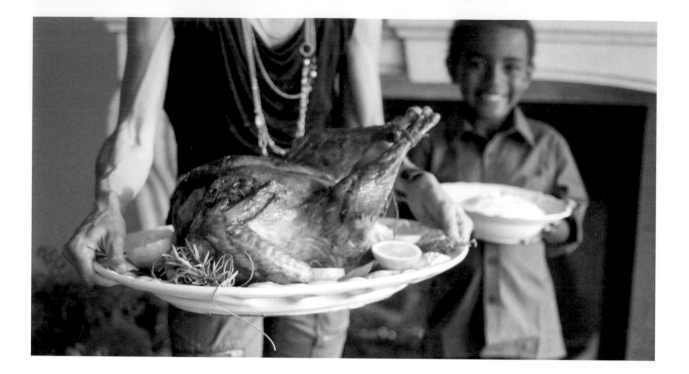

proteins

It's always best to choose humanely raised, grass-fed or pastured meat and eggs and wild-caught seafood. Not only do they offer more nutrients, but they also haven't been exposed to added hormones, antibiotics, or other potential toxins.

For help choosing sustainably sourced seafood, check out the Monterey Bay Aquarium Seafood Watch app and website, seafoodwatch.org.

BEEF	WILD MEATS	POULTRY	EGGS	FISH	SEAFOOD/SHELLFISH
BUFFALO	· Bear	· Chicken	· Chicken eggs	· Ahi/mahi mahi	· Clams
GOAT	· Boar	· Duck	· Duck eggs	· Catfish	· Crab
LAMB	· Elk	· Game hen	· Goose eggs	· Halibut	· Langostino
PORK	· Rabbit	· Goose	· Ostrich eggs	· Herring	· Lobster
	· Venison	· Ostrich	· Quail eggs	· Mackerel	· Mussels
		· Partridge		· Salmon	· Oysters
		· Pheasant		· Sardines	· Prawns
		· Quail		· Snapper	· Scallops
		· Squab		· Swordfish	· Shrimp
		· Turkey		· Trout	· Snails
				· Tuna	
				· Walleye	
				· Whitefish (cod, bluegill)	

| NUTRITIONAL INFO (per 4 ounces) | | | | | | | | |
Beef Cuts	CALORIES	FAT (G)	PROTEIN (G)	CARBS (G)	FIBER (G)	% FAT	% PROTEIN	% CARBS
Rib-eye steak	310	25.0	20.0	0	0	73%	26%	0%
Rib roast	373	28.0	27.0	0	0	69%	30%	0%
Beef back ribs	310	26.0	19.0	0	0	75%	25%	0%
Porterhouse steak	280	22.0	21.0	0	0	70%	30%	0%
T-bone steak	170	12.2	15.8	0	0	64%	36%	0%
Top loin steak	270	20.0	21.0	0	0	67%	31%	0%
Tenderloin roast	180	8.0	25.0	0	0	40%	56%	0%
Tenderloin steak	122	3.0	22.2	0	0	60%	40%	0%
Tri-tip roast	340	29.0	18.0	0	0	77%	21%	0%
Tri-tip steak	200	11.0	23.0	0	0	50%	46%	0%
Top sirloin steak	240	16.0	22.0	0	0	60%	37%	0%
Top round steak	180	9.0	25.0	0	0	45%	56%	0%
Bottom round roast	220	14.0	23.0	0	0	57%	42%	0%
Bottom round steak	220	14.0	23.0	0	0	57%	42%	0%
Eye round roast	253	13.4	32.0	0	0	48%	51%	0%
Eye round steak	182	9.0	25.0	0	0	45%	55%	0%
Round tip roast	199	12.0	22.9	0	0	54%	46%	0%
Round tip steak	150	6.0	23.5	0	0	36%	63%	0%
Sirloin tip center roast	190	7.0	31.0	0	0	33%	65%	0%
Sirloin tip center steak	190	7.0	31.0	0	0	33%	65%	0%
Sirloin tip side steak	190	6.0	34.0	0	0	28%	72%	0%
Skirt steak	255	16.5	27.0	0	0	58%	42%	0%
Flank steak	200	8.0	32.0	0	0	36%	64%	0%
Shank cross cut	215	6.7	38.7	0	0	28%	72%	0%
Brisket flat cut	245	14.7	28.0	0	0	54%	46%	0%
Chuck 7-bone pot roast	240	14.0	28.0	0	0	53%	47%	0%
Chuck boneless pot roast	240	14.0	28.0	0	0	53%	47%	0%
Chuck steak boneless	160	8.0	22.0	0	0	45%	55%	0%
Chuck eye steak	250	18.0	21.0	0	0	65%	34%	0%
Shoulder top blade steak	204	13.0	22.0	0	0	57%	43%	0%
Shoulder top blade flat iron	204	13.0	22.0	0	0	57%	43%	0%
Shoulder pot roast	185	7.0	30.7	0	0	34%	66%	0%
Shoulder steak	204	12.0	24.0	0	0	53%	47%	0%
Shoulder center ranch steak	152	8.0	24.0	0	0	40%	60%	0%
Shoulder petite tender	150	7.0	22.0	0	0	42%	59%	0%
Shoulder petite tender medallions	150	7.0	22.0	0	0	42%	59%	0%
Boneless short ribs	440	41.0	16.0	0	0	84%	15%	0%

| NUTRITIONAL INFO (per 4 ounces) | | | | | | | | |
Pork Cuts	CALORIES	FAT (G)	PROTEIN (G)	CARBS (G)	FIBER (G)	% FAT	% PROTEIN	% CARBS
Chop	241	12.0	33.0	0	0	45%	55%	0%
Loin	265	15.5	30.8	0	0	53%	46%	0%
Pork hocks	285	24.0	17.0	0	0	76%	24%	0%
Leg ham	305	20.0	30.4	0	0	59%	40%	0%
Rump	280	16.2	32.8	0	0	52%	47%	0%
Tenderloin	158	4.0	30.0	0	0	23%	76%	0%
Middle ribs (country style)	245	16.0	25.0	0	0	59%	41%	0%
Loin back ribs (baby back ribs)	315	27.0	10.0	0	0	77%	22%	0%
Belly	588	60.0	10.4	0	0	92%	7%	0%
Shoulder	285	23.0	19.0	0	0	73%	27%	0%
Butt	240	18.0	19.0	0	0	68%	32%	0%
Bacon	600	47.2	41.8	0	0	71%	28%	0%

NUTRITIONAL INFO (per 4 ounces)

Poultry	CALORIES	FAT (G)	PROTEIN (G)	CARBS (G)	FIBER (G)	% FAT	% PROTEIN	% CARBS
Chicken breast, skinless	138	4.0	25.0	0	0	26%	72%	0%
Chicken breast, skin-on	200	8.4	31.0	0	0	38%	62%	0%
Chicken leg, skinless	210	9.5	30.7	0	0	41%	58%	0%
Chicken leg, skin-on	255	15.2	29.4	0	0	54%	46%	0%
Chicken thigh, skinless	165	10.0	19.0	0	0	55%	46%	0%
Chicken thigh, skin-on	275	17.6	28.3	0	0	58%	41%	0%
Chicken wings	320	22.0	30.4	0	0	62%	38%	0%
Chicken drums	178	9.9	22.0	0	0	50%	49%	0%
Game hen	220	16.0	19.0	0	0	65%	35%	0%
Pheasant	200	10.5	25.7	0	0	47%	51%	0%
Turkey	175	9.9	21.0	0	0	51%	48%	0%
Goose	340	24.9	28.5	0	0	66%	34%	0%
Duck	228	13.9	26.3	0	0	55%	46%	0%

NUTRITIONAL INFO (per 4 ounces)

Fish	CALORIES	FAT (G)	PROTEIN (G)	CARBS (G)	FIBER (G)	% FAT	% PROTEIN	% CARBS
Tuna (yellowfin)	150	1.5	34.0	0	0	9%	91%	0%
Tuna (canned)	123	0.8	27.5	1.5	0	6%	89%	5%
Salmon	206	9.0	31.0	0	0	39%	60%	0%
Anchovies	256	15.9	28.0	0	0	56%	44%	0%
Sardines	139	7.5	18.0	0	0	49%	52%	0%
Barramundi	110	2.0	23.0	0	0	16%	84%	0%
Trout	190	8.6	28.0	0	0	41%	59%	0%
Walleye	156	7.5	22.0	0	0	43%	56%	0%
Cod	113	1.0	26.0	0	0	8%	92%	0%
Sea bass	135	3.0	27.0	0	0	20%	80%	0%
Halibut	155	3.5	30.7	0	0	20%	79%	0%
Mackerel	290	20.3	27.0	0	0	63%	37%	0%
Arctic char	208	10.0	29.0	0	0	43%	56%	0%

NUTRITIONAL INFO (per 4 ounces)

Seafood/Shellfish	CALORIES	FAT (G)	PROTEIN (G)	CARBS (G)	FIBER (G)	% FAT	% PROTEIN	% CARBS
Scallops	97	1.0	19.0	3.0	0	9%	78%	12%
Mussels	97	2.8	13.5	4.5	0	26%	56%	19%
Clams	82	1.1	15.0	3.0	0	12%	73%	15%
Shrimp	135	2.0	25.8	1.7	0	18%	78%	4%
Oysters	58	1.9	6.5	3.1	0	29%	33%	38%
Crab	107	2.0	22.0	0.0	0	17%	82%	0%
Lobster	116	1.8	25.0	0.0	0	14%	86%	0%
Caviar	260	12.0	31.0	8.0	0	42%	48%	12%

FINDING THE BEST-QUALITY EGGS

Eggs are an amazingly nutritious food, especially the yolks, which are full of choline, healthy fats, and a ton of flavor. And high-quality eggs—those from healthy, happy, humanely raised hens—are even more nourishing and tastier. So which eggs are the best quality?

Brown or White Eggs: There's absolutely no difference in quality between brown and white eggs; the only thing that determines the color of an egg is the breed of the hen. Do not choose eggs based on color.

Egg Grades: Eggs can be grade AA, A, or B. There is little to no difference in the taste, though, and no difference in nutritional value. Grade AA eggs have the thickest, firmest whites and high, round yolks. This grade of egg is virtually free of defects and is best for frying, poaching, or methods where presentation is important. Grade A eggs are the same quality as grade AA, but the whites are categorized as "reasonably" firm. Most grade B eggs are sold to restaurants, bakeries, and other food institutions and are used to make liquid, frozen, and dried egg products.

Vegetarian-Fed: The only thing this label means is that the hens are fed a diet based on corn (which is usually genetically modified). To ensure that the hens consume a strictly vegetarian diet, they are kept in cages. But chickens are natural omnivores. they evolved to eat insects, worms, and grubs as well as grass and grains. They weren't meant to be vegetarians!

Certified Organic: This label means that the hens are not kept in cages but in barns. They are required to have access to the sun, but that doesn't necessarily mean they can go outside; there may be a small window in the barn for sunlight. The hens are fed an organic, vegetarian diet that is free from antibiotics and pesticides. This label is regulated with inspections.

Free-Range or Cage-Free: This sounds like a good choice, right? Well, all this label really means is that the hens are not caged. However, there is no requirement to let the hens outside, there are no mandatory inspections to regulate this claim, and there are no guidelines for what the birds are fed.

Omega-3 Enriched: This label indicates that the hens' feed has extra omega-3 fatty acids added to it in the form of flaxseed. But eggs already are a good source of omega-3s, so there's no need to seek out eggs bearing this label.

Since most of the terms used on egg labels don't really help us figure out which eggs are healthiest, here are some guidelines to follow when egg shopping:

1. Be conscious of antibiotic and hormone use. While the USDA prohibits the use of hormones for egg production and the use of therapeutic antibiotics is illegal unless the hens are ill, these rules aren't always enforced. The only way to ensure that the hens were not given antibiotics is to purchase organic eggs.

2. To guarantee that you get truly free-range eggs, purchase eggs from pastured hens. Pastured hens are able to eat their natural diet of greens, seeds, worms, and bugs, and studies show that their eggs may contain more omega-3 fatty acids, vitamins, and minerals.

3. Smaller eggs tend to have thicker shells than larger eggs and therefore are less likely to become contaminated by bacteria.

4. Be cautious of unregulated labels. Terms like "natural" and "cage-free" are frequently used, but these claims may not necessarily be valid. Claims on egg packaging with the USDA shield have been verified by the United States Department of Agriculture, so look for the shield when purchasing eggs from a store.

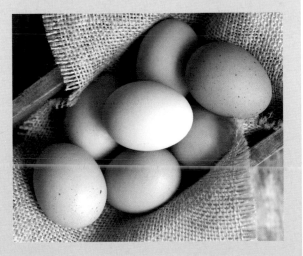

nuts and seeds

Most nuts and seeds are fine on a keto diet, but they can take some people with metabolic syndrome out of ketosis. If you are extremely metabolically damaged and your goal is to lose weight, I highly recommend that you consume ketogenic dishes that use nuts, seeds, or nut flour in moderation, not every day. There are so many recipes to choose from in this book that you should never feel deprived! Nuts are also constipating, so if you suffer from lack of stool elimination, I suggest that you limit or cut out nuts, as well as dairy.

- Almonds
- Brazil nuts
- Hazelnuts
- Macadamia nuts
- Pecans
- Pumpkin seeds
- Sesame seeds
- Sunflower seeds
- Walnuts

Cashews, chestnuts, and pistachios have too many carbohydrates and therefore are not allowed on a ketogenic diet.

veggies

Fresh vegetables are packed with nutrients and are an important part of a ketogenic diet, but to make sure you stay in ketosis, it's important to choose nonstarchy vegetables, which are lower in carbs than starchy vegetables. The following are some of the nonstarchy vegetables that I use most:

- Arugula
- Asparagus
- Bok choy
- Broccoli
- Cabbage
- Cauliflower
- Celery
- Collard greens
- Endive
- Garlic
- Kale
- Kelp
- Lettuces: red leaf, Boston, romaine, radicchio
- Mushrooms
- Onions: green, yellow, white, red
- Peppers: bell peppers, jalapeños, chiles
- Seaweed
- Swiss chard
- Watercress

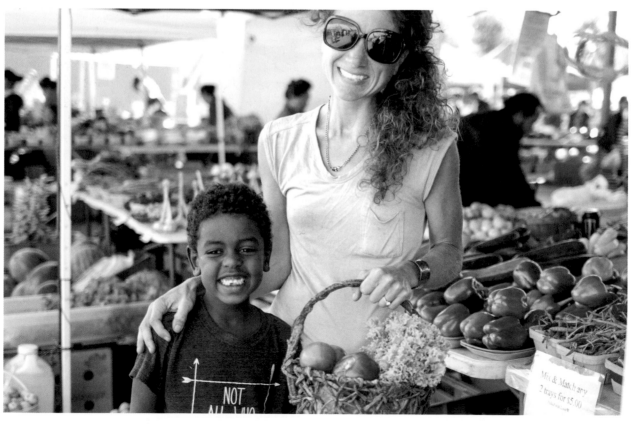

herbs and spices

Spices and fresh herbs are the most nutritious plants you can consume. For example, everyone thinks spinach is an amazingly nutritious food, but fresh oregano has eight times the amount of antioxidants! Sure, we don't eat a cup of oregano, but it goes to show that a little bit of an herb provides a huge benefit. Here are some of my favorite herbs and spices:

- Anise
- Annatto
- Basil
- Bay leaf
- Black pepper
- Caraway
- Cardamom
- Cayenne pepper
- Celery seed
- Chervil
- Chili pepper
- Chives
- Cilantro
- Cinnamon
- Cloves
- Coriander
- Cumin
- Curry
- Dill
- Fenugreek
- Galangal
- Garlic
- Ginger
- Lemongrass
- Licorice
- Mace
- Marjoram
- Mint
- Mustard seeds
- Oregano
- Paprika
- Parsley
- Peppermint
- Rosemary
- Saffron
- Sage
- Spearmint
- Star anise
- Tarragon
- Thyme
- Turmeric
- Vanilla beans

fruit

We tend to think of fruit as a health food, but in reality, most fruits are full of carbs and sugar. In fact, studies prove that the produce we consume today is lower in nutrients and much higher in sugar than it was in Paleolithic times. In general, high-sugar fruits like bananas, grapes, and mangoes should be avoided on a ketogenic diet.

But that doesn't mean you have to avoid *all* fruits! I once made a keto fruit salad filled with cucumbers, olives, eggplant, and capers, all covered in a Greek vinaigrette. So yes, fruits are certainly allowed; just seek out those that are low in sugar.

- Avocados
- Cucumbers
- Eggplants
- Lemons
- Limes
- Olives
- Seasonal wild berries (in moderation)
- Tomatoes

beverages

It probably goes without saying that sodas and fruit juices should be avoided—they're full of sugar that will raise your blood glucose and kick you out of ketosis. But that doesn't mean you're limited to drinking just water! The following are all liquids that you can consume on a ketogenic diet.

- Unsweetened almond milk
- Unsweetened cashew milk
- Unsweetened coconut milk
- Unsweetened hemp milk
- Decaf coffee (make sure it is not chlorinated)
- Decaf caffè Americano (espresso with water)
- Decaf green tea
- Mineral water
- Water (reverse osmosis is best)

the pantry

In addition to the whole foods discussed above, some pantry items are essential for making the recipes in this book.

baking products

See page 23 for recommended sweeteners.

- Baking powder
- Baking soda
- Blanched almond flour
- Coconut flour
- Egg white protein powder (check carbs and added ingredients—I recommend Jay Robb brand)
- Extracts and essential oils, including pure vanilla extract, for flavoring
- Guar gum
- Pecan meal
- Maca powder
- Unsweetened baking chocolate
- Unsweetened cocoa powder

sauces and flavor enhancers

- Coconut aminos
- Coconut vinegar
- Fish sauce

EGG REPLACER

The only keto egg replacer that I recommend is unflavored gelatin. Chia and flax seeds are not recommended because of their estrogenic properties as well as their high total carb count.

pantry foods

It is always better to buy fresh, but here are some keto-friendly foods that are also great jarred, canned, or prepackaged:

- Banana peppers
- Boxed beef and chicken broth
- Canned full-fat coconut milk
- Canned salmon
- Canned tuna
- Capers
- EPIC bars (made from grass-fed meat—but check for added sugars)
- Fermented pickles*
- Fermented sauerkraut*
- Marinara sauce (check for unhealthy oils and added sugar)**
- Mikey's English Muffins
- Nori wraps
- Olives (choose jars over cans)
- Organic dried spices
- Paleo mayo
- Pickled eggs
- Pickled herring
- Pizza sauce (check for unhealthy oils and added sugar)**
- Pure Wraps
- Roasted bell peppers
- Sardines
- Tomato paste**
- Tomato sauce**

Not only is fermenting a great way to preserve food, but it also creates beneficial gut bacteria and helpful digestive enzymes. Fermented sauerkraut is particularly rich in B vitamins.

**When it comes to tomato products, opt for jarred (the best choice) or BPA-free canned products. The linings of cans often contain BPA, a chemical that's associated with several health problems and may affect children's development, and tomatoes' high acidity can cause more BPA to leach into the food.*

natural sweeteners

In my recipes, I always use natural sweeteners. Just as sugarcane and honey are found in nature, so are erythritol and the stevia herb.

However, I prefer not to use sweeteners such as honey, maple syrup, and agave in my recipes because, even though they're natural, they raise blood sugar, which not only causes inflammation but will also take you out of ketosis.

Fructose is particularly problematic. More than glucose, it promotes a chemical reaction called glycation, which results in advanced glycation end products (AGEs). AGEs form a sort of crust around cells that has been linked to a wide range of diseases, from diabetes and heart disease to asthma, polycystic ovary syndrome, and Alzheimer's. Fructose also contributes to nonalcoholic fatty liver disease. For these reasons, I avoid sweeteners that are high in fructose: table sugar, high-fructose corn syrup, honey, agave, and fruit.

The following is a list of the natural sweeteners that I recommend, all of which have little effect on blood sugar.

- **Erythritol:** A sugar alcohol that is found naturally in some fruits and fermented foods. Erythritol is generally available in granulated form, though sometimes you can find it powdered. If you purchase a granulated product, such as Sukrin or Wholesome! All-Natural Zero, I recommend grinding it to a powder before use.

- **Swerve and other blended sweeteners:** These products combine two zero-calorie natural sweeteners, usually erythritol (see above) and oligosaccharides, which are found in many plants. They do not affect blood sugar and measure cup for cup just like table sugar. I use the powdered form of Swerve (the one labeled "confectioners") because it dissolves particularly well. Other blends I recommend are Pyure (erythritol and stevia), Norbu (erythritol and monk fruit), Natvia (erythritol and stevia), Lakanto (erythritol and monk fruit), and Zsweet (erythritol and stevia).

- **Stevia:** Available as a powder or a liquid. Because stevia is so concentrated, many companies add bulking agents like maltodextrin to the powdered form so that it's easier to bake with. Stay away from those products. Look for products that contain just stevia or stevia combined with another natural, keto-friendly sweetener.

- **Stevia glycerite:** A thick liquid form of stevia that is similar in consistency to honey. Do not confuse it with liquid stevia, which is much more concentrated. Stevia glycerite is about twice as sweet as sugar, making it a bit less sweet than liquid or powdered stevia. I prefer stevia glycerite because, unlike powdered and liquid stevia, it has no bitter aftertaste. Stevia glycerite is great for cooking because it maintains its flavor when heated. However, it doesn't caramelize or create bulk, so most baking recipes call for combining it with another sweetener.

- **Monk fruit:** Also known as lo han kuo, monk fruit comes in pure liquid and powdered forms. Since it is 300 times sweeter than sugar, the powdered form is typically bulked up with another sweetener so that it measures cup for cup like sugar. Check the ingredients for things like maltodextrin, and buy brands that add only keto-friendly sweeteners, such as erythritol.

- **Xylitol:** A naturally occurring low-calorie sweetener found in fruits and vegetables. It has a minimal effect on blood sugar and insulin. Xylitol has been known to kick some people out of ketosis, so if you're using it in baking or cooking, monitor your ketones closely and stop using it if you find that you're no longer in ketosis.

- **Yacón syrup:** A thick syrup that is pressed from the yacón root and tastes a bit like molasses. I use yacón syrup sparingly—a tablespoon here and there to improve the texture and flavor of my sauces—both because it is very expensive and because it has some fructose in it.

using sweeteners in the recipes in this book

If you're trying keto for the first time, the recipes in this book should have just the right amount of sweetness. But as you continue with a ketogenic lifestyle, you may find that food naturally begins to taste sweeter, and you may want to reduce the amount of sweetener used in the recipes.

Whenever a recipe requires a powdered sweetener, my go-to choice is the powdered (confectioners) form of Swerve because it gives a smoother finished product and better overall results. That said, you can always pulverize a granular form of erythritol, such as Wholesome! All-Natural Zero, in a blender or coffee grinder to get a powdered texture.

If a recipe calls for a specific sweetener or type of sweetener (such as powdered or liquid), do not substitute any other sweeteners; these recipes rely on these particular sweeteners. For example, in recipes where the sweetener has to melt, some products won't work—so it's important to use exactly what's called for.

If a sweetener in an ingredient list is followed by "or equivalent," such as "¼ cup Swerve confectioners'-style sweetener or equivalent amount of liquid or powdered sweetener," you are free to use any keto-friendly sweetener, liquid or powdered. For example, you could use liquid stevia, stevia glycerite, monk fruit, Zsweet, or xylitol.

If you prefer to use a keto-friendly sweetener other than Swerve, here are the conversions:

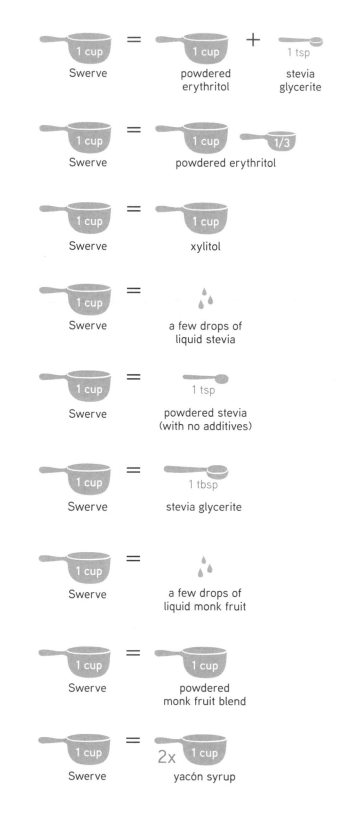

1 cup Swerve = 1 cup powdered erythritol + 1 tsp stevia glycerite

1 cup Swerve = 1 cup powdered erythritol 1/3

1 cup Swerve = 1 cup xylitol

1 cup Swerve = a few drops of liquid stevia

1 cup Swerve = 1 tsp powdered stevia (with no additives)

1 cup Swerve = 1 tbsp stevia glycerite

1 cup Swerve = a few drops of liquid monk fruit

1 cup Swerve = 1 cup powdered monk fruit blend

1 cup Swerve = 2x 1 cup yacón syrup

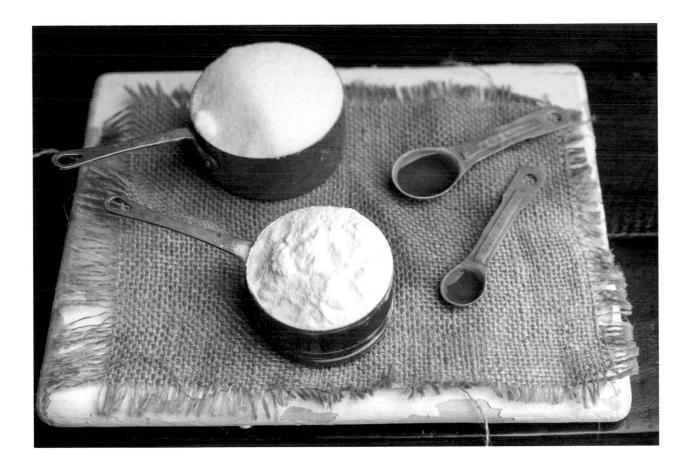

advanced tip: blending sweeteners for the tastiest keto treats

For newcomers to the keto lifestyle, I try to keep my recipes as simple as possible and to limit the number of ingredients I use. For example, in recipes that are sweetened, I usually just call for Swerve or an equivalent. But the truth is, you'll get better results if you use a blend of different natural sweeteners.

For example, if a recipe calls for 1 cup of confectioners'-style Swerve, I use:

   ½ cup confectioners'-style Swerve

   1 teaspoon stevia glycerite

   10 to 15 drops liquid monk fruit

Adding a pinch of salt will also increase the sweetness because salt is a flavor enhancer.

So if you think that desserts made with Swerve have too much of an aftertaste or a cooling effect on your mouth, I highly recommend that you try making baked goods and keto ice cream with this combination of sweeteners.

The less Swerve/erythritol you use in keto ice cream, the less hard your ice cream will freeze. Sometimes the divine taste of natural organic heavy cream is enough, and all you need to add is a teaspoon of stevia glycerite. Then your ice cream won't harden like a rock. Slowly add the natural sweetener to the ice cream and adjust the sweetness before churning or making ice pops or push pops.

substitutions for high-carb foods

Many everyday foods are high in sugar and carbs, which is why I've found healthier substitutions to use in my recipes. I was that girl who could never stop at ½ cup of pasta or one chip, so I loved putting together this information—all the foods in each photo have the same amount of carbs, so they make it shockingly clear just how much healthier these replacements are. As Craig and I prepped the ingredients to photograph, Craig had to keep making more and more and more zucchini noodles just to equal the carbs in a measly ½ cup of whole-wheat pasta!

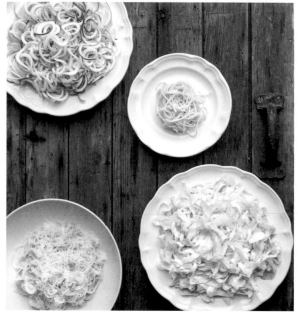

½ cup whole-wheat pasta = noodles from 3 stalks broccoli OR 5 cups zucchini noodles (page 363) OR 5 cups cabbage pasta

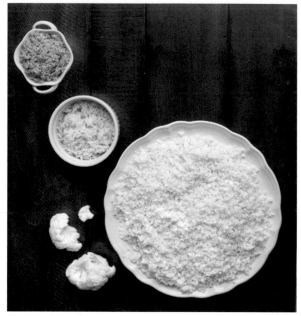

⅔ cup white rice = ½ cup quinoa = 4 cups Cauliflower Rice (page 362)

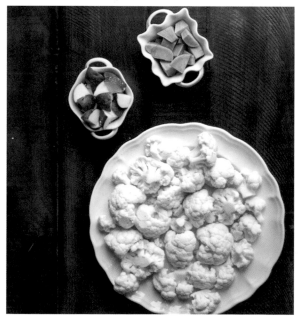

¾ cup diced sweet potato = 1 cup diced white potato = 4 cups mashed cauliflower

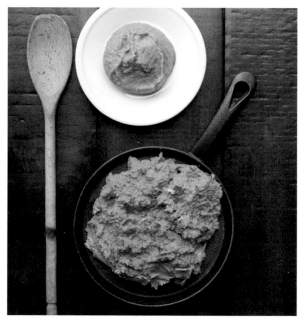

½ cup refried beans = 1½ cups of my healthified refried "beans" made with eggplant or zucchini (visit my site, MariaMindBodyHealth.com, for the recipe)

avoiding foods that contain gluten

As you're probably well aware, a ketogenic diet typically omits gluten. But you may not realize that gluten lurks in many unexpected places!

Once when we were visiting family, someone asked if I wanted a Bloody Mary, explaining that the mix she had bought was gluten-free. I don't drink alcohol, so I passed, but the offer prompted my brother to ask if Bloody Marys typically contain gluten. Yep, many mixes include Worcestershire sauce (or the bartender will add a few drops to the mix), and Worcestershire sauce contains gluten.

During that same visit, my aunt made stuffed mushrooms and claimed that they were gluten-free because she hadn't added any crackers or breadcrumbs, but when I asked her for her recipe, she said that she adds a few dashes of Worcestershire sauce. This hidden gluten can be quite problematic for people with serious allergies! So I put a list together for you, whether you want to get rid of all gluten from your diet or you have a guest coming for dinner who suffers from a gluten allergy.

Foods You Wouldn't Expect to Contain Gluten, but Sometimes Do

· Beverage mixes
· Bologna
· Candy (even sugar-free candy)
· Chewing gum
· Cold cuts
· Commercially prepared broth
· Commercially prepared soup
· Custard
· Enchilada sauce
· Gravy
· Hot dogs
· Ice cream (even low-carb ice cream)
· Nondairy creamer
· Pudding (even sugar-free pudding)
· Root beer (even sugar-free root beer)
· Salad dressings
· Soy sauce
· Taco seasoning
· Vegetables with commercially prepared sauces, such as Alfredo

Ingredients That Often Contain Hidden Gluten

· Barley
· Barley grass
· Binders
· Some blue cheese
· Bouillon
· Bran
· Brewer's yeast
· Bulgur
· Chilton
· Couscous
· Durum
· Emulsifiers
· "Fillers"
· Hydrolyzed plant protein
· Hydrolyzed vegetable protein
· Kamut
· Kasha
· Malt

· Malt flavoring
· Malt vinegar
· Matzo
· Modified food starch
· Monosodium glutamate (MSG)
· "Natural" flavor
· Rye
· Seitan
· Semolina
· Soy sauce
· Spelt
· Some spice mixes
· Stabilizer
· Suet
· Teriyaki sauce
· Textured vegetable protein (TVP)
· Wheat grass
· Wheat protein

Tools

For the most part, the recipes in this book require tools that are part of a basic kitchen setup: standard pots, pans, baking sheets, and so on. However, some of the recipes, particularly the desserts, rely on specialized tools, and there are some tools that will simply make your life in the kitchen easier.

Spiral slicer

For: vegetable noodles, especially zucchini noodles

A spiral slicer makes it easy to cut vegetables into noodles—see, for instance, the recipe for Zoodles on page 363.

I'm often asked what my favorite spiral slicer is. It depends on the thickness of the noodle. For a thicker noodle, I love the Veggetti Pro Table-Top Spiralizer. If you prefer a thin, angel hair–like noodle, I recommend the Joyce Chen Saladacco Spiral Slicer.

8-inch crepe pan or nonstick skillet

For: crepes, omelets, and wraps

Does such a thing as a healthy nonstick pan exist? Nonstick cookware can be very handy when cooking crepes, omelets, or wraps, but most nonstick pans are coated with Teflon and other chemicals that we want to avoid. Instead, you can use a well-seasoned cast-iron pan or a stainless-steel pan coated with lots of keto-friendly oil.

I've also found that the glazed ceramic pans from Ceramcor have a great nonstick surface without any chemicals. They can be cleaned as you would any other pan—the surface is very hard to scratch. They are super-durable and heavy-duty. However, there is a little learning curve with these pans. Because they are ceramic, they take longer to heat up. For omelets, I turn my burner on low for 2 or 3 minutes to warm the pan, then I add my cooking fat; I turn off the heat when I flip the omelet (ceramic pans, like cast-iron pans, hold heat longer). The omelet slides right out!

High-speed blender

For: pureeing and making shakes, salad dressings, dips, and ice cream

A high-speed blender is perfect for processing liquids. High-powered blenders, such as those from Blendtec and Vitamix, have better performance, durability, and speed—but they're also more expensive than regular blenders.

Ice cream maker

For: making ice cream and sorbet

Ice cream treats are my favorite! You will always find keto ice cream and other frozen treats in my freezer. I adore my Cuisinart ICE-21 1.5 Quart Frozen Yogurt/Ice Cream Maker. About ten years ago, I got my first ice cream maker from Cuisinart, and when it broke due to overuse, they sent me a new motor for free!

Immersion (stick) blender

For: pureeing and blending

I can't believe I went so long without an immersion blender! I'm not a gadget person like my husband is—I like simplicity and I'm not a fan of clutter—so when Craig first asked if I wanted an immersion blender (also known as a stick blender), I politely said, "No thank you." But I have to tell you, when I started to use one, I was immediately hooked! It is so easy to use, and I can't believe the power behind this little tool. I love to use it for making pureed soups, shakes, and homemade mayo, sauces, and salad dressings.

Waffle maker

For: making waffles

I love to keep grain-free waffles in the freezer for easy breakfasts. My advice is to spend the money on a quality waffle maker. I adore my Waring Pro WMK600 Double Belgian Waffle Maker.

Slow cooker (6-quart)

For: slow cooking over low heat over several hours

If you don't have a lot of time for hands-on cooking, a slow cooker is a great tool that can save you time and effort. You can prep the ingredients the night before, turn it on before you leave for work in the morning, and come home to a wonderful home-cooked meal. A 4-quart slow cooker can be handy for smaller quantities.

Double boiler

For: making and reheating sauces

A double boiler is a great tool for making sure you don't overheat sauces and cause them to separate or burn. I often reheat my Easy Basil Hollandaise (page 358) in a double boiler. But if you don't have a double boiler, you can use a heat-safe bowl set over a pot of simmering water. I even reheat my hollandaise this way when we go camping.

Whipped cream canister

For: making sweetened whipped cream

This is definitely a frivolous gadget, but also one of the most fun to use! I keep mine filled with heavy cream presweetened with a keto sweetener (see page 298 for the suggested ratio) so I always have whipped cream at the ready. The brand I use is iSi.

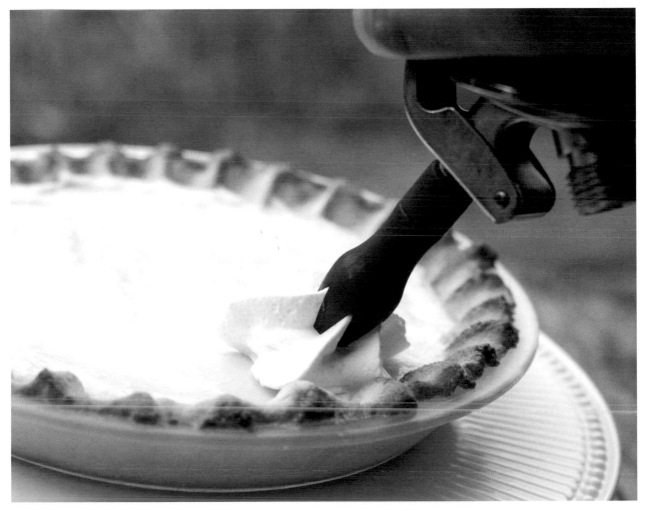

How to Use
the Recipes in This Book

In addition to 175 delicious keto comfort food recipes, this book has some handy features to help you along your keto journey.

icons

I've marked the recipes with a number of icons, as applicable.

First, there are icons highlighting those recipes that are free of dairy, nuts, and/or eggs, which are problematic for some people:

If a recipe isn't free of a particular allergen but there's a substitution to make the recipe free of that allergen, you will see the word OPTION below the icon, like this:

OPTION   OPTION   OPTION

keto meters and
nutritional information

Keto meters indicate where each recipe ranks on the keto "scale": low, medium, or high. Note that in a few cases, a dish's ranking can vary based on whether you include an optional ingredient or component, such as a keto salad dressing.

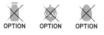

I have also included nutritional information for each recipe, listing the total calories along with the fat, protein, carbohydrate, and fiber counts in grams. You'll find this information helpful as you fine-tune your personal keto targets for these macronutrients.

nutritional info (per serving)				
calories	fat	protein	carbs	fiber
255	22g	9g	4g	2g

If you're wondering whether the recipes in this book are recipes that you can enjoy every day on your ketogenic diet, the answer is yes, most of them are. There are a few dishes, such as Brussels Sprouts with Soft-Boiled Eggs and Avocado (page 132), that I would eat only on special occasions. The keto meters can help you decide when and how often to make certain recipes; dishes marked as High are everyday comfort foods to enjoy anytime, while dishes marked as Low should be reserved for holidays and other special occasions. Those recipes marked as Medium are generally for weekends or overfeeding days.

Some recipes, such as Mashed Fauxtatoes (page 129), are higher in carbohydrates. This dish is still a great ketogenic comfort food, and it's much lower in carbs than mashed potatoes, so I felt it was a great fit for this book. Plus, many of my clients can have more carbs than others. I see very metabolically damaged clients in my practice, and in their case I limit carbohydrates to less than 20 to 30 grams a day. But I've also worked with athletes who can eat closer to 50 grams of carbs a day and remain in ketosis. This is where you and your testing come into play. Depending on your goals—remember, ketosis isn't just about weight loss—you can determine which recipes to incorporate into your menus by using the keto meter at the top of each recipe. For more on testing, overfeeding, and other keto strategies, see my previous book, *The 30-Day Ketogenic Cleanse.*

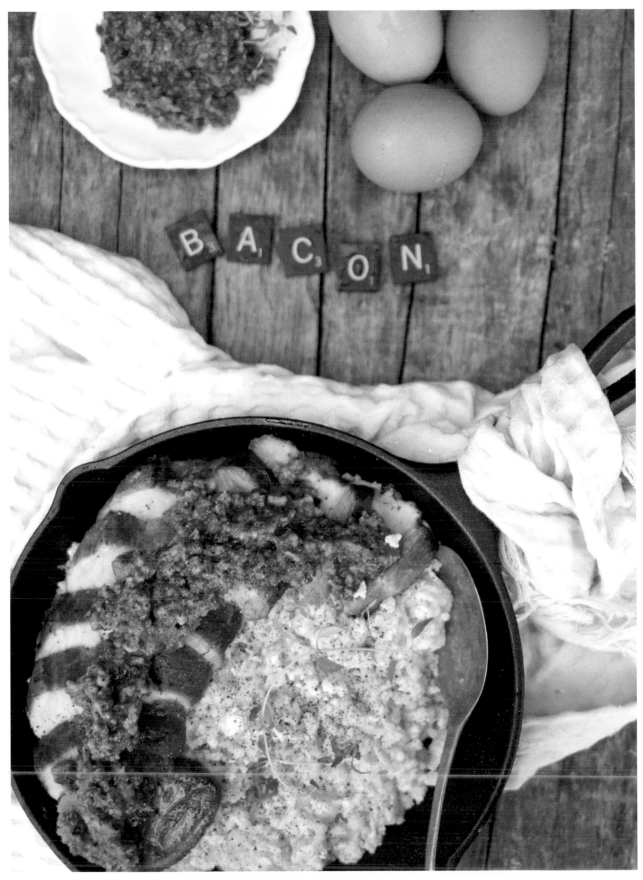

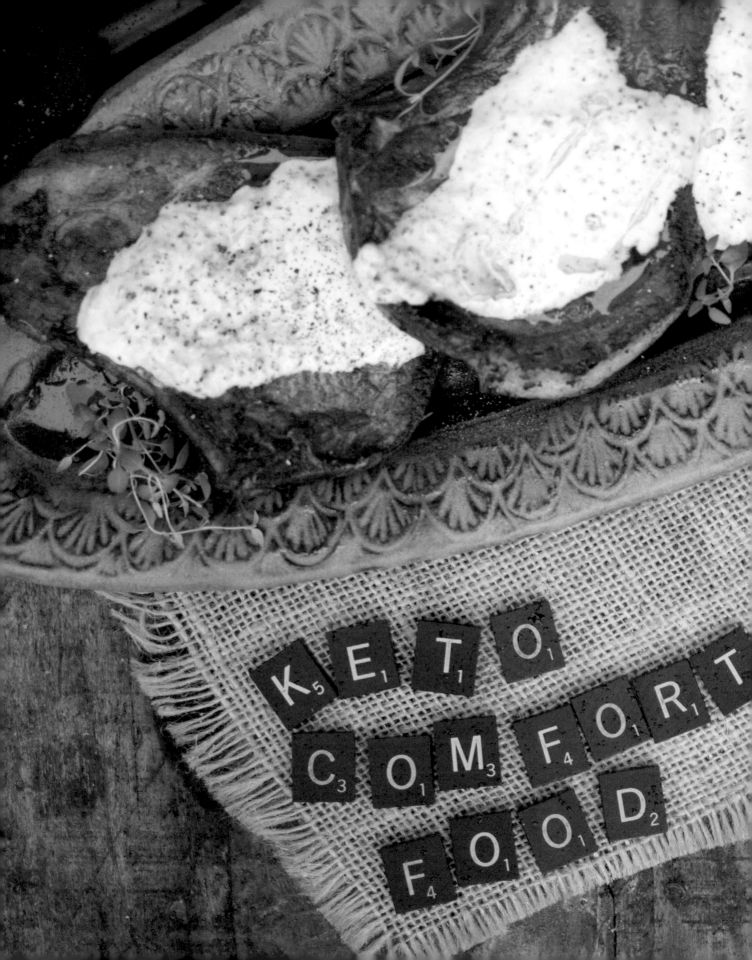

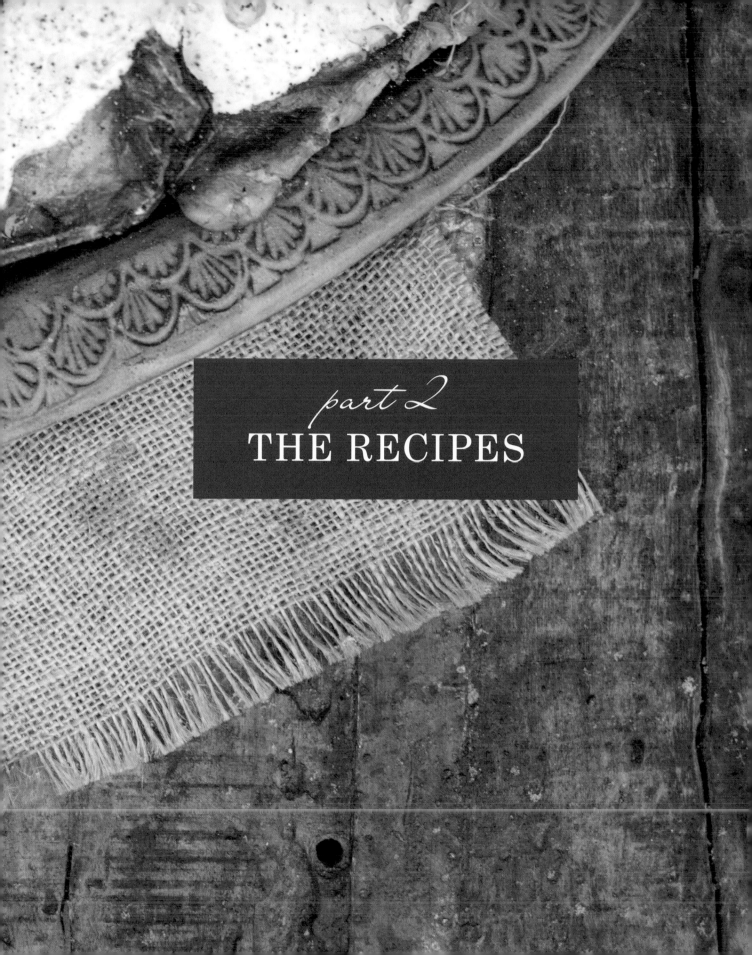

part 2
THE RECIPES

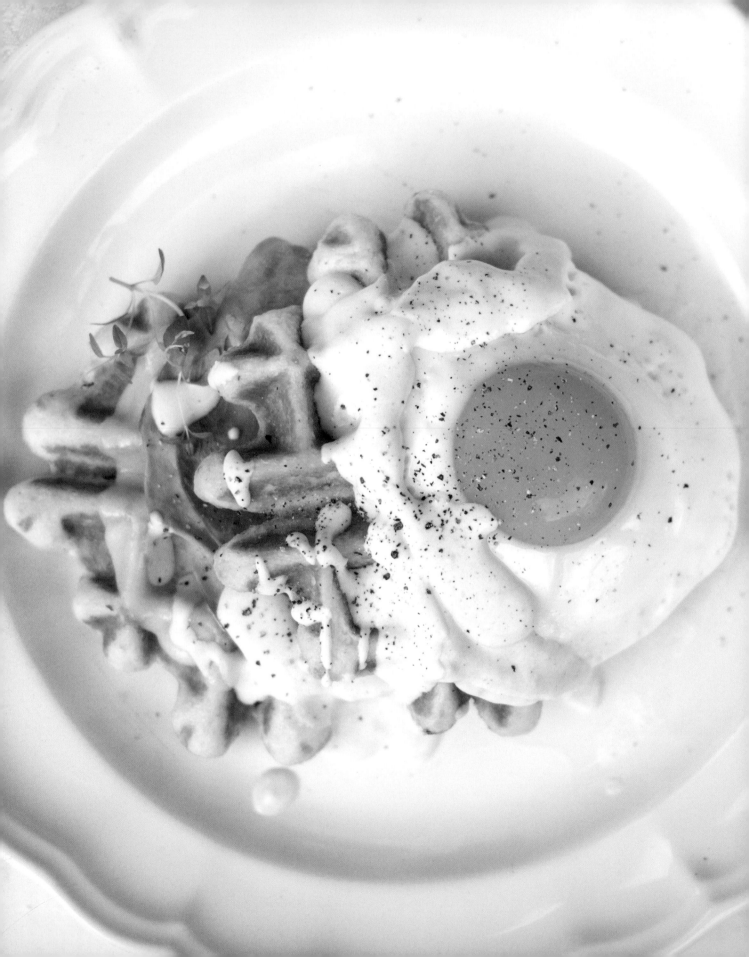

Breakfast

If I opened a diner, I would call it "Thyme for Break-Fast." The reason I adore that name for a diner is that I love herbs, especially thyme. Herbs are one of the most wonderfully nutrient-filled foods and enhance flavor more than anything!

I also love the play on Break-Fast. Breakfast isn't the most important meal of the day..."breaking your fast" is! And breakfast foods are my favorite foods!

Browned Butter Mocha Latte

When I was in high school, I worked at the cutest coffee shop called Uncommon Ground. I loved that job. I often dream about opening my own little coffee shop someday. If I did, this latte would for sure be on my menu!

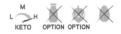

KETO   OPTION OPTION

2 tablespoons unsalted butter (or butter-flavored coconut oil if dairy-free)

1¼ cups unsweetened cashew milk (or hemp milk if nut-free)

2 tablespoons unsweetened cocoa powder, plus extra for garnish (optional)

2 tablespoons Swerve confectioners'-style sweetener or equivalent amount of liquid or powdered sweetener (see page 24)

3 tablespoons hot brewed decaf espresso or other strong brewed decaf coffee

Whipped cream, for garnish (optional)

special equipment (optional)

Immersion blender

prep time: 3 minutes (not including time to brew coffee or whip cream)

cook time: 10 minutes *yield:* 1 serving

1. Place the butter in a saucepan over high heat, stirring, until the butter froths and brown flecks begin to appear, about 5 minutes; this is browned butter. If using butter-flavored coconut oil, heat the oil just until melted.

2. Reduce the heat to medium and slowly whisk in the cashew milk; it will sizzle as you add it to the browned butter. Heat until warmed through. (At Uncommon Ground, we heated it to between 145°F and 165°F.) Stir in the cocoa powder and sweetener. If desired, insert an immersion blender and blend until the mixture resembles a frothy latte, about 1 minute.

3. Pour the espresso into a large mug. Add the hot milk mixture and stir well. Serve immediately, garnished with whipped cream and a sprinkle of unsweetened cocoa powder, if desired.

nutritional info (per serving)				
calories	*fat*	*protein*	*carbs*	*fiber*
273	27g	4g	5g	2g

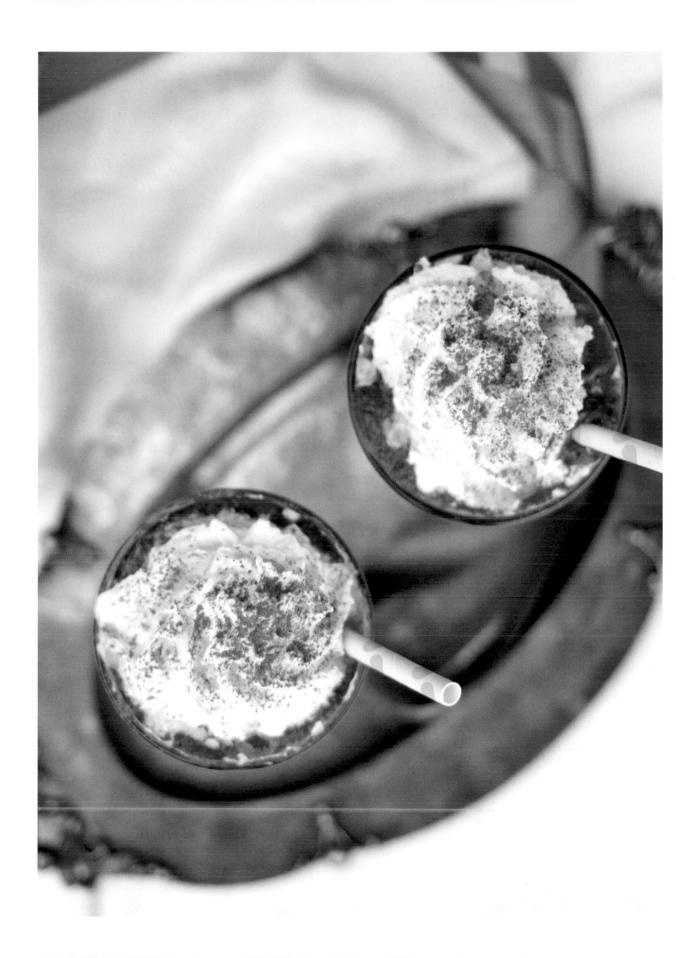

Lovers' Omelet

This omelet is no joke: it is so large that it is meant to feed two people!

prep time: 15 minutes   *cook time:* 15 minutes   *yield:* 2 servings

1 tablespoon plus 1 teaspoon ghee or unsalted butter, divided

¼ cup diced onions

¼ cup sliced mushrooms

2 tablespoons diced green or red bell peppers

¼ cup ground pork or beef

¼ teaspoon fine sea salt, divided

4 large eggs, beaten

¼ cup diced Canadian bacon

¼ cup shredded sharp cheddar cheese, plus extra for garnish

Sliced green onions, for garnish

¼ cup salsa, for serving

¼ cup sour cream, for serving

1. Melt 1 tablespoon of the ghee in a saucepan over medium-low heat. Add the onions, mushrooms, and bell peppers and cook, stirring, until the onions and peppers are soft and the mushrooms are golden. Add the ground meat and sauté until cooked through, about 3 minutes. Season with ⅛ teaspoon of the salt.

2. In a mixing bowl, combine the eggs, Canadian bacon, 2 tablespoons of water, and remaining ⅛ teaspoon of salt and stir well. Set aside.

3. Heat a 12-inch skillet over medium-low heat. Add the remaining teaspoon of ghee and swirl to coat the pan. Pour in the egg mixture. Cover and cook until the eggs are almost set. Remove the lid and sprinkle in the cheese to cover the entire omelet. Place the vegetable filling on top of the cheese.

4. Fold the omelet in half and place on a serving platter. Sprinkle with additional cheese and green onions. Serve with the salsa and sour cream.

5. Store extras in an airtight container in the refrigerator for up to 3 days. Reheat in a sauté pan over medium heat for a minute or two, until warmed through.

nutritional info (per serving)				
calories	fat	protein	carbs	fiber
576	46g	30g	6g	1g

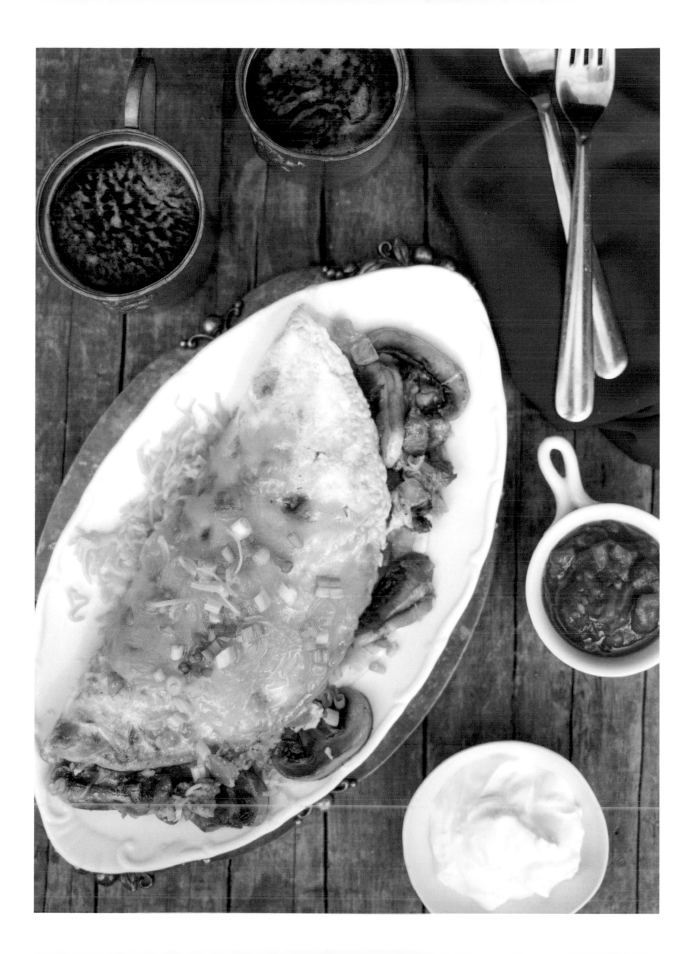

Quiche Lorraine Dutch Baby

L · M · H
KETO · OPTION · OPTION

prep time: 5 minutes   *cook time:* 25 minutes   *yield:* 2 servings

2 strips bacon, diced

3 large eggs

¾ cup unsweetened cashew milk or almond milk (or hemp milk if nut-free)

¼ cup unflavored egg white protein powder (or other protein powder, such as beef)

1 teaspoon baking powder

1 teaspoon fine sea salt

2 teaspoons diced fresh chives

½ cup sharp cheddar cheese (or nutritional yeast if dairy-free), divided

1. Preheat the oven to 425°F.

2. Place the diced bacon in a medium-sized cast-iron skillet or other oven-safe skillet. Set the pan over medium heat and cook until the bacon is crisp, about 5 minutes. Leave the bacon drippings and half of the bacon in the pan; remove the other half of the bacon and set aside.

3. In a blender, combine the eggs, cashew milk, protein powder, baking powder, and salt. Blend for about 1 minute, until foamy. Add the chives and ¼ cup of the cheese. Pour the mixture into the hot skillet over the bacon.

4. Transfer the skillet to the oven and bake for 10 minutes. Remove from the oven and top with more cheese.

5. Bake for another 10 minutes or until the Dutch baby crust is puffed and golden brown. Cut into wedges, garnish with the reserved bacon, and enjoy!

6. Store extras in an airtight container in the refrigerator for up to 3 days. Reheat on a rimmed baking sheet in a preheated 350°F oven for 5 minutes or until warmed through.

nutritional info (per serving)				
calories	fat	protein	carbs	fiber
365	25g	33g	2g	0.2g

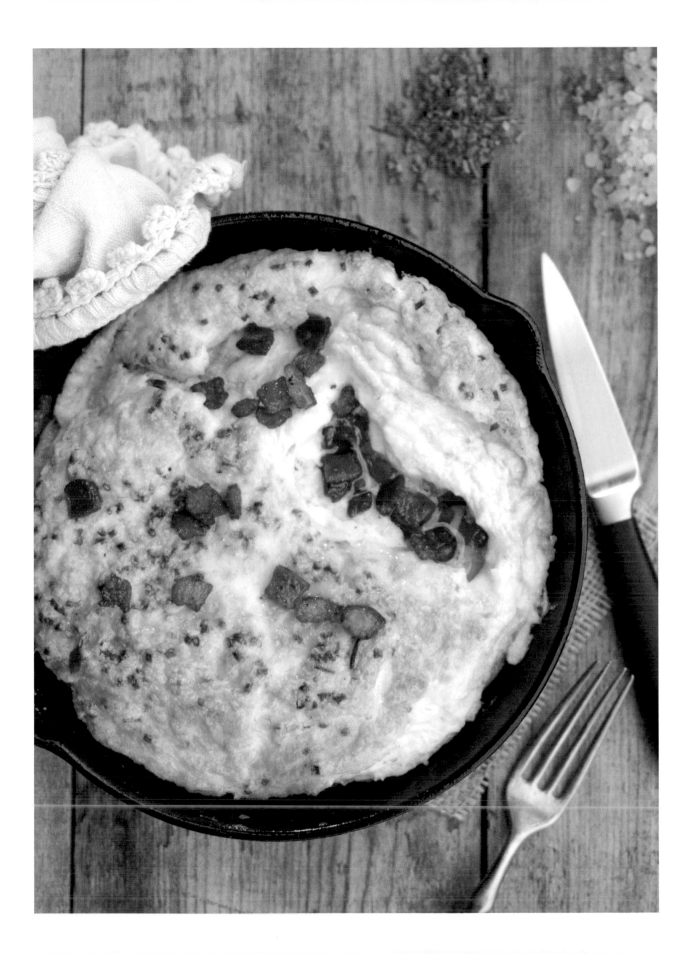

Garlicky Cheddar Biscuits and Gravy

L M H
KETO   OPTION

biscuits

3 large egg whites

2 cloves garlic, minced

1 cup blanched almond flour, plus extra if needed

1 teaspoon baking powder

¼ teaspoon fine sea salt

2 tablespoons very cold unsalted butter (or lard if dairy-free), cut into ¼-inch dice

½ cup sharp cheddar cheese cut into ¼-inch dice (omit for dairy-free)

gravy

10 ounces bulk pork sausage, crumbled

¼ cup minced onions

2 cloves garlic, minced

1 (8-ounce) package cream cheese (Kite Hill brand cream cheese style spread if dairy-free), softened

1 cup beef or chicken bone broth, homemade (page 356) or store-bought

Fine sea salt and ground black pepper

1. To make the biscuits, preheat the oven to 400°F. Grease a baking sheet or 8 wells of a standard-size 12-well muffin pan with coconut oil spray.

2. In a medium-sized bowl, whip the egg whites until very stiff, then gently mix in the garlic. Set aside.

3. In a separate medium-sized bowl, stir together the almond flour, baking powder, and salt until well combined. Cut in the cold diced butter until the butter pieces are pea-sized or smaller. Gently fold the dry mixture into the egg whites. Fold in the cheese. If the dough is too wet to form into mounds, add a few tablespoons of almond flour until the dough holds together well.

4. Using a large spoon, dollop the dough onto the greased baking sheet (or into the greased muffin cups), making 8 biscuits total. Bake for 11 to 15 minutes, until golden brown.

5. Meanwhile, make the gravy: Place the sausage, onions, and garlic in large skillet over medium heat. Cook for 5 to 6 minutes, stirring frequently, until the sausage is browned. Gradually add the cream cheese and broth; cook, stirring constantly, until the mixture comes to a gentle simmer, thickens, and becomes smooth. Reduce the heat to medium-low and simmer for 2 minutes to thicken the gravy further, stirring constantly. Season to taste with salt and pepper.

6. To serve, split the biscuits in half. Place 2 halves on a plate, then top with about ⅓ cup of the sausage gravy. Repeat with the rest of the biscuits and gravy.

7. Store extras in separate airtight containers in the refrigerator for up to 3 days. Reheat the biscuits on a baking sheet in a preheated 350°F oven for 5 minutes or until warmed through. Reheat the gravy in a saucepan over medium-low heat until warmed, stirring constantly. If the gravy has become too thick, add a little water when reheating it.

tip : *When making these biscuits, it's very important that the butter be very cold; if it's not, the biscuits won't turn out.*

nutritional info (per serving)				
calories	*fat*	*protein*	*carbs*	*fiber*
359	31g	14g	5g	2g

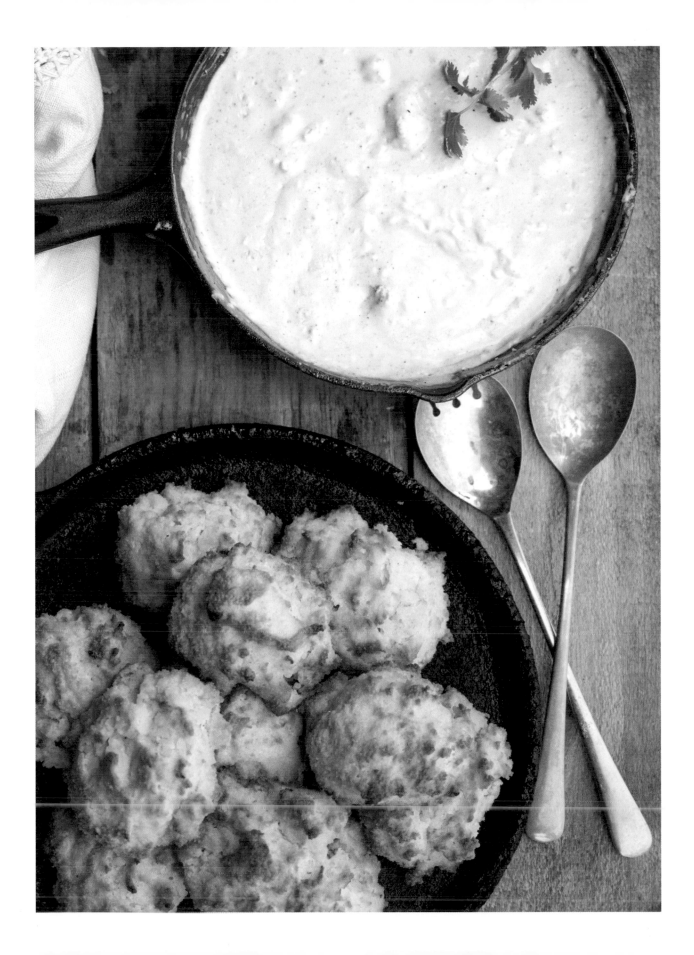

Creamy Stuffed Blintzes

L M H
KETO   OPTION   OPTION

batter

2 large eggs

2 hard-boiled eggs

4 ounces cream cheese (½ cup) (Kite Hill brand cream cheese style spread if dairy-free), softened

1 tablespoon Swerve confectioners'-style sweetener or equivalent amount of liquid or powdered sweetener (see page 24)

½ teaspoon vanilla or almond extract

Pinch of fine sea salt

filling

4 ounces cream cheese (½ cup) (Kite Hill brand cream cheese style spread if dairy-free), softened

¼ cup Swerve confectioners'-style sweetener or equivalent amount of liquid or powdered sweetener (see page 24)

1 large egg

⅛ teaspoon vanilla extract

2 tablespoons unsalted butter (or avocado oil if dairy-free), for the pan

optional garnishes

Chocolate Sauce (page 311)

Fresh mint leaves

special equipment

8-inch crepe pan or nonstick skillet (see page 28)

prep time: 5 minutes (not including time to hard-boil eggs or make chocolate sauce) *cook time:* 18 minutes *yield:* 6 blintzes (3 per serving)

1. To make the batter, place the raw eggs, hard-boiled eggs, cream cheese, sweetener, extract, and salt in a blender and blend until very smooth.

2. Grease an 8-inch crepe pan or nonstick skillet with coconut oil spray and place it over medium-high heat. When hot, pour ¼ cup of the batter into the skillet and swirl to spread the batter to the edges of the pan. Cook until golden brown, about 2 minutes, then flip and cook for another 2 minutes. Remove from the pan and repeat with the remaining batter, regreasing the skillet after cooking each blintz. Place the finished blintzes on a platter and cover with a towel to keep them from drying out while you cook the rest.

3. To make the filling, place the cream cheese, sweetener, egg, and vanilla in a small bowl and beat with a hand mixer until smooth.

4. Preheat the oven to 400°F. Spread 2 heaping tablespoons of the filling in the center of each blintz. Fold in the edges, then roll it up like a tight burrito.

5. Melt the butter in a large cast-iron skillet or other oven-safe skillet over medium heat. Place the blintzes seam side down in the hot butter and cook until golden brown, about 2 minutes. Flip and cook for another 2 minutes or until golden brown.

6. Transfer the skillet to the oven. Bake for 6 minutes or until the outsides of the blintzes are golden brown and the cheese filling is heated through. Serve with a drizzle of chocolate sauce and some mint leaves, if desired.

7. Store extras in an airtight container in the refrigerator for up to 3 days. Reheat on a rimmed baking sheet in a preheated 350°F oven for 5 minutes or until warmed through.

---

busy family tip:

I make the batter and store the blender jar, covered, in the refrigerator overnight for an easy breakfast the next morning. Or you can make the blintzes, then stuff and fold them and store them in an airtight container in the refrigerator for up to 3 days before cooking them.

nutritional info (per serving)				
calories	*fat*	*protein*	*carbs*	*fiber*
685	60g	24g	5g	0g

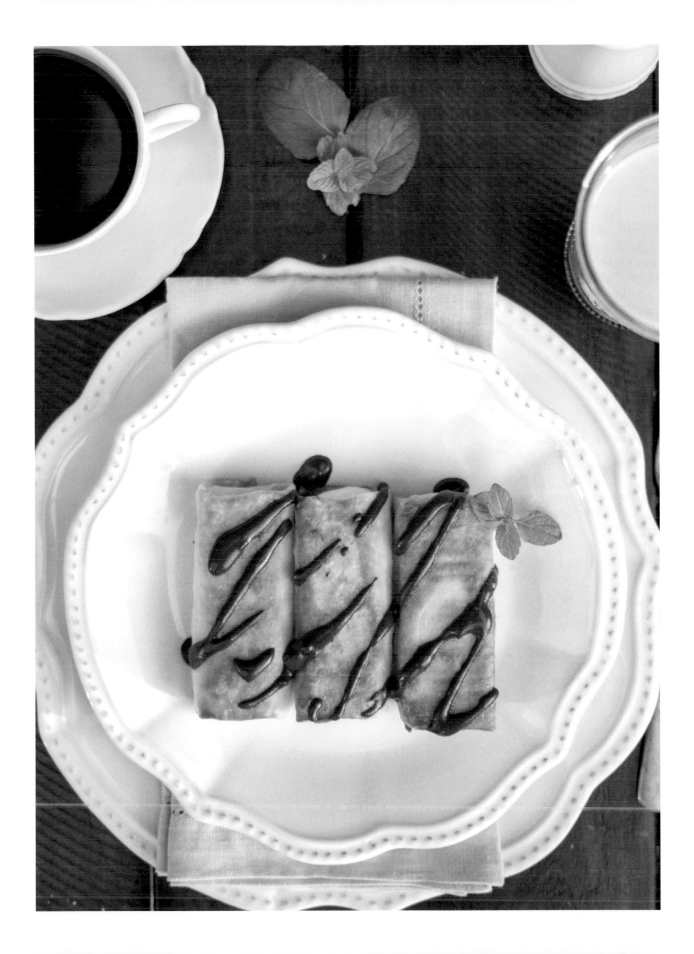

Flappers

I love taking my son Micah out on dates on Saturday mornings. We found a gem of a place in Minnesota called the Colossal Cafe. I saw that it was featured on the TV show *Diners, Drive-Ins and Dives*! One of the restaurant's specialties is flappers: fluffy pancakes served with warm Brie cheese, walnuts, and a walnut sauce. This is my keto-friendly interpretation of that dish.

L ⟍ H
M
KETO

prep time: 10 minutes *cook time:* 6 minutes per batch
yield: 16 flappers (2 per serving)

pancakes

½ cup coconut flour, or 2 cups blanched almond flour

¼ cup Swerve confectioners'-style sweetener or equivalent amount of liquid or powdered sweetener (see page 24)

½ teaspoon baking powder

½ teaspoon fine sea salt

1 cup unsweetened almond milk

2 tablespoons melted unsalted butter (or coconut oil if dairy-free)

7 large eggs (4 eggs if using almond flour), beaten

1 teaspoon apple or vanilla extract (apple tastes great with Brie)

Coconut oil, for the pan

sauce

½ cup (1 stick) unsalted butter

½ cup Swerve confectioners'-style sweetener or equivalent amount of liquid or powdered sweetener (see page 24)

½ cup unsweetened cashew milk or almond milk

1 teaspoon maple extract

toppings

1 cup raw walnut pieces

8 ounces Brie cheese, sliced

1. Make the pancakes: In a large bowl, combine the flour, powdered sweetener (if using powdered), baking powder, and salt. In a separate bowl, combine the almond milk, melted butter, eggs, extract, and liquid sweetener (if using liquid). Stir the wet mixture into the dry mixture.

2. Grease a large skillet with coconut oil and place it over medium-high heat. Pour 3 tablespoons of the batter into the hot skillet, making a circle about 3½ inches in diameter. Cook the pancakes until the bottoms are golden brown, about 2 minutes, then carefully flip and cook on the other side until golden. Repeat with the remaining batter, greasing the pan as needed between batches.

3. Meanwhile, make the sauce: Before you begin, make sure you have the sweetener, cashew milk, and extract next to the pan, ready to go in. Work fast or the sweetener will burn. Heat the butter in a heavy-bottomed saucepan over high heat. As soon as it comes to a boil, watch for brown flecks; this is browned butter (so good on veggies!). Immediately add the sweetener, milk, and extract to the pan. Whisk until the sauce is smooth, then slide the pan off the heat. (*Note:* The sauce can be made up to 2 weeks ahead.)

4. To serve, place 2 pancakes on each plate and top with walnuts, Brie, and sauce. Enjoy!

5. Store extra pancakes in an airtight container in the refrigerator for up to 3 days. Store cooled sauce in a glass jar in the fridge for up to 2 weeks. Reheat the pancakes on a baking sheet in a preheated 350°F oven for 5 minutes or until warmed through. Reheat the sauce in a saucepan over medium heat for 3 minutes or until warmed through.

---

variation:

Extremely Keto Pancakes. To make this style of pancake, you need a nonstick skillet (see page 28). Place 4 large eggs, 4 hard-boiled eggs, one 8-ounce package of cream cheese (Kite Hill brand cream cheese style spread if dairy-free), softened, 2 to 3 tablespoons Swerve confectioners'-style sweetener or equivalent amount of liquid or powdered sweetener, 1 teaspoon apple, vanilla, or almond extract, and a pinch of fine sea salt in a blender and process until very smooth. Grease a nonstick skillet with coconut oil and place it over medium-high heat. Once hot, place 2½ tablespoons of the batter in the skillet. Cook until golden brown, about 2 minutes, then flip and cook for another 2 minutes. Remove from the pan and repeat with the remaining batter. Make the sauce and serve the pancakes as described above.

nutritional info (per serving of coconut flour pancakes with toppings and sauce)				
calories	fat	protein	carbs	fiber
437	38g	13g	6g	3g

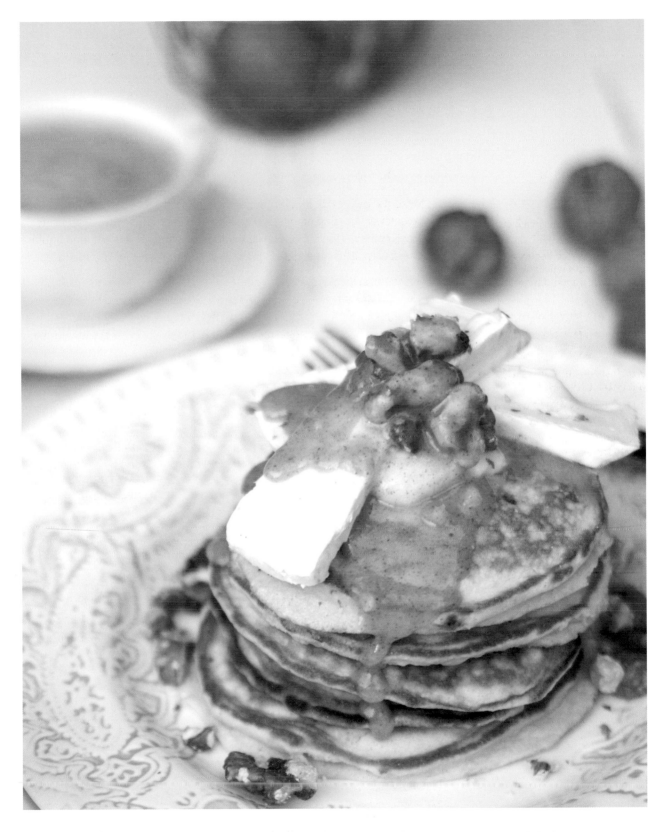

nutritional info (per serving of almond flour pancakes with toppings and sauce)				
calories	fat	protein	carbs	fiber
375	35.8g	13.4g	3g	1.6g

nutritional info (per serving of coconut flour pancakes only)				
calories	fat	protein	carbs	fiber
116	7.9g	6g	5.7g	3.1g

nutritional info (per serving of almond flour pancakes only)				
calories	fat	protein	carbs	fiber
102	9g	4.4g	1.1g	0.9g

Buttery Scones

While I was in high school and college, I worked at two different coffee shops: maybe that's where my love of baking came about. Both places served amazing scones, but they were totally different. In high school I was taught to make European scones, which are lighter, drier, and not very sweet and taste awesome dipped in espresso. In college I was taught to make drop scones, which are more "Americanized" and much sweeter. This recipe makes the sweeter, denser type—more of a drop scone. I hope you enjoy them!

M
L ⬧ H
KETO

2 cups blanched almond flour

½ cup Swerve confectioners'-style sweetener or equivalent amount of liquid or powdered sweetener (see page 24)

1 teaspoon baking powder

½ teaspoon fine sea salt

6 tablespoons (¾ stick) unsalted butter, frozen

¼ cup unsweetened cashew milk or heavy cream

1 large egg

Seeds scraped from 1 vanilla bean (about 8 inches long), or 1 teaspoon vanilla extract

1 teaspoon ground cinnamon

prep time: 5 minutes   *cook time:* 15 minutes
yield: 8 scones (1 per serving)

1. Preheat the oven to 400°F. Line a baking sheet with parchment paper.

2. In a medium-sized bowl, mix together the almond flour, powdered sweetener (if using powdered), baking powder, and salt. Cut the butter into ½-inch squares, then use your fingers to work the butter into the dry ingredients. When you are done, the mixture should still have chunks of butter.

3. In a small bowl, whisk the cashew milk, egg, and liquid sweetener (if using liquid) until blended. Using a fork, stir the milk and egg mixture into the flour mixture until large clumps form. Use your hands to press the dough against the side of the bowl, forming 8 balls.

4. Place the balls of dough on the prepared baking sheet, spacing them about 2 inches apart. Bake until golden, 13 to 15 minutes. Let cool on the pan for at least 5 minutes. Serve warm or at room temperature.

5. Store extras in an airtight container in the refrigerator for up to 3 days. Reheat on a baking sheet in a preheated 350°F oven for 5 minutes or until warmed through.

nutritional info (per scone)				
calories	fat	protein	carbs	fiber
246	23g	7g	6g	3g

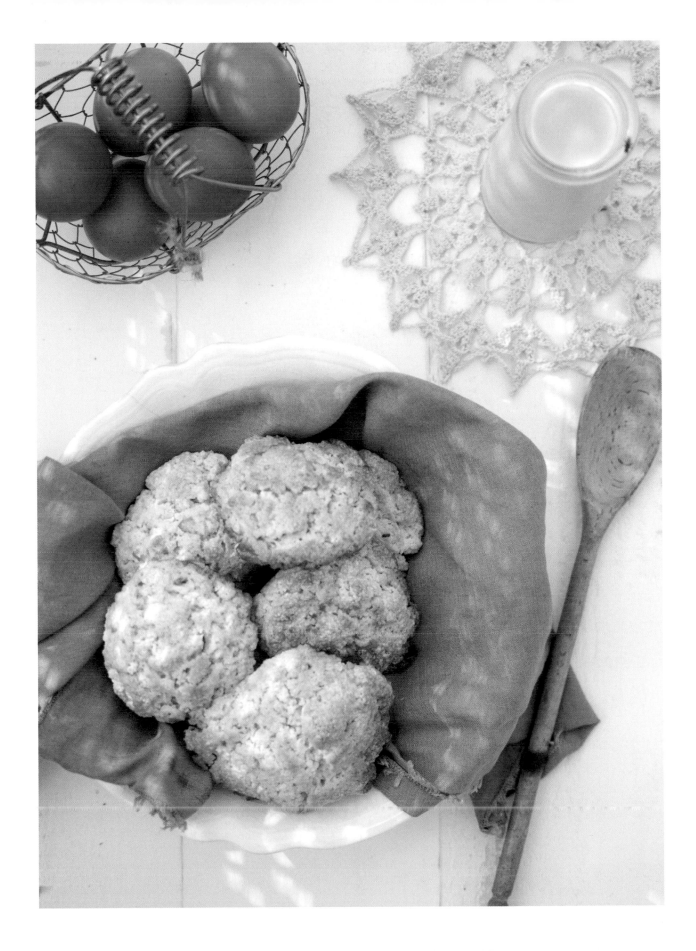

Cinnamon Roll Bread Pudding

L M H
KETO   OPTION OPTION

This bread pudding is not only super-tasty, but also extremely low in carbs because there are no nut flours in it. And this recipe is friendly to those who need to remain dairy-free.

prep time: 15 minutes, plus time to cool bread and bread pudding
cook time: 1 hour 20 minutes *yield:* 12 servings

bread

½ cup vanilla egg white protein powder or beef protein powder

½ cup Swerve confectioners'-style sweetener or equivalent amount of powdered stevia or erythritol (see page 24)

12 large egg whites

2 teaspoons cream of tartar

1 teaspoon vanilla extract

2 teaspoons ground cinnamon

pudding

1 cup unsweetened cashew milk or almond milk (or full-fat coconut milk if nut-free)

½ cup heavy cream (or full-fat coconut milk if dairy-free)

3 large eggs

⅔ cup Swerve confectioners'-style sweetener or equivalent amount of liquid or powdered sweetener (see page 24)

Seeds scraped from 1 vanilla bean (about 8 inches long), or 1 teaspoon vanilla extract

1 teaspoon ground cinnamon

½ teaspoon fine sea salt

glaze

1 cup (2 sticks) unsalted butter (or coconut oil if dairy-free), softened

½ cup strong-brewed cinnamon tea (or unsweetened cashew milk or hemp milk), warmed

¾ cup Swerve confectioners'-style sweetener or equivalent amount of liquid or powdered sweetener (see page 24)

1 teaspoon ground cinnamon

1. To make the bread, preheat the oven to 350°F. Grease an 11 by 7-inch baking dish.

2. Sift the protein powder and sweetener and set aside. In a large clean bowl, whip the egg whites until foamy (save the yolks for making ice cream). Add the cream of tartar and continue to beat until the whites are very stiff (when sufficiently stiff, you will be able to turn the bowl upside down and the whites won't fall out). Add the vanilla, then quickly fold in the protein powder mixture and cinnamon.

3. Pour the batter into the prepared baking dish. Bake for 40 minutes, until golden brown. Let cool completely, preferably in the refrigerator overnight. When completely cool, cut the bread into 1-inch cubes and place them in a large mixing bowl.

4. To make the bread pudding, preheat the oven to 350°F. Grease an 11 by 7-inch baking dish. Cover the bread cubes with the cashew milk and cream; set aside. In another bowl, combine the eggs, sweetener, vanilla, cinnamon, and salt; blend well. Pour the egg mixture over the soaked bread and stir to combine. Pour the mixture into the prepared baking dish. Bake for 30 to 40 minutes, until set. Let cool in the pan.

5. To make the glaze, place all the ingredients in a blender or food processor and process until smooth. Once the bread pudding is cool, cut it into 12 pieces and pour about 2 tablespoons of the glaze over each piece. *Note:* The glaze will separate if it sits out and gets too warm. If that happens, puree the glaze again until smooth.

6. Store extras in an airtight container in the refrigerator for up to 3 days. Reheat on a rimmed baking sheet in a preheated 350°F oven for 5 minutes or until warmed through.

busy family tip:
The bread can be made a day ahead, saving you time the day you bake the bread pudding.

nutritional info (per serving)				
calories	fat	protein	carbs	fiber
223	20g	8g	2g	0.3g

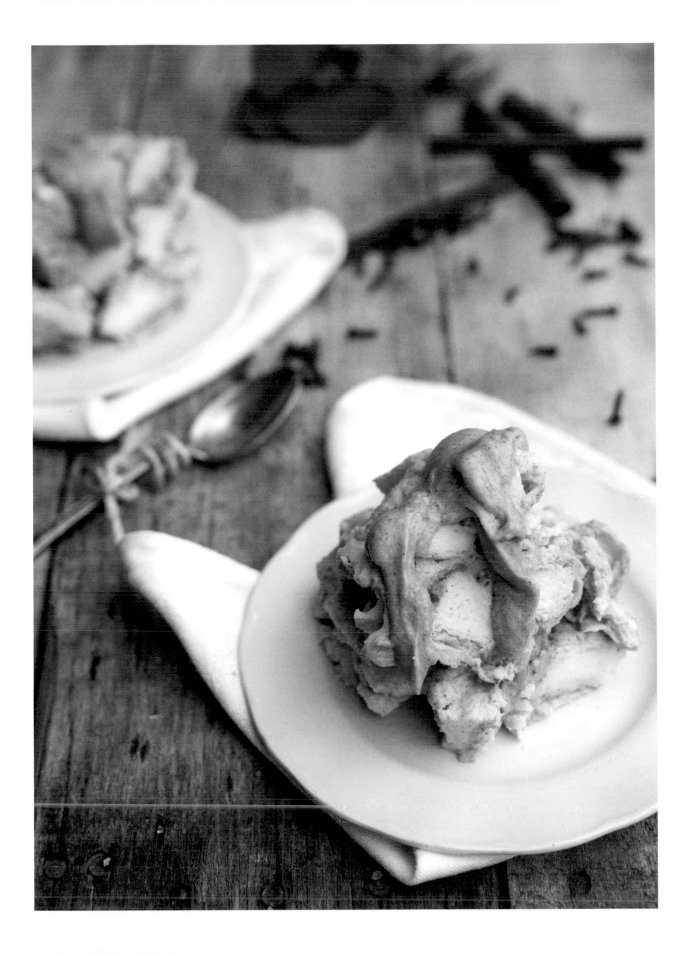

Cream Cheese Pumpkin Muffins

When I worked at Uncommon Ground, we made the absolute best pumpkin cream cheese muffins in the fall. They usually sold out before 8 a.m. Once I was asked to do a presentation at a large company in Stillwater, Minnesota, and the woman coordinating the event asked me to bring a few food samples. I thought "'tis the season," so I made my equally tasty keto-friendly version of the coffee shop's pumpkin muffins. They disappeared within minutes!

KETO   OPTION

prep time: 7 minutes   *cook time:* 40 minutes
yield: 6 muffins (1 per serving)

muffin batter

1½ cups blanched almond flour

½ teaspoon baking soda

¼ teaspoon fine sea salt

1 teaspoon ground cinnamon

½ teaspoon ground nutmeg

¼ teaspoon ground ginger

⅛ teaspoon ground cloves

2 tablespoons unsalted butter (or coconut oil if dairy-free), softened

½ cup Swerve confectioners'-style sweetener or equivalent amount of liquid or powdered sweetener (see page 24)

3 large eggs

1 cup fresh or canned pumpkin puree

cream cheese filling

1 (8-ounce) package cream cheese (Kite Hill brand cream cheese style spread if dairy-free), softened

¼ cup Swerve confectioners'-style sweetener or equivalent amount of liquid or powdered sweetener (see page 24)

1 large egg yolk

2 teaspoons vanilla extract

1. Preheat the oven to 325°F. Grease or place paper liners in 6 wells of a standard-size muffin pan.

2. In a large mixing bowl, stir the almond flour, baking soda, salt, and spices until well combined. In another bowl, mix together the butter, sweetener, eggs, and pumpkin until smooth. Stir the wet ingredients into the dry. Spoon the batter into the prepared muffin cups, filling each about two-thirds full.

3. To make the filling, using a hand mixer, beat the cream cheese in a medium-sized bowl until smooth. Add the sweetener, egg yolk, and vanilla and beat until well combined. Top each muffin with about 1 tablespoon of the cream cheese filling and use a toothpick to swirl it into the batter.

4. Bake the muffins for 30 to 40 minutes, until a toothpick inserted into the center of a muffin comes out clean. Allow to cool before removing from the pan. Store extras in an airtight container in the refrigerator for up to 3 days. Reheat on a baking sheet in a preheated 350°F oven for 5 minutes or until warmed through.

nutritional info (per muffin)				
calories	fat	protein	carbs	fiber
399	33g	13g	12g	4g

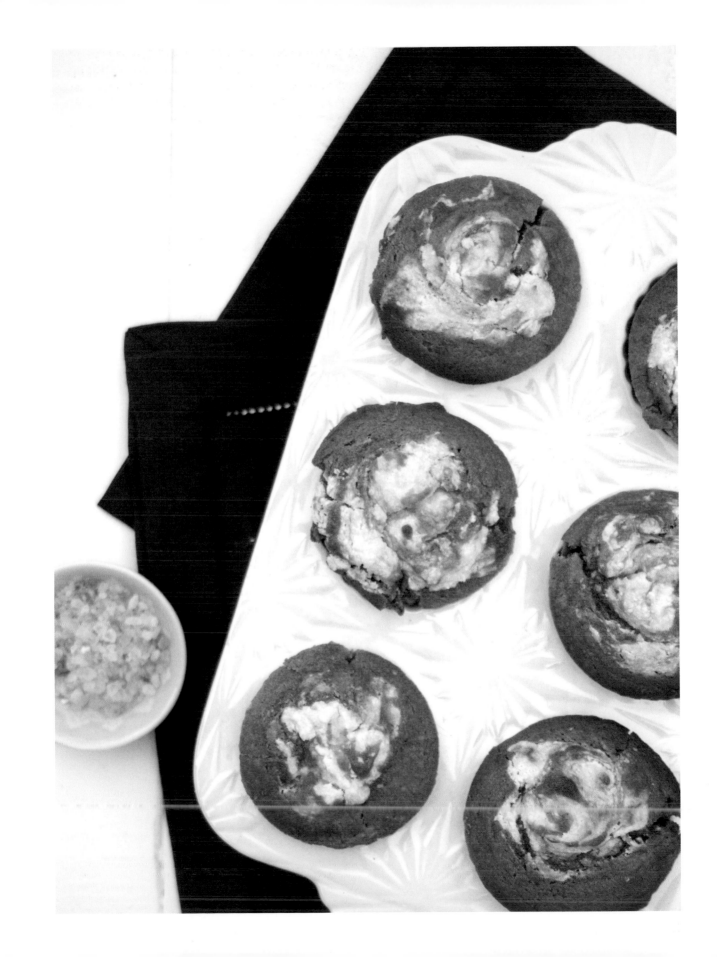

Grandma Suzie's Kringle

When Craig and I first met (and our diet and lifestyle were quite different than they are today), we adored camping up on the south shore of Lake Superior in the adorable town of Bayfield, Wisconsin. Every morning we went to a cute bakery in town and ordered the almond kringle. It was ooey and gooey and stuffed with a decadent cream cheese mixture. It has been more than a decade, but this keto-friendly kringle reminds me of those early-morning trips to the bakery in Bayfield. My recipe is named after my mother-in-law, Sue (my boys call her Grandma Suzie), who also makes an amazing kringle.

This recipe may seem daunting, but let me tell you some tricks that I learned while working at coffee shop bakeries, where I needed to get multiple confections ready and into the display case before 5 a.m.:

• You can make the dough, fillings, and glaze up to 2 days ahead and store them in the refrigerator. Then all you have to do is assemble and bake the kringle on the day you want to consume it.

• You can make multiple batches of the dough and store them in airtight containers in the freezer for future use.

• You can bake the kringle and freeze it, but it is much better fresh!

M
L ⤳ H
KETO

dough

1¾ cups shredded mozzarella cheese

1 ounce cream cheese (2 tablespoons)

¾ cup blanched almond flour

1 large egg, beaten

⅛ teaspoon fine sea salt

cinnamon filling

2 tablespoons melted unsalted butter

2 tablespoons Swerve confectioners'-style sweetener or equivalent amount of liquid or powdered sweetener (see page 24)

2 tablespoons ground cinnamon

cream cheese filling

1 (8-ounce) package cream cheese, softened

¼ cup Swerve confectioners'-style sweetener or equivalent amount of liquid or powdered sweetener (see page 24)

1 large egg yolk

prep time: 15 minutes, plus 1 hour to chill dough, if needed
cook time: 15 minutes   *yield:* 8 servings

1. Preheat the oven to 400°F.

2. To make the dough, place the mozzarella and cream cheese in a microwave-safe bowl and microwave for 1 to 2 minutes, until the cheese is entirely melted. Stir well.

3. To the bowl, add the almond flour, egg, and salt and combine well using a hand mixer. Use your hands and work it like a traditional dough, kneading for about 3 minutes. (*Note:* If the dough is too sticky, chill it in the refrigerator for an hour or overnight.)

4. Grease a 14-inch-long piece of parchment paper and place it on a pizza stone (or a baking sheet, but a pizza stone will bake the bottom of the kringle better). Place the dough on the greased parchment and use a rolling pin or your hands to form it into a large oval, about 12 inches by 8 inches. Position the oval so that one of the short sides is facing you.

5. To make the cinnamon filling, place the melted butter, sweetener, and cinnamon in a small bowl and use a fork to combine well. Place this mixture on top of the dough and spread it out, covering as much of the surface of the dough as possible.

6. To make the cream cheese filling, place the softened cream cheese, sweetener, and egg yolk in a bowl and mix well to combine. Starting 3 inches from the top of the dough oval and working your way toward you, pour this mixture down the middle of the oval, ending 3 inches from the edge nearest you. Now spread the filling into an oval shape, leaving 1½ inches along the left and right edges exposed.

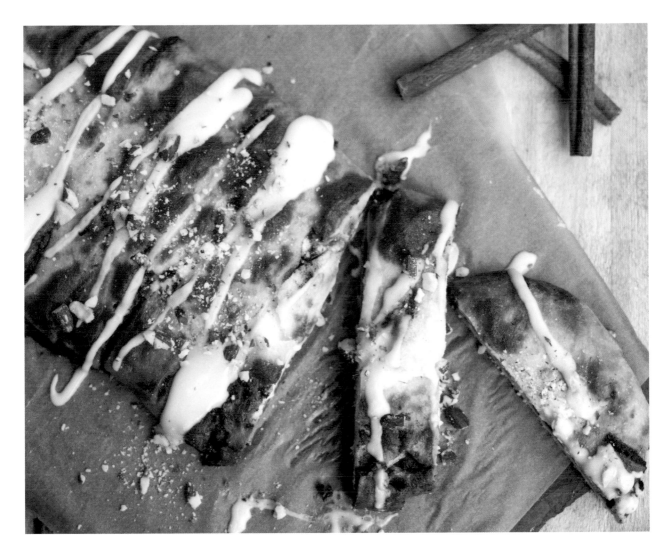

glaze

¼ cup Swerve confectioners'-style sweetener or equivalent amount of powdered stevia or erythritol (see page 24)

1 to 2 tablespoons unsweetened cashew milk or heavy cream

optional garnish

Crushed almonds

7. Cut 1½-inch long, ¾-inch-wide flaps along the long sides of the kringle, cutting only into the part that doesn't have any cream cheese filling on it. Fold the top and bottom ends in, on top of the cream cheese filling. Then, starting at the top of the oval, fold the right flap over the cream cheese filling, then the left flap; continue folding the flaps over the filling until the whole kringle is wrapped and a zipper like kringle is made. Some of the cream cheese will be exposed.

8. Place the pizza stone with the kringle in the oven to bake for 15 minutes or until the kringle is golden brown and the dough is fully cooked. Remove from the oven and allow to cool on the stone for 10 minutes.

9. Meanwhile, make the glaze: Place the sweetener in a small bowl and add just enough cashew milk to make a thin glaze. If it gets too thin, add a tablespoon of sweetener, and if it is still too thick, add another splash of milk.

10. Once the kringle is cool, drizzle the glaze over it and sprinkle with crushed almonds, if desired. Store extras in an airtight container in the refrigerator for up to 3 days. Reheat on a baking sheet in a preheated 350°F oven for 5 minutes or until warmed through.

nutritional info (per serving)				
calories	fat	protein	carbs	fiber
271	23g	11g	5g	2g

Sour Cream Coffee Cake
with Browned Butter Glaze

There's nothing more special than setting out a huge coffee cake for a Saturday breakfast or brunch. If you are pressed for time in the morning, you can prepare the batter, filling, and glazes a night or two beforehand. Pour the batter and filling into the pan and place the pan in the refrigerator. Then all you have to do in the morning is place the pan in the oven, then pour the glaze over the top after baking. Your house will be filled with the wonderful aroma of cinnamon and browned butter!

KETO

prep time: 15 minutes   *cook time:* 45 minutes
yield: 1 Bundt cake (14 servings)

cake batter

1 cup coconut flour, or 4 cups blanched almond flour

1 tablespoon ground cinnamon

2 teaspoons baking powder

1 teaspoon fine sea salt

¾ cup (1½ sticks) unsalted butter or coconut oil, softened

1½ cups Swerve confectioners'-style sweetener or equivalent amount of liquid or powdered sweetener (see page 24)

1½ teaspoons vanilla extract

8 large eggs (4 eggs if using almond flour)

1½ cups sour cream

cinnamon filling

½ cup Swerve confectioners'-style sweetener or equivalent amount of liquid or powdered sweetener (see page 24)

6 tablespoons (¾ stick) melted unsalted butter or coconut oil

1 tablespoon ground cinnamon

1 teaspoon vanilla extract

browned butter glaze

¾ cup (1½ sticks) unsalted butter or coconut oil

¼ cup Swerve confectioners'-style sweetener or equivalent amount of liquid or powdered sweetener (see page 24)

cream cheese glaze

1 (8-ounce) package cream cheese, softened

¼ cup unsweetened cashew milk

¼ cup Swerve confectioners'-style sweetener or equivalent amount of liquid or powdered sweetener (see page 24)

Seeds scraped from 1 vanilla bean (about 8 inches long), or 1 teaspoon vanilla extract

Chopped nuts of choice, for garnish (optional)

1. Preheat the oven to 350°F. Grease a 9-cup Bundt pan.

2. To make the cake batter, stir together the coconut flour, cinnamon, baking powder, and salt in a medium-sized bowl; set aside. In a large bowl, using a hand mixer, beat the softened butter, sweetener, and vanilla until light and fluffy. Add the eggs one at a time, beating for at least 1 minute after each addition. Beat in the flour mixture alternately with the sour cream. Pour half of the batter into the prepared pan.

3. To make the cinnamon filling, place the sweetener, melted butter, cinnamon, and vanilla in a small bowl and stir well to combine. Pour the filling evenly over the batter in the pan, using a knife to swirl it into the batter. Pour the rest of the batter into the pan.

4. Bake for 40 to 45 minutes, until a toothpick inserted in the center of the cake comes out clean. Let it cool in the pan for 10 minutes, then turn it out onto a wire rack to cool completely.

5. Meanwhile, make the browned butter glaze: Place the butter in a saucepan over medium-high heat and cook, whisking constantly, until brown (but not black!) flecks appear. Keep heating and whisking; the butter will froth up and then settle down. Remove the pan from the heat. (If using coconut oil, simply heat the oil in the pan until melted.)

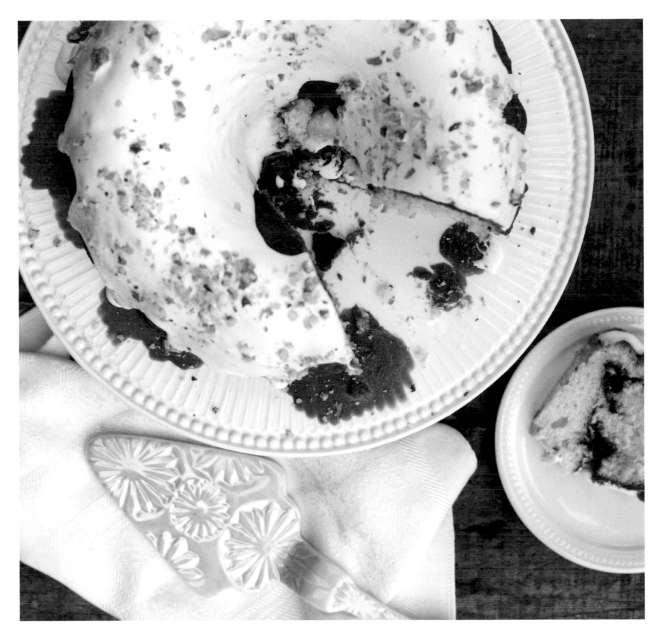

nutritional info (per serving of cake made with almond flour)				
calories	fat	protein	carbs	fiber
536	51g	11g	9g	4g

nutritional info (per serving of cake made with coconut flour)				
calories	fat	protein	carbs	fiber
403	37g	7g	7g	3g

Add the sweetener and whisk until smooth. Set in the refrigerator to cool for 5 to 8 minutes.

6. Once the browned butter glaze has cooled and thickened a bit, pour it over the cooled cake and place the cake in the refrigerator to set the glaze, about 8 minutes.

7. Meanwhile, make the cream cheese glaze: Using the hand mixer, beat the softened cream cheese, cashew milk, and sweetener in a medium-sized bowl. Add the vanilla and stir well; taste and add more sweetener, if desired.

8. Remove the cake from the fridge. Drizzle the cream cheese glaze over the cake and garnish with chopped nuts, if desired. Store extras in an airtight container in the refrigerator for up to 3 days.

Tiramisu Muffins

L M H
KETO OPTION OPTION

prep time: 10 minutes cook time: 20 minutes
yield: 12 muffins (1 per serving)

muffins

½ cup coconut flour, or 2 cups blanched almond flour

½ cup Swerve confectioners'-style sweetener or equivalent amount of liquid or powdered sweetener (see page 24)

2 tablespoons unsweetened cocoa powder

¼ teaspoon fine sea salt

¼ teaspoon baking soda

6 large eggs (2 eggs if using almond flour), beaten

½ cup (1 stick) unsalted butter (or coconut oil if dairy-free), melted but not hot

½ cup brewed decaf espresso or other strong brewed decaf coffee

2 teaspoons rum extract

frosting

1 (8-ounce) package mascarpone cheese (or Kite Hill brand cream cheese style spread if dairy-free), softened

¼ cup Swerve confectioners'-style sweetener or equivalent amount of liquid or powdered sweetener (see page 24)

1 ounce brewed decaf espresso or other strong brewed decaf coffee

1 teaspoon rum extract

Unsweetened cocoa powder, for dusting

1. Preheat the oven to 350°F. Grease a standard-size 12-well muffin pan, or line the wells with paper liners.

2. In a medium-sized bowl, sift together the dry ingredients for the muffin batter. Slowly add the wet ingredients to the dry ingredients and stir until very smooth. Fill each well of the muffin pan about two-thirds full with the batter. Bake for 18 to 20 minutes, until a toothpick inserted in the center of a muffin comes out clean. Allow to cool in the pan before removing.

3. Meanwhile, make the frosting: Combine all the ingredients and mix until smooth. Set aside until the muffins are cool, then frost the muffins. Dust the frosted muffins with cocoa powder.

4. Store extras in an airtight container in the refrigerator for up to 1 week. The muffins can be frozen if unfrosted, but do not freeze the frosting.

nutritional info (per muffin)				
calories	fat	protein	carbs	fiber
209	19g	5g	3g	2g

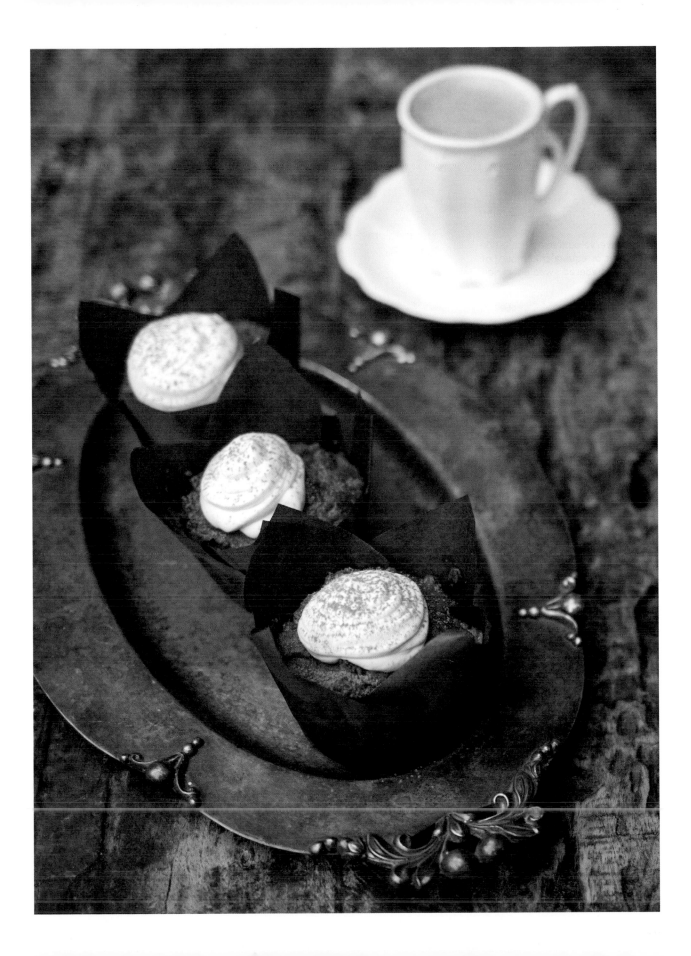

Amazing Breakfast Sausage Bake

There is a fantastic little brunch place near us that makes the juiciest, most flavorful sausage bake. If you're looking for a fast yet amazing brunch dish, you must try this recipe! If you plan on serving four people, it's easy to double the recipe.

½ pound bulk pork sausage

½ teaspoon fine sea salt

⅓ cup beef bone broth, homemade (page 356) or store-bought

2 strips bacon, diced

¼ cup shredded cheddar cheese

¼ cup thinly sliced green onions, for garnish

prep time: 5 minutes *cook time:* 8 minutes *yield:* 2 servings

1. Preheat the broiler. Form the sausage into four 1½ by 2½-inch oval-shaped patties. Season on all sides with the salt.

2. Place the sausage patties in an 8-inch square casserole dish. Pour the broth over the patties and place the dish in the oven. Broil for 7 minutes or until the patties are cooked through.

3. Meanwhile, cook the diced bacon in a skillet over medium heat, stirring often, for 5 minutes or until the bacon is cooked through and crispy. Remove from the heat and set aside.

4. Remove the dish from the oven and top the sausage patties with the cheese and cooked bacon. Return the pan to the oven for 1 minute or until the cheese is melted. Garnish with the green onions.

5. Store extras in an airtight container in the refrigerator for up to 3 days. Reheat on a baking sheet in a preheated 350°F oven for 5 minutes or until warmed through.

nutritional info (per serving)				
calories	fat	protein	carbs	fiber
493	42g	26g	1g	0.4g

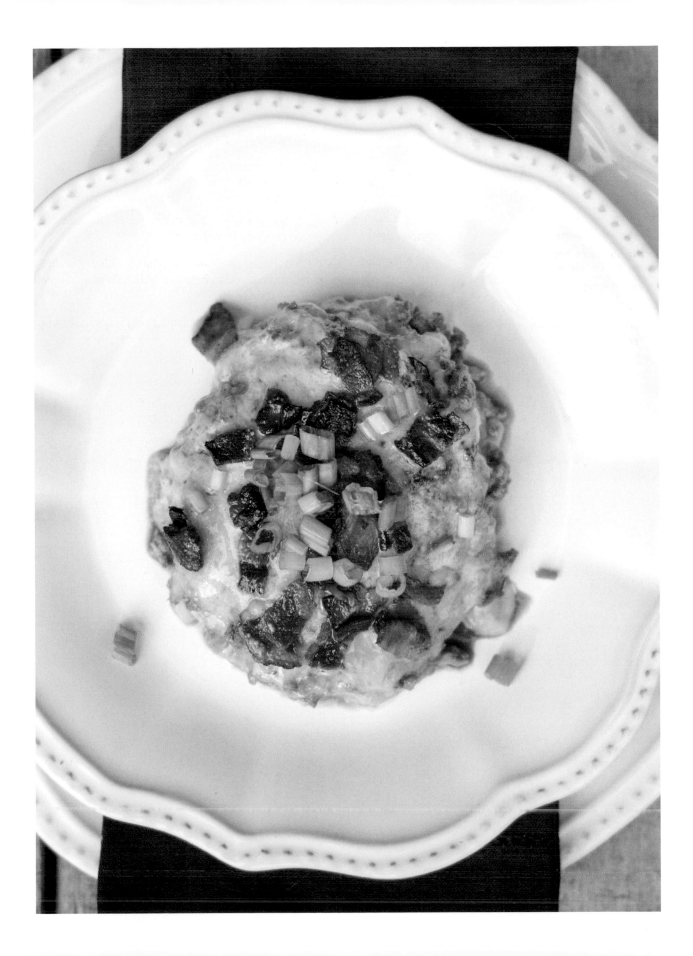

Monte Cristo Crepes

I always store hard-boiled eggs in the refrigerator so I can easily whip up a batch of crepes!

KETO   OPTION OPTION

prep time: 10 minutes (not including time to hard-boil eggs)
cook time: 8 minutes   *yield:* 2 servings

crepes

2 large eggs

2 hard-boiled eggs

4 ounces cream cheese (½ cup) (Kite Hill brand cream cheese style spread if dairy-free), softened

1 tablespoon Swerve confectioners'-style sweetener or equivalent amount of liquid or powdered sweetener (see page 24)

½ teaspoon vanilla or almond extract

Pinch of fine sea salt

Coconut oil, for the pan

filling

2 very thin slices ham

2 thin slices (1 ounce) Swiss cheese (omit for dairy-free)

raspberry glaze

1½ ounces cream cheese (3 tablespoons) (Kite Hill brand cream cheese style spread if dairy-free), softened

2 tablespoons unsweetened cashew milk (or hemp milk if nut-free), warmed

2 tablespoons Swerve confectioners'-style sweetener or equivalent amount of liquid or powdered sweetener (see page 24)

½ teaspoon raspberry extract

special equipment

8-inch crepe pan or nonstick skillet (see page 28)

1. To make the crepe batter, place the raw eggs, hard-boiled eggs, cream cheese, sweetener, extract, and salt in a blender and blend until very smooth.

2. Grease an 8-inch crepe pan or nonstick skillet with coconut oil or coconut oil spray and set it over medium-high heat. When hot, pour ¼ cup of the batter into the skillet and swirl the skillet to spread the batter to the edges of the pan. Cook until golden brown, about 2 minutes, then flip and cook for another 2 minutes. Remove from the pan and repeat with the remaining batter.

3. Place 1 slice of ham and 1 slice of cheese in the center of each crepe. Fold the crepe in half, then fold it again into quarters.

4. Make the glaze: Place all the ingredients in a small bowl and whisk until well combined. Taste and add more sweetener and/or extract, if desired. Serve the crepes drizzled with the glaze.

5. Store extra crepes and glaze in separate airtight containers in the refrigerator for up to 3 days. Reheat the crepes on a baking sheet in a preheated 350°F oven for 5 minutes or until warmed through. Bring the glaze to room temperature, then drizzle it over the crepes.

nutritional info (per serving)				
calories	fat	protein	carbs	fiber
452	38g	20g	4g	0g

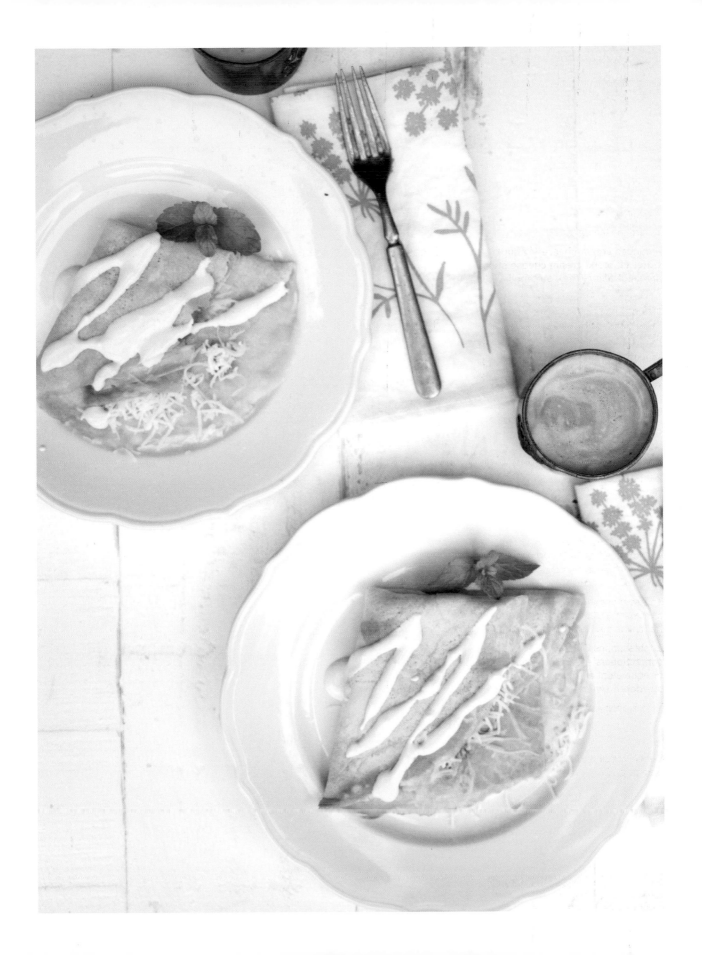

Chicken and Waffles
with Hollandaise

L M H
KETO OPTION

chicken

1 cup coconut oil or bacon fat, for frying

2 large eggs

1½ cups grated Parmesan cheese (or pork dust if dairy-free)

¼ teaspoon ground black pepper

1 pound boneless, skinless chicken thighs

waffles

3 cups shredded zucchini

Fine sea salt

1 cup powdered Parmesan cheese (see page 13) (or pork dust if dairy-free)

2 tablespoons unsalted butter (or coconut oil if dairy-free), softened

2 large eggs, beaten

½ cup Hollandaise (page 358), for serving

1. To make the chicken, place 1 cup of coconut oil in a 4-inch-deep (or deeper) cast-iron skillet over medium heat and heat it to 350°F.

2. Meanwhile, prepare the egg wash and breading: In a medium-sized bowl, beat the eggs. In another medium-sized bowl, mix together the 1½ cups of Parmesan cheese and the pepper.

3. Cut the chicken into bite-sized nuggets. Dip the nuggets into the egg mixture, then into the cheese mixture, coating each nugget well.

4. When the oil is hot, fry the nuggets in batches for about 5 minutes or until the chicken is no longer pink inside and the batter has a nice golden color. The exact timing will depend on how big you make the nuggets.

5. To make the waffles, heat a waffle iron to high heat. Place the shredded zucchini in a colander over the sink and sprinkle with salt. Allow to drain for 4 minutes. Squeeze out the excess moisture.

6. Place the zucchini in a medium-sized bowl. Add the 1 cup of Parmesan, butter, and eggs and mix well.

7. Grease the hot waffle iron. Place 3 tablespoons of the zucchini mixture in the center of the iron and close. Cook for 3 to 4 minutes, until the waffle is golden brown and crisp.

8. To serve, place 2 waffles on each plate and top with 2 chicken nuggets. Serve smothered in hollandaise.

9. Store extras in separate airtight containers in the refrigerator for up to 3 days. Reheat on a baking sheet in a preheated 350°F oven for 5 minutes or until warmed through, then top with the hollandaise. To reheat the hollandaise, see page 358.

tip : *If you prefer not to fry the chicken nuggets, you can bake them instead. Preheat the oven to 350°F. Place the breaded nuggets on a greased baking sheet and bake for 20 to 30 minutes, until they're golden brown and cooked through. Again, the exact timing will depend on how big you make the nuggets.*

nutritional info (per serving)				
calories	fat	protein	carbs	fiber
639	48g	60g	2g	1g

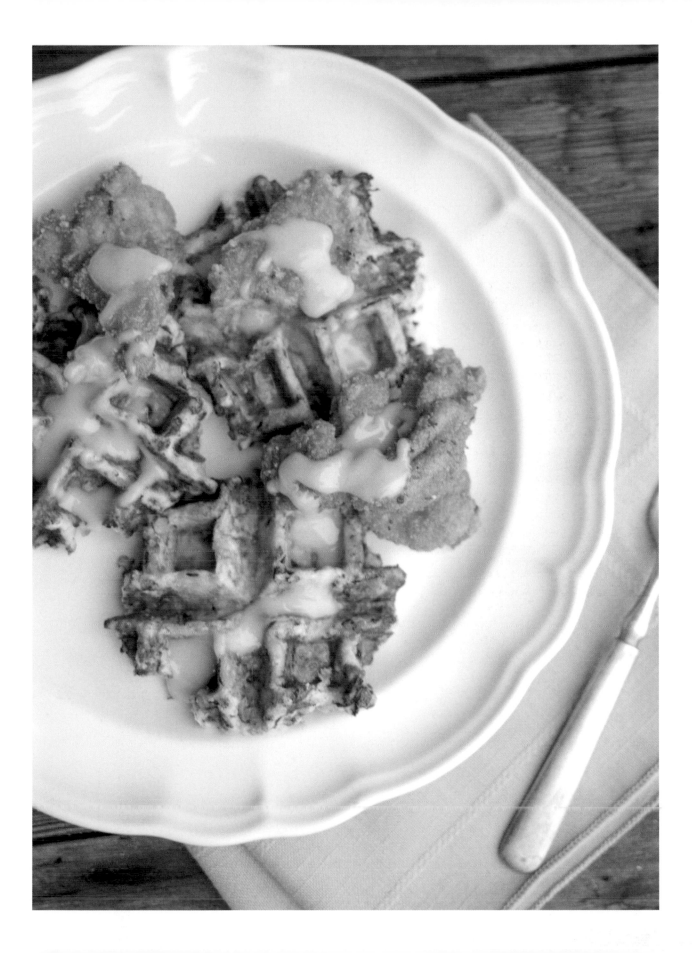

Glazed Chocolate Donuts

L M H
KETO OPTION OPTION

chocolate donuts

½ cup coconut flour

½ cup Swerve confectioners'-style sweetener or equivalent amount of liquid or powdered sweetener (see page 24)

⅓ cup unsweetened cocoa powder

½ teaspoon baking soda

½ teaspoon ground cinnamon

⅛ teaspoon fine sea salt

5 large eggs

½ cup unsweetened almond milk (or hemp milk if nut-free)

½ cup (1 stick) unsalted butter (or coconut oil if dairy-free), softened

1 teaspoon vanilla extract

chocolate glaze

¾ cup full-fat coconut milk (or heavy cream if not dairy-sensitive)

⅓ cup Swerve confectioners'-style sweetener or equivalent amount of liquid or powdered sweetener (see page 24)

2 ounces unsweetened chocolate, finely chopped

Seeds scraped from 1 vanilla bean (about 8 inches long), or 1 teaspoon vanilla extract

special equipment (optional)

6-cavity donut pan (see note)

prep time: 5 minutes *cook time:* 20 minutes
yield: 6 donuts (1 per serving)

1. Preheat the oven to 350°F. Grease a 6-cavity donut pan.

2. To make the donuts, combine all the dry ingredients in a mixing bowl and stir together until well combined. Add the wet ingredients to the bowl and use a hand mixer to combine until smooth.

3. Fill each well of the donut pan two-thirds full with the batter. Bake for about 20 minutes, until a toothpick inserted in the center of a donut comes out clean. Let the donuts cool in the pan before glazing them.

4. To make the glaze, place the coconut milk, sweetener, and chopped chocolate in a double boiler or a heat-safe bowl set over a pan of simmering water. Heat on low, stirring, just until the chocolate melts. Remove from the heat. Add the vanilla and stir well to combine. Dip the cooled donuts in the glaze.

5. Store extras in an airtight container in the refrigerator for up to 3 days.

note: If you don't own a donut pan, you can also make these in a muffin pan. Simply grease 6 wells of a standard-size muffin pan and follow the instructions above.

nutritional info (per donut)				
calories	*fat*	*protein*	*carbs*	*fiber*
332	28g	9g	9g	5g

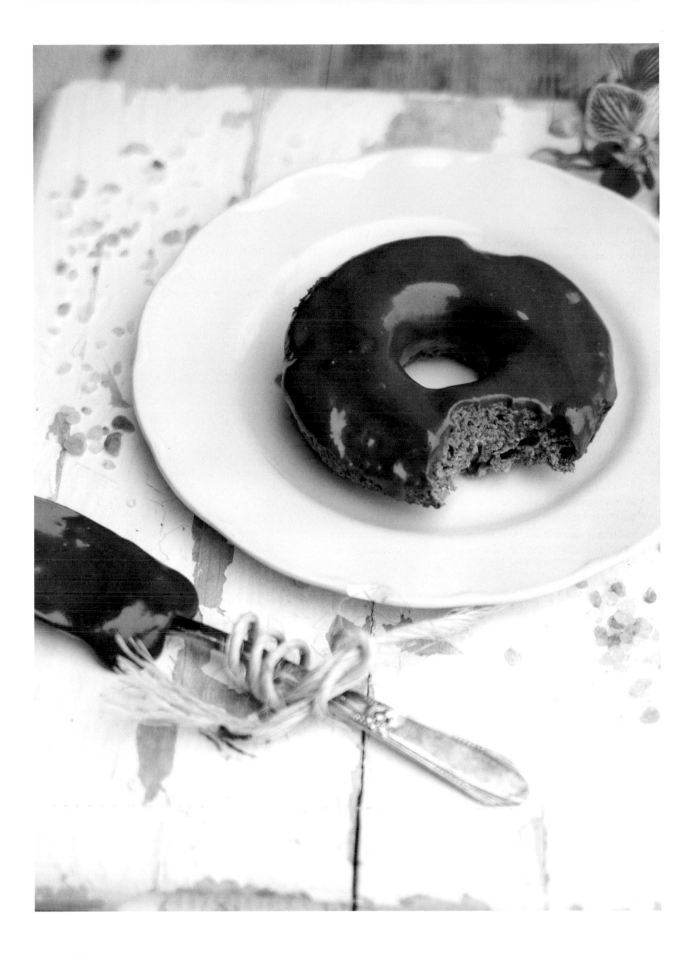

Chocolate Donut Bread Pudding

I love listening to cooking podcasts for inspiration while I run. One podcaster talked about how she would pick up donuts at the gas station, leave them out to get dry, and then make bread pudding out of them for Christmas morning. She prepared the bread pudding on Christmas Eve, so all she had to do was throw the pan in the oven while the kids were unwrapping their gifts. I thought, "Hmm, I can do that!"

For an even more indulgent breakfast, make a double batch of the chocolate glaze when making the donuts and drizzle each piece of bread pudding with 1 to 2 tablespoons of the extra glaze.

1 batch Glazed Chocolate Donuts (page 66), preferably a day old, cut into 1-inch cubes

pudding

1 cup unsweetened cashew milk or almond milk (or hemp milk if nut-free)

½ cup heavy cream (or full-fat coconut milk if dairy-free)

3 large eggs

⅔ cup Swerve confectioners'-style sweetener or equivalent amount of liquid or powdered sweetener (see page 24)

1 teaspoon ground cinnamon

Seeds scraped from 1 vanilla bean (about 8 inches long), or 1 teaspoon vanilla extract

½ teaspoon fine sea salt

optional topping

Extra Chocolate Glaze (page 66), for drizzling

prep time: 10 minutes (not including time to make donuts)

cook time: 45 minutes to 1 hour (less if using a muffin pan) *yield:* 12 servings

1. Preheat the oven to 350°F. Grease an 11 by 7-inch baking dish or a standard-size 12-well muffin pan.

2. In a bowl, cover the cubed donuts with the milk and cream; set aside. In another bowl, combine the eggs, sweetener, cinnamon, and vanilla; blend well. Pour the egg mixture over the soaked donuts and stir to blend. Pour the combined mixture into the prepared baking dish or muffin pan (if using a muffin pan, fill each well about two-thirds full).

3. Bake for 45 minutes to 1 hour, until set. If making muffins, bake for 25 to 30 minutes, until set. Allow to cool completely in the pan. Cut bread pudding made in a baking dish into 12 equal-size pieces. If desired, drizzle each piece (or "muffin") with 1 to 2 tablespoons of extra chocolate glaze.

4. Store extras in an airtight container in the refrigerator for up to 3 days. Reheat on a baking sheet in a preheated 350°F oven for 5 minutes or until warmed through.

nutritional info (per serving)				
calories	fat	protein	carbs	fiber
220	19g	6g	5g	3g

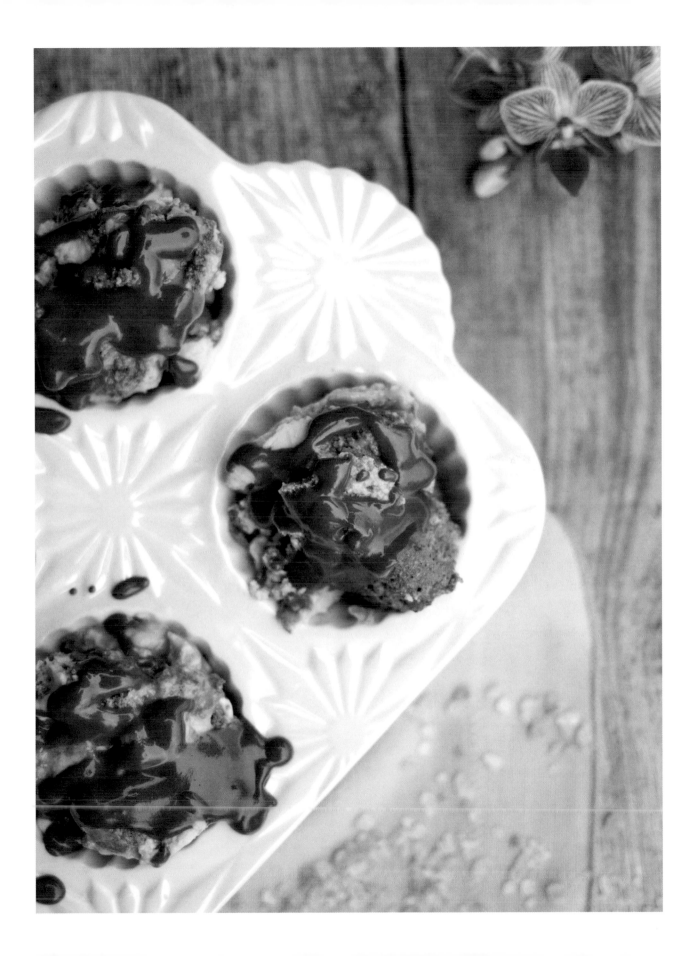

Red Velvet Pancakes
with Cream Cheese Syrup

prep time: 5 minutes (not including time to hard-boil eggs)

cook time: 8 minutes   yield: four 3-inch pancakes (2 per serving)

pancakes

2 large eggs

2 hard-boiled eggs

4 ounces cream cheese (½ cup) (Kite Hill brand cream cheese style spread if dairy-free)

1 tablespoon Swerve confectioners'-style sweetener or equivalent amount of liquid or powdered sweetener (see page 24)

1 tablespoon natural red food dye

1½ teaspoons unsweetened cocoa powder

½ teaspoon vanilla or almond extract

Pinch of fine sea salt

Coconut oil or spray, for the pan

cream cheese syrup

1½ tablespoons cream cheese (Kite Hill brand cream cheese style spread if dairy-free), softened

¼ cup unsweetened cashew milk (or unsweetened hemp milk if nut-free), plus more if needed

2 tablespoons Swerve confectioners'-style sweetener or equivalent amount of liquid or powdered sweetener (see page 24)

Seeds scraped from 1 vanilla bean (about 8 inches long), or 1 teaspoon vanilla extract

1. Place the ingredients for the pancakes in a blender and blend until very smooth.

2. Grease a large nonstick skillet with coconut oil or coconut oil spray and place over medium-high heat. When hot, pour ¼ cup of the batter into the skillet, forming a 3-inch round pancake; repeat to cook 2 pancakes at a time. Cook until cooked through on the bottom, about 2 minutes, then flip and cook for another 2 minutes. Remove the pancakes from the pan and repeat with the remaining batter.

3. To make the syrup, place the softened cream cheese, cashew milk, sweetener, and vanilla in a small bowl and beat with a hand mixer until smooth. Add more or less milk depending on how thick or thin you prefer the syrup. Serve the pancakes drizzled with the syrup.

4. Store extra pancakes and syrup in separate airtight containers in the refrigerator for up to 3 days. Reheat the pancakes on a baking sheet in a preheated 350°F oven for 5 minutes or until warmed through. Heat the syrup in a saucepan over medium heat for about 2 minutes.

busy family tip:

I make the batter and store the blender jar in the refrigerator overnight for an easy breakfast the next morning.

nutritional info (per serving)				
calories	fat	protein	carbs	fiber
401	33g	19g	5g	1g

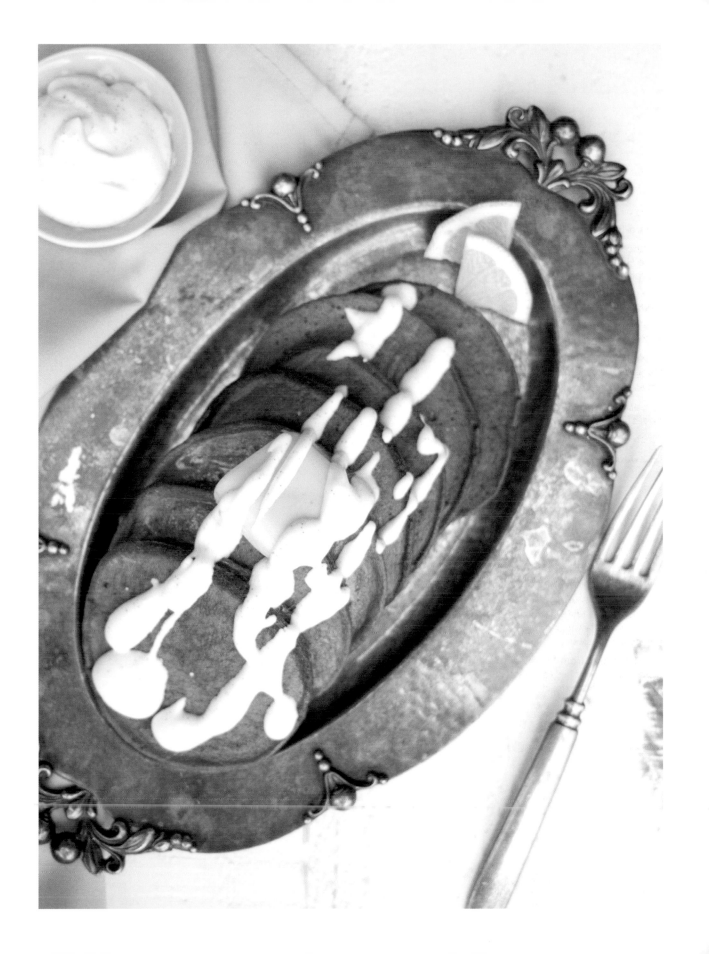

Snickerdoodle Breakfast Pots de Crème

Whenever I make these pots de crème—or crème brûlée or ice cream, for that matter—I save the whites for making Keto Buns (page 362).

L M H KETO   OPTION   OPTION

2 cups heavy cream (or full-fat coconut milk if dairy-free)

¾ cup unsweetened cashew milk or almond milk (or hemp milk if nut-free)

Seeds scraped from 1 vanilla bean (about 8 inches long), or 1 teaspoon vanilla extract

6 large egg yolks

½ cup Swerve confectioners'-style sweetener or equivalent amount of liquid or powdered sweetener (see page 24)

2 teaspoons ground cinnamon

prep time: 10 minutes, plus 3 hours to chill   *cook time:* 1 hour
yield: 6 servings

1. Preheat the oven to 325°F.

2. Bring the cream, milk, and vanilla just to a simmer in a medium-sized heavy saucepan over medium heat. Remove from the heat.

3. In a large bowl, whisk the egg yolks, sweetener, and cinnamon. Gradually whisk the egg mixture into the cream mixture.

4. Use a fine-mesh strainer to strain the mixture into another bowl. Let cool for 10 minutes, skimming any foam from the surface.

5. Divide the mixture among six 6-ounce custard cups. Place the cups in a large baking dish that is at least 2 inches deep. Add hot water to the baking dish to come halfway up the sides of the cups. Cover the baking dish with a lid or foil to trap the steam.

6. Bake until the custards are set but the center of each still moves slightly when gently shaken, about 55 minutes. Remove from the water. Chill the custards until cold, about 3 hours.

7. Store extras in an airtight container in the refrigerator for up to 3 days.

nutritional info (per serving)				
calories	fat	protein	carbs	fiber
326	37g	3g	1g	0.2g

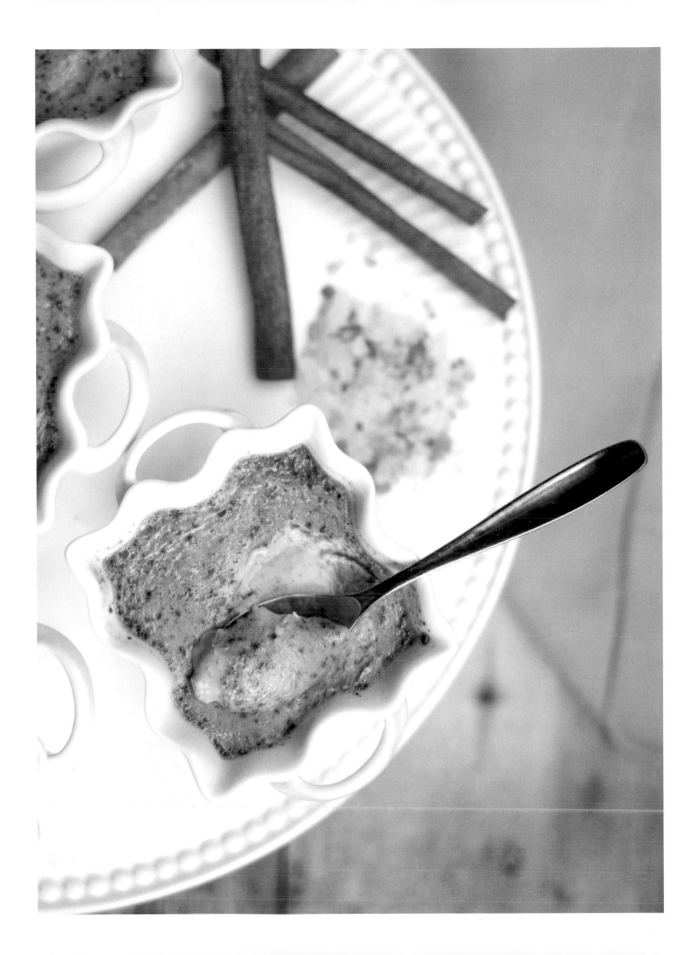

BBQ Pulled Pork Hash
with Eggs

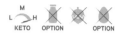

prep time: 5 minutes (not including time to make pulled pork)
cook time: 15 minutes *yield:* 4 servings

1 tablespoon ghee or unsalted butter (or coconut oil if dairy-free)

½ cup chopped red onions

1½ cups shredded red or green cabbage

2 cups leftover BBQ Pulled Pork (page 258), plus sauce from the slow cooker

¾ teaspoon fine sea salt

¼ teaspoon ground black pepper

¼ teaspoon cayenne pepper (optional)

4 large eggs (omit for egg-free)

Melted ghee, for serving

Chopped fresh cilantro or parsley, for garnish

Finely diced red onions, for garnish

1. Melt the ghee in a skillet over medium heat. Add the onions and cook, stirring, until slightly softened, about 2 minutes. Add the cabbage and continue to cook for 5 minutes or until the cabbage is very soft.

2. Add the pulled pork to the skillet and stir well to combine. Make 4 wells in the hash and crack an egg into each well. Season with the salt, black pepper, and cayenne pepper, if using.

3. Cover and cook for 3 minutes or until the egg whites are cooked but the yolks are still soft.

4. Drizzle with extra BBQ sauce and melted ghee and garnish with cilantro or parsley and diced red onions.

5. Store extras in an airtight container in the refrigerator for up to 3 days. Reheat on a baking sheet in a preheated 350°F oven for 5 minutes or until warmed through.

nutritional info (per serving)				
calories	*fat*	*protein*	*carbs*	*fiber*
482	36g	29g	7g	2g

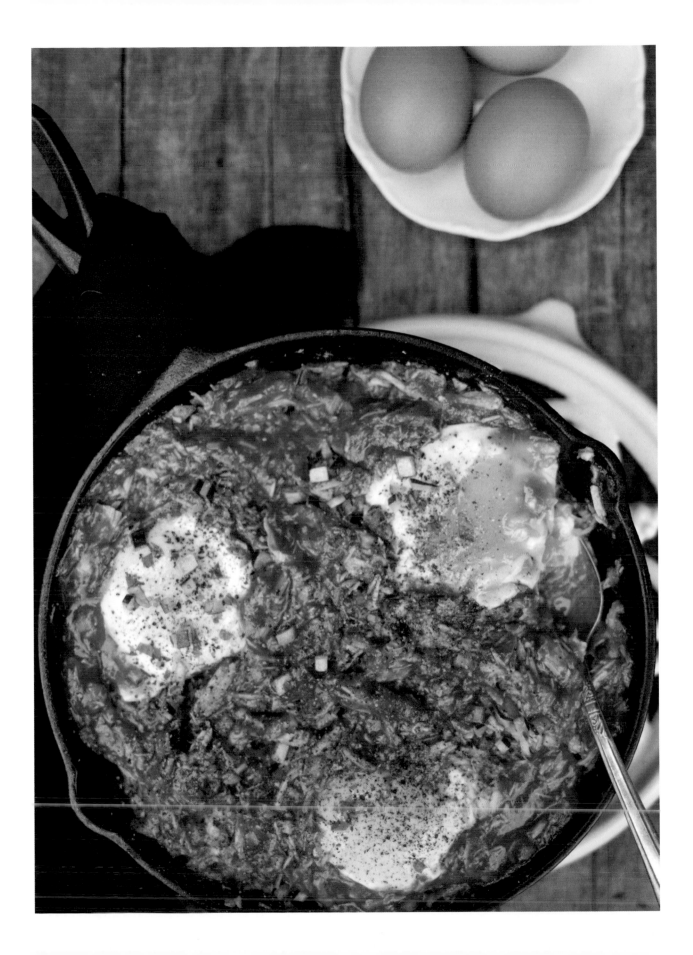

Maple Bacon Waffle Breakfast Sundaes

Even the *International Business Times* wrote about how eating ice cream for breakfast may improve mental performance and alertness.

There aren't a lot of foods that I am tempted by anymore. There was a time when I would have to excuse myself at dinner if someone ordered a decadent dessert, but now I do not feel deprived given all the tasty desserts I can make at home. But walking by an ice cream shop that makes its own waffle cones must bring back special memories or something, because I *love* that smell! When we were vacationing in Hawaii, Craig said the same thing as we walked by this cute ice cream shop. That smell inspired me to come home and create this delicious creation of ice cream over waffles!

L M H
KETO   OPTION

prep time: 10 minutes (not including time to hard-boil eggs, make ice cream or glaze, or cook bacon) *cook time:* about 20 minutes *yield:* 6 servings

waffles

4 large eggs

4 hard-boiled eggs

¼ cup Swerve confectioners'-style sweetener or equivalent amount of liquid or powdered sweetener (see page 24)

2 tablespoons egg white protein powder

2 tablespoons ground cinnamon

¾ teaspoon baking powder

¼ teaspoon fine sea salt

¼ cup coconut oil, plus extra for the waffle iron

2 teaspoons vanilla extract

1 batch Maple Bacon Ice Cream (page 322)

½ batch Browned Butter Glaze (page 56), for drizzling (optional; omit for dairy-free)

Cooked diced bacon, for garnish (optional)

1. Heat a waffle iron to high heat. Place the raw eggs, hard-boiled eggs, sweetener, protein powder, cinnamon, baking powder, and salt in a blender or food processor and blend until smooth and thick. Add the coconut oil and vanilla and combine well.

2. Grease the hot waffle iron. Place 3 tablespoons of the batter in the center of the iron and close. Cook for 3 to 4 minutes, until the waffle is golden brown and crisp. Repeat with the remaining batter, making a total of 6 waffles.

3. To serve, place a waffle on a serving plate or bowl and top with a scoop of Maple Bacon Ice Cream. Garnish with a drizzle of browned butter glaze and diced cooked bacon, if desired.

4. Store extra waffles in an airtight container in the refrigerator for up to 3 days or in the freezer for up to 1 month. Reheat in a preheated 375°F oven or toaster oven for 3 minutes or until warmed through.

tip : *To change up the flavor of the waffles a bit, substitute 1 teaspoon of almond extract for 1 teaspoon of the vanilla extract.*

nutritional info (per serving)				
calories	fat	protein	carbs	fiber
712	70g	18g	3g	0.5g

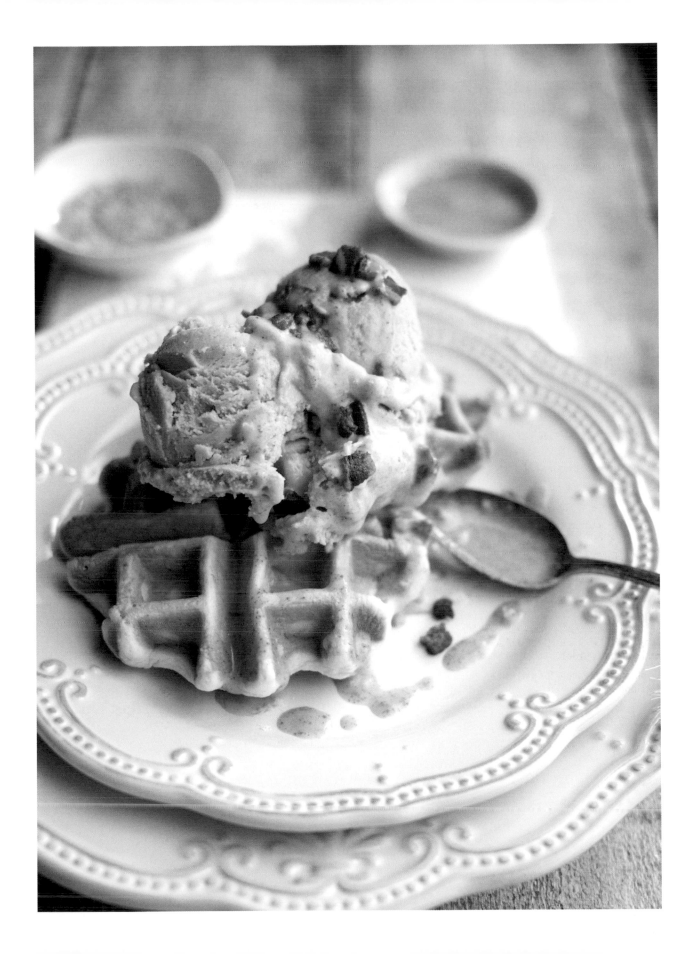

Croque Madame Waffles

prep time: 10 minutes (not including time to hard-boil eggs)
cook time: about 30 minutes   *yield:* 8 servings

waffles

8 large eggs

4 hard-boiled eggs

¼ cup powdered Parmesan cheese (see page 13)

1 teaspoon baking powder

1 teaspoon onion powder (optional)

½ teaspoon fine sea salt

½ cup ghee or coconut oil, melted but not hot

mornay sauce

¼ cup beef or chicken bone broth, homemade (page 356) or store-bought

¼ cup (½ stick) unsalted butter

1 ounce cream cheese (2 tablespoons)

1 cup shredded Gruyère or cheddar cheese

⅛ teaspoon fine sea salt

sandwich fillings

12 slices ham

½ cup shredded Gruyère or cheddar cheese

4 large eggs

1 teaspoon ghee or unsalted butter

for garnish (optional)

Ground black pepper

Fresh thyme leaves

1. To make the waffles, heat a waffle iron to high heat. Place the raw eggs, hard-boiled eggs, Parmesan cheese, baking powder, onion powder (if using), and salt in a blender or food processor and combine until smooth and thick. Add the melted ghee and combine well.

2. Grease the hot waffle iron. Place a heaping ¼ cup of the batter in the center of the iron and close. Cook for 3 to 4 minutes, until golden brown and crisp. Repeat with the remaining batter, making a total of 8 waffles.

3. To make the Mornay sauce, place the broth, butter, cream cheese, and shredded cheese in a saucepan over medium-high heat, whisking often, just until the cheese is melted. Add the salt, then slide the pan off the heat. Using an immersion blender, blend until very smooth (or transfer the mixture to a countertop blender and blend until smooth); set aside.

4. When you are ready to make the Croques Madames, preheat the oven to broil. Place the waffles on a rimmed baking sheet. Top 4 of the waffles with 3 slices of ham and 2 tablespoons of shredded cheese each. Set aside.

5. To fry the eggs, heat the ghee in a cast-iron skillet over medium heat. When hot, crack the 4 eggs into the pan and fry on one side for about 2 minutes, until the whites are cooked and the yolks are still runny. Place the waffles under the broiler at this point (see Step 6). Season the eggs with salt and pepper and remove the skillet from the heat.

6. While the eggs are cooking, broil the waffles for 1 to 2 minutes, until the cheese is melted and the waffles are warm.

7. To assemble the Croques Madames, place 1 ham and cheese–topped waffle on a serving plate. Top with a plain waffle, then add a sunny-side-up egg and smother with Mornay sauce. Sprinkle with freshly ground pepper and garnish with thyme leaves, if desired. Repeat with the remaining waffles, eggs, and Mornay sauce.

8. Store plain waffles in an airtight container in the refrigerator for up to 3 days or in the freezer for up to 1 month. Reheat the waffles in a preheated 375°F oven or toaster oven for 3 minutes or until warmed through. Store the Mornay sauce in an airtight container in the refrigerator for up to 3 days; it will thicken overnight. Reheat the sauce in a saucepan over medium heat, stirring, until warm, about 2 minutes. Add a few tablespoons of broth if the sauce is too thick.

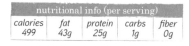

nutritional info (per serving)				
calories	fat	protein	carbs	fiber
499	43g	25g	1g	0g

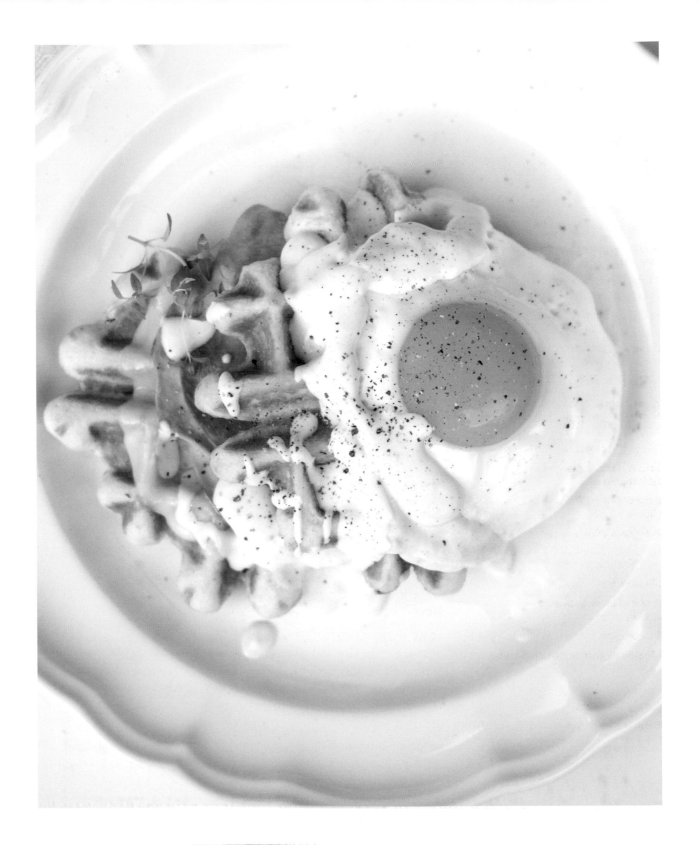

tip : The waffles and Mornay sauce can be made up to 3 days
ahead and stored in separate airtight containers in the
refrigerator. The waffles can be frozen for up to a month.

Sweet Breakfast Biscuits
with Chocolate or Caramel Mocha Gravy

prep time: 10 minutes   *cook time:* 15 minutes   *yield:* 8 servings

biscuits

3 large egg whites

1 cup blanched almond flour

2 tablespoons Swerve confectioners'-style sweetener or equivalent amount of powdered stevia or erythritol (see page 24)

1 teaspoon baking powder

¼ teaspoon fine sea salt

2 tablespoons very cold unsalted butter, cut into ¼-inch pieces, or cold coconut oil

Seeds scraped from 1 vanilla bean (about 8 inches long), or 1 teaspoon vanilla extract

option 1: chocolate gravy

¾ cup heavy cream

⅓ cup Swerve confectioners'-style sweetener or equivalent amount of liquid or powdered sweetener (see page 24)

2 ounces unsweetened chocolate, finely chopped

Seeds scraped from 1 vanilla bean (about 8 inches long), or 1 teaspoon vanilla extract

option 2: caramel mocha gravy

¾ cup (1½ sticks) unsalted butter

6 ounces cream cheese or mascarpone cheese (¾ cup)

¾ cup Swerve confectioners'-style sweetener or equivalent amount of liquid or powdered sweetener (see page 24)

3 tablespoons unsweetened cocoa powder

4 to 5 tablespoons brewed decaf espresso or other strong brewed decaf coffee, to thin the sauce

Seeds scraped from 1 vanilla bean (about 8 inches long), or 1 teaspoon vanilla extract

Fresh mint leaves, for garnish

1. Preheat the oven to 400°F. Grease a baking sheet or 8 wells of a standard-size muffin pan with coconut oil spray.

2. To make the biscuits, whip the egg whites in a medium-sized bowl until very stiff. In a separate medium-sized bowl, stir together the almond flour, sweetener, baking powder, and salt until well combined. Then cut the chilled butter into the flour mixture. (If the butter isn't chilled, the biscuits won't turn out.) Gently fold the dry mixture into the whites. If the dough is too wet to form into mounds, add a few tablespoons of almond flour until the dough holds together well.

3. Using a large spoon, dollop the dough into 8 mounds on the greased baking sheet (or into the greased muffin cups) and bake for 11 to 15 minutes, until golden brown.

4. If making the chocolate gravy, place the cream, sweetener, and chopped chocolate in a double boiler or in a heat-safe bowl set over a pan of simmering water. Heat on low, stirring, just until the chocolate melts. Remove from the heat and stir in the vanilla.

   If making the caramel mocha gravy, place the butter in a saucepan over medium-high heat. Cook, stirring often, until the butter foams up and brown (but not black!) flecks appear. Remove from the heat and allow to cool a bit. Using a hand mixer, cream the browned butter, cream cheese, and sweetener in a medium-sized bowl. Add the cocoa powder, espresso, and vanilla and beat until combined.

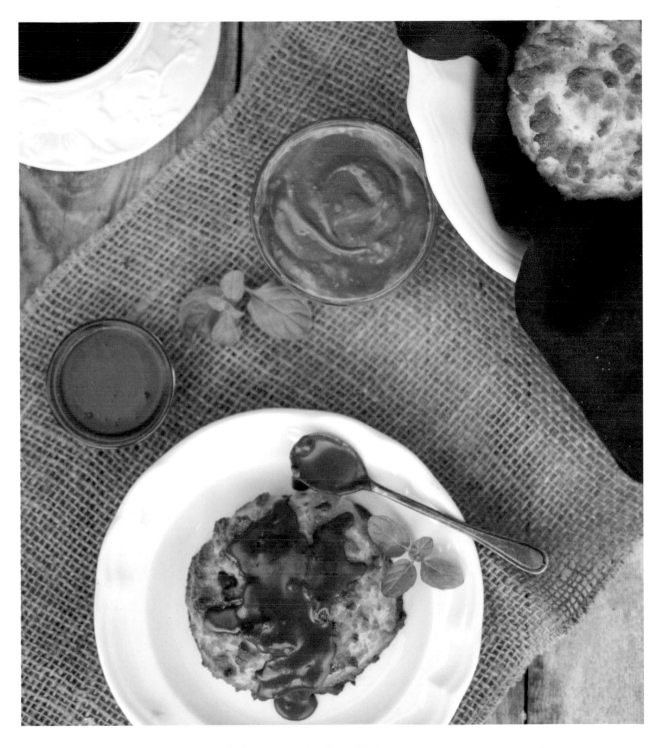

nutritional info (per biscuit with caramel mocha gravy)				
calories	fat	protein	carbs	fiber
345	34g	6g	5g	2g

5. Serve the biscuits with the warm gravy poured over them.

6. Store extra biscuits and gravy in separate airtight containers in the refrigerator for up to 3 days. The biscuits can be frozen for up to 1 month. Reheat the biscuits on a baking sheet in a preheated 350°F oven for 3 minutes or until warmed through. Reheat the gravy in a saucepan over low heat, whisking often, for 1 minute or until the gravy loosens a bit. Do not overheat or the chocolate will separate. Pour the warm gravy over the biscuits.

Crab Cake Eggs Benedict

prep time: 7 minutes (not including time to make hollandaise)
cook time: 10 minutes   *yield:* 4 servings

crab cakes

1 pound canned lump crabmeat

1 tablespoon mayonnaise, homemade (page 359) or store-bought

5 tablespoons powdered Parmesan cheese (see page 13) (or 2 tablespoons coconut flour if dairy-free)

2 large eggs

2 teaspoons seafood seasoning

2 tablespoons lard or coconut oil, for frying

poached eggs

8 large eggs

½ cup Hollandaise (page 358), for serving

1. Make the crab cakes: In a large bowl, mix together all the ingredients except the lard until well blended. Heat the lard in a large skillet over medium-high heat. With a spoon, place 2-tablespoon dollops of the crab mixture in the pan to form 8 mini-cakes. Cook until golden brown, about 2 minutes, and then flip each crab cake and cook for another minute, until golden brown on the other side.

2. Poach the eggs: Fill a large saucepan with about 4 inches of water. Bring to a simmer. Swirl the water in one direction and gently crack in the eggs. Poach the eggs until the whites are just cooked but the yolks are still soft and runny. Poach in 2 batches if needed to avoid overcrowding.

3. To serve, place 2 crab cakes on each plate, then top each crab cake with a poached egg and a drizzle of hollandaise.

4. Store the crab cakes and poached eggs in separate airtight containers in the refrigerator for up to 3 days. Store the hollandaise in a covered jar in the refrigerator for up to 5 days. Reheat the crab cakes in a greased skillet over medium heat, frying for a minute or two on each side until heated through. Reheat the poached eggs in a pot of simmering water for 1 minute or until warmed through. To reheat the hollandaise, see page 358.

nutritional info (per serving)				
calories	fat	protein	carbs	fiber
554	41g	40g	1g	0g

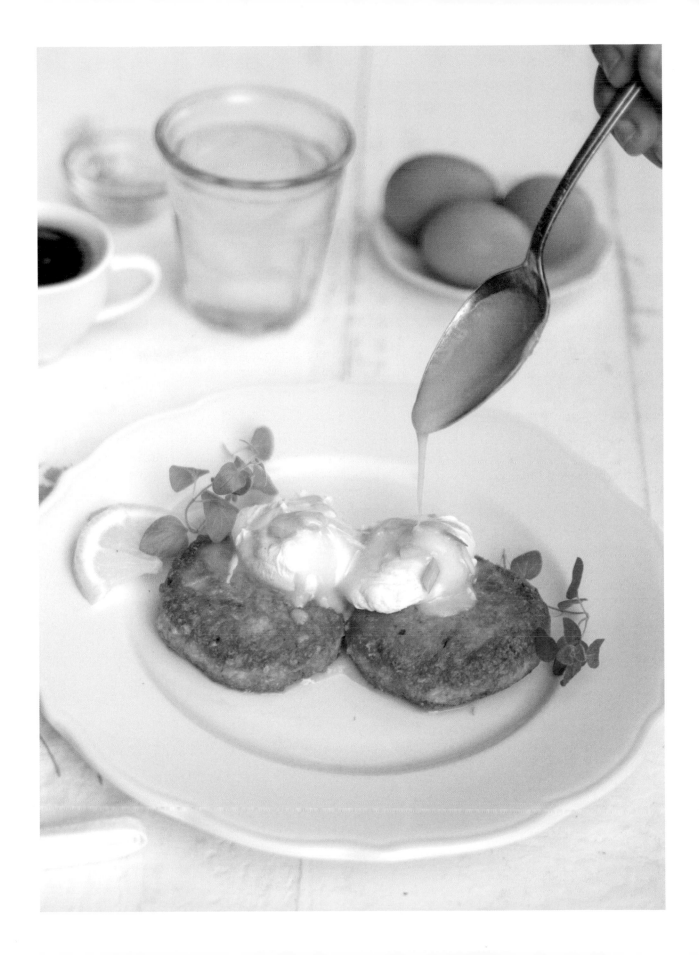

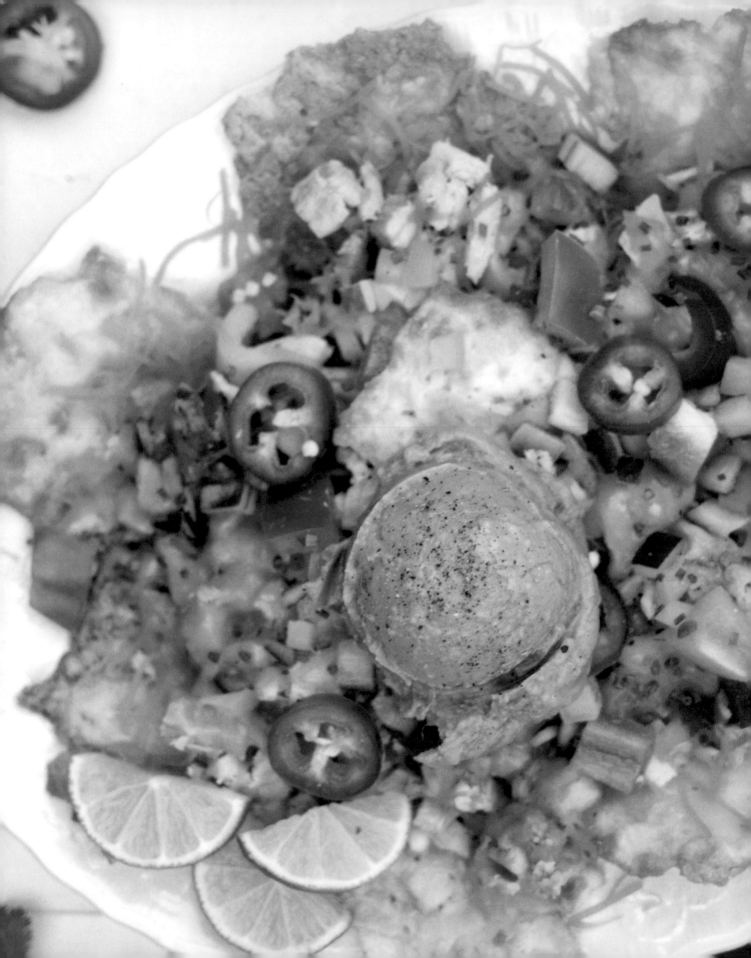

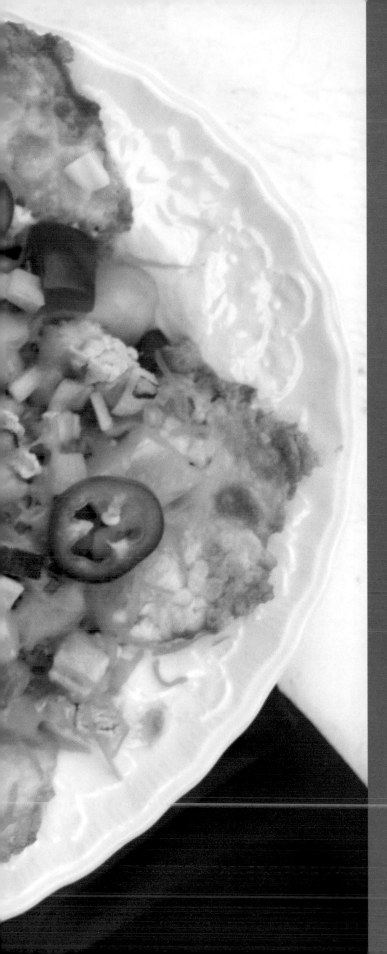

Appetizers
and Snacks

BLT Party Cheese Ball

1 (8-ounce) package cream cheese, softened

½ cup sour cream

1 cup crumbled blue cheese or shredded sharp cheddar cheese

½ cup diced tomatoes (fresh or canned)

¼ teaspoon fine sea salt

3 strips bacon, finely diced

Crispy lettuce leaves, such as iceberg or romaine, for serving

1. In a medium-sized bowl, combine the cream cheese, sour cream, blue cheese, tomatoes, and salt. Form the mixture into a ball, wrap in parchment paper, and place in the refrigerator to chill for 1 hour.

2. Meanwhile, cook the bacon: Place it in a skillet and fry over medium heat until golden and crispy, about 4 minutes. Remove the bacon from the skillet (reserving the fat for another use) and place in a shallow bowl.

3. When the cheese ball is set, roll it in the bacon pieces. Place on a serving platter and serve with crispy lettuce leaves cut into cracker-like squares. Store leftovers in an airtight container in the refrigerator for up to 4 days.

nutritional info (per serving)				
calories	fat	protein	carbs	fiber
268	22g	12g	2g	0g

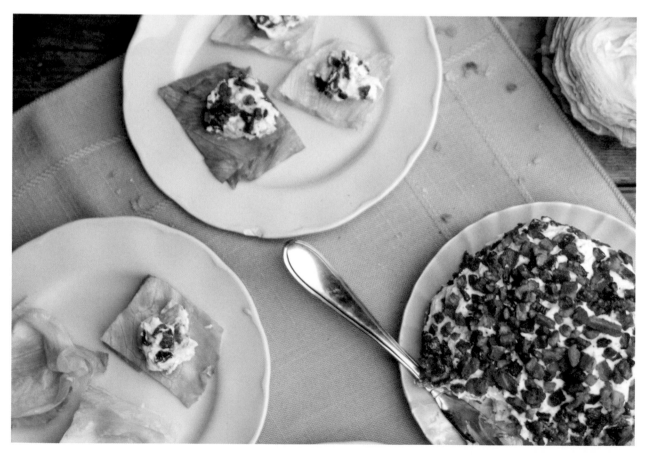

BLT Stuffed Mushrooms

prep time: 5 minutes *cook time:* about 30 minutes *yield:* 4 servings

20 large button mushrooms

1 tablespoon unsalted butter or coconut oil

¼ cup diced onions

2 cloves garlic, minced

½ pound bacon, cut into tiny pieces

4 ounces cream cheese (½ cup), softened

¼ cup shredded sharp cheddar cheese

½ teaspoon fine sea salt

½ teaspoon ground black pepper

2 cups chopped lettuce

nutritional info (per serving)				
calories	fat	protein	carbs	fiber
520	43g	25g	6g	1g

1. Preheat the oven to 350°F.

2. Wash the mushrooms and remove the stems. Set the caps aside on a paper towel to dry. Finely chop the stems.

3. Melt the butter in a skillet over medium heat, then add the onions, garlic, and mushroom stems. Cook for 2 to 3 minutes, until the onions begin to soften. Add the bacon and cook until crispy, about 4 minutes.

4. Transfer the bacon mixture to a mixing bowl. Stir in the cheeses. Stuff 1 tablespoon of the bacon and cheese mixture into each mushroom cap.

5. Place the stuffed mushrooms in an 8-inch square baking dish (a pie pan also works), then season them with the salt and pepper. Bake for 25 minutes or until the mushrooms are soft and the cheese is melted. Place the chopped lettuce on a serving platter. Serve the baked mushrooms on top of the bed of lettuce.

6. These are best served fresh, but any leftovers can be covered and refrigerated for up to 3 days. Reheat in a preheated 350°F oven or toaster oven for 5 minutes or until the cheese is melted.

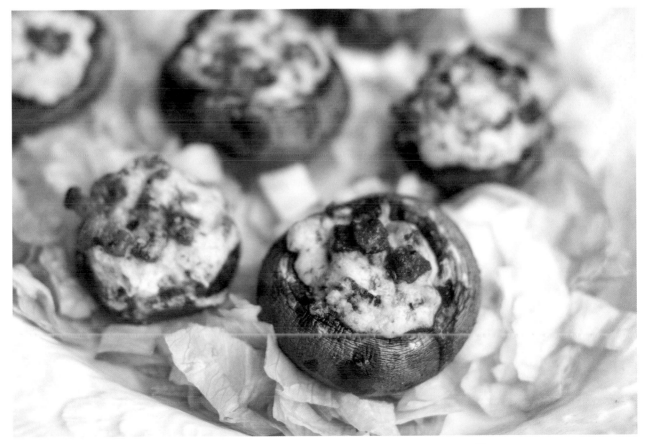

Twice-Baked Mashed Fauxtato Bites

If you are a visual learner like me, check out the video about how to make these bites on my site, MariaMindBodyHealth.com (type the word *video* in the search field).

prep time: 5 minutes (not including time to make fauxtatoes or cook bacon)

cook time: 15 to 30 minutes *yield:* 24 mini bites or 12 larger bites (6 mini bites or 3 larger bites per serving)

1 batch Mashed Fauxtatoes (page 129)

2 large eggs

for garnish

Sour cream

Shredded sharp cheddar cheese

Cooked diced bacon

Chopped fresh or dried chives

nutritional info (per serving)				
calories	fat	protein	carbs	fiber
354	25g	19g	14g	6g

1. Preheat the oven to 350°F.

2. Place the fauxtatoes in a large bowl. Add the eggs and mix well to combine.

3. Grease a 24-well mini muffin pan or a standard-size 12-well muffin pan. Fill each well two-thirds full with the fauxtato mixture. Bake for 15 to 20 minutes for mini muffins or 25 to 30 minutes for standard-size muffins, until they are turning golden brown.

4. Garnish each bite with a dot of sour cream and a sprinkle of shredded cheese, diced bacon, and chives. Store extra bites, ungarnished, in an airtight container in the refrigerator for up to 3 days. Reheat in a preheated 350°F oven for 4 minutes or until warmed through, then garnish and serve.

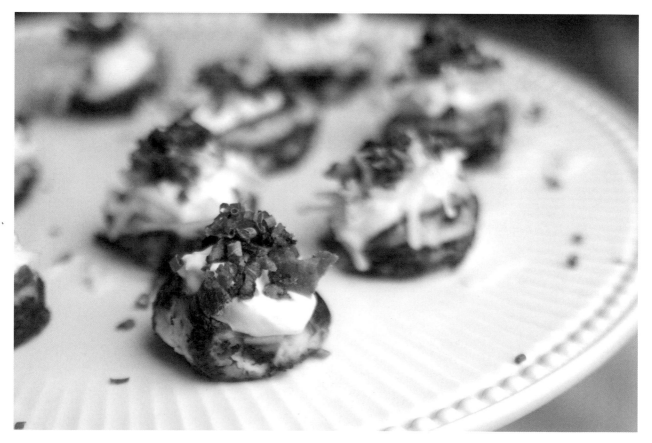

Bacon Poppers

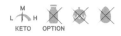
KETO   OPTION

prep time: 10 minutes (not including time to make dressing)
cook time: 30 minutes   yield: 6 servings

36 jalapeño peppers

1 (8-ounce) package cream cheese (Kite Hill brand cream cheese style spread if dairy-free), softened

1 clove garlic, smashed to a paste

1 teaspoon fine sea salt

¼ teaspoon ground black pepper

2 tablespoons chopped fresh cilantro, chives, or other herbs of choice (optional)

18 strips bacon

½ batch The Best Blue Cheese Dressing (page 360), for serving

1. Preheat the oven to 375°F.

2. Wash the jalapeños, cut off the stems, and cut the peppers in half lengthwise. Clean out the insides of the peppers.

3. In a medium-sized bowl, combine the cream cheese, garlic, salt, and pepper. Stir in the herbs, if using. Using a butter knife, stuff the peppers with the cream cheese mixture.

4. Cut the strips of bacon in half crosswise, then wrap one half strip around each stuffed pepper and secure with a toothpick.

5. Place the poppers on a rimmed baking sheet and bake for 25 to 30 minutes, until the bacon is fully cooked. Let cool slightly before eating. Serve with blue cheese dressing.

6. These are best served fresh, but any extra poppers and dressing can be stored in separate airtight containers in the refrigerator for up to 3 days. Reheat the poppers in a preheated 350°F oven until warmed through.

nutritional info (per serving)				
calories	fat	protein	carbs	fiber
478	39g	21g	9g	3g

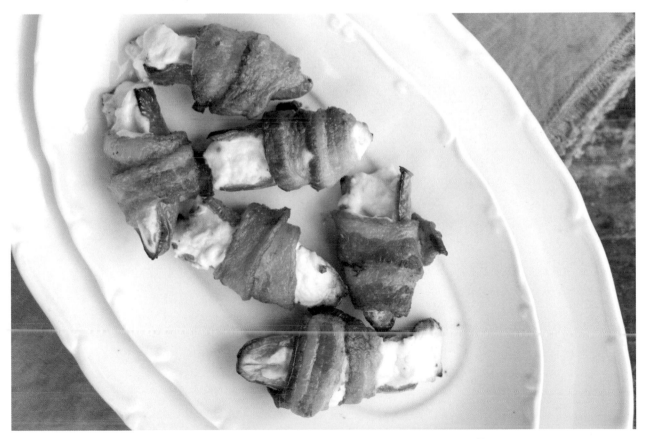

Buffalo Chicken Cannoli

To make this recipe even easier, use leftover cooked chicken or organic rotisserie chicken from the grocery store.

prep time: 10 minutes   *cook time:* 1 hour 45 minutes   *yield:* 4 servings

buffalo chicken

3 tablespoons bacon fat, lard, or ghee

4 chicken leg quarters (about 3 pounds)

1½ teaspoons fine sea salt

½ teaspoon ground black pepper

¼ cup diced onions

1 teaspoon minced garlic

1 cup chicken bone broth, homemade (page 356) or store-bought

¼ cup wing sauce or other medium-hot hot sauce

cannoli tubes

1 cup grated hard cheese, divided such as Parmesan, Asiago, or aged Gouda

for garnish

4 tablespoons wing sauce or other medium-hot hot sauce, divided

4 tablespoons crumbled blue cheese, divided

Celery sticks, for serving

1. To make the chicken, heat the fat in a deep sauté pan over medium-high heat. Season the leg quarters with the salt and pepper, place them in the hot fat, and sauté for about 8 minutes, until golden brown on all sides.

2. Add the onions and garlic and cook over medium heat for about 8 minutes, stirring occasionally, until the onions are golden brown.

3. Add the broth and hot sauce and simmer, covered, over medium heat for about 1½ hours, until the chicken is almost falling off the bone.

4. About 25 minutes before the chicken is done, make the cannoli tubes: Preheat the oven to 375°F. Have on hand 2 cylindrical objects, about 1 inch in diameter (I use spice jars). Place a sheet of parchment paper on a rimmed baking sheet and grease the parchment with coconut oil spray. Place ¼ cup of the cheese in a circle about 4 inches in diameter. Repeat with another ¼ cup of cheese to make a second 4-inch circle, leaving at least 2 inches of space between them. Bake for 4 to 5 minutes, until golden brown.

5. When you remove the baking sheet from the oven, you will need to move quickly. Using a spatula or knife, transfer the rounds of cheese to the cylindrical objects and form them around the molds. Allow to cool for 10 minutes before removing from the molds. Repeat with the remaining cheese to make a total of 4 tubes. (*Note:* Once you're practiced at making cheese tubes, you can make up to four at time.) Once cool, fill with the chicken filling.

6. When the chicken is done, remove the leg quarters from the pan and allow them to cool until you can handle them. Pull the meat off the bones, then chop it.

7. To serve, fill the cooled cheese tubes with the chopped chicken. Place each cannoli on a serving plate, drizzle with 1 tablespoon of hot sauce, and top with 1 tablespoon of blue cheese crumbles. Serve with celery sticks.

8. These are best served fresh, but any extra buffalo chicken and cannoli tubes can be stored in separate airtight containers in the refrigerator for up to 3 days.

nutritional info (per serving)				
calories	fat	protein	carbs	fiber
441	31g	36g	3g	0.4g

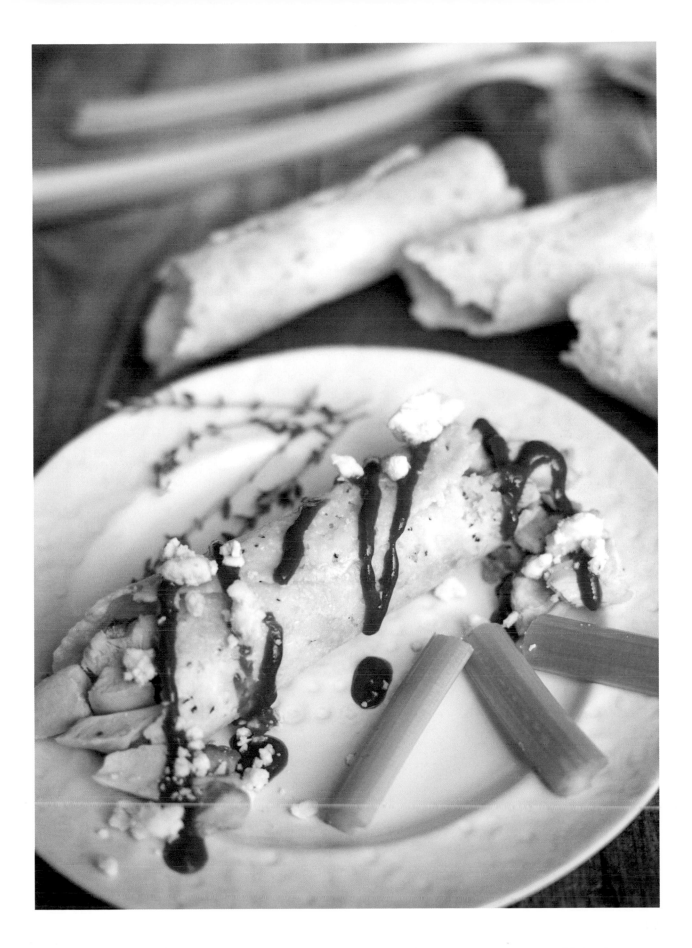

Loaded Fries
with Ranch

L M H
KETO ✖

prep time: 7 minutes *cook time:* about 20 minutes *yield:* 8 servings

3 medium zucchini

1 large egg

½ cup powdered Parmesan cheese (see page 13)

¾ cup diced bacon (about 4 strips)

¾ cup shredded Colby Jack cheese

Sliced green onions, for garnish

½ cup ranch dressing, homemade (page 359) or store-bought, for serving

1. Preheat the oven to 450°F. Line a rimmed baking sheet with parchment paper. Grease the parchment with coconut oil spray and set aside.

2. Cut the zucchini into French fry shapes about ½ inch by ½ inch by 4 inches.

3. Whisk the egg in a large bowl. Place the zucchini fries in the bowl and mix well with your hands, coating all sides of the zucchini with the egg.

4. Place the Parmesan cheese in a large resealable plastic bag.

5. Place half of the egg-coated zucchini in the bag with the Parmesan. Seal the bag with some air inside it and shake well to coat the zucchini. Place the coated fries on the prepared baking sheet.

6. Repeat Step 5 with the remaining zucchini. Bake the fries for 13 to 15 minutes, until golden brown.

7. Meanwhile, fry the diced bacon in a cast-iron skillet for about 4 minutes, until crispy.

8. Top the fries with the shredded cheese, then the crispy bacon. Return to the oven for 4 minutes or until the cheese is melted. Garnish with sliced green onions. Serve with ranch dressing.

9. These fries are best served fresh, but any extras can be stored in an airtight container in the refrigerator for up to 3 days. Reheat on a rimmed baking sheet in a preheated 375°F oven until the fries are crispy and heated through, about 5 minutes.

nutritional info (per serving)				
calories	fat	protein	carbs	fiber
191	16g	9g	3g	1g

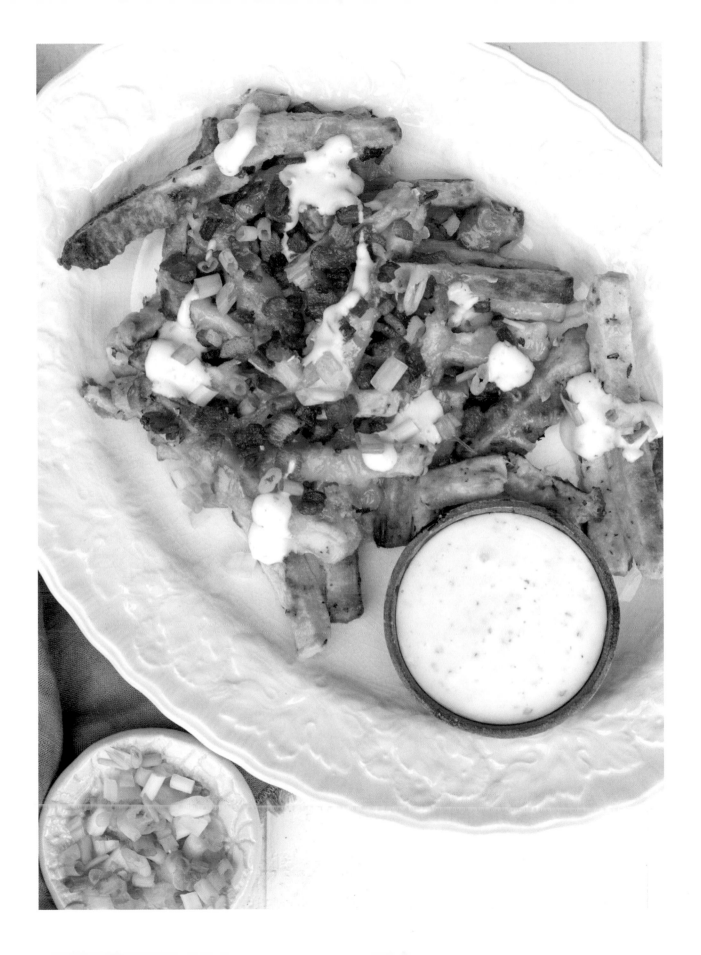

Pizza Fat Bombs

L M H
KETO ✕ ✕

1 (8-ounce) package cream cheese, softened

¼ cup powdered Parmesan cheese (see page 13)

3 tablespoons pizza sauce, homemade (page 358) or store-bought, plus extra for serving (optional)

1 teaspoon Italian seasoning, plus extra for garnish (optional)

¼ teaspoon red pepper flakes (optional)

1 cup mini pepperoni slices or finely diced pepperoni

Extra-virgin olive oil or avocado oil, for drizzling (optional)

1. Place the cheeses, pizza sauce, Italian seasoning, and red pepper flakes, if using, in a bowl. Mix until smooth. Cover and place in the refrigerator to thicken overnight.

2. Remove the cheese mixture from the fridge. Take 2 tablespoons of the mixture and roll it into a golf ball–sized ball. Repeat with the remaining cheese mixture, making a total of 8 balls.

3. Roll the balls in the pepperoni. Garnish with a sprinkle of Italian seasoning and a drizzle of olive oil and serve with additional pizza sauce, if desired.

4. Store extras in an airtight container in the refrigerator for up to 3 days.

nutritional info (per fat bomb)				
calories	fat	protein	carbs	fiber
142	13g	4g	1g	0g

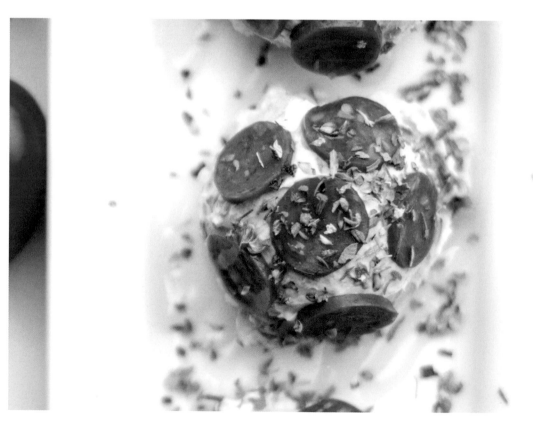

Bacon-Wrapped Stuffed Portobellos

prep time: 5 minutes (not including time to make dressing)
cook time: 10 minutes   *yield:* 6 servings

6 large baby portobello (aka cremini) mushrooms, about 3 inches in diameter

4 ounces cream cheese (½ cup), softened

½ teaspoon fine sea salt

3 dashes hot sauce, or to taste

2 ounces blue cheese, crumbled

6 strips bacon, cut in half lengthwise

½ batch The Best Blue Cheese Dressing (page 360), for serving

1. Preheat the oven to 400°F. Line a rimmed baking sheet with parchment paper.

2. Remove the stems from the mushrooms and finely chop the stems (I use a food chopper for this task). Place the chopped stems in a small bowl. Add the softened cream cheese, salt, and hot sauce. Taste and add more hot sauce, if desired.

3. Place the mushroom caps on the lined baking sheet, cavity side up. Stuff the cream cheese mixture into the mushroom caps. Top the filling with the blue cheese crumbles.

4. Wrap 2 bacon halves around each mushroom cap, forming a cross, and secure the bacon ends with a toothpick; otherwise, the bacon will curl up as it cooks.

5. Bake the stuffed mushrooms for 10 minutes or until the bacon is cooked to your liking. Serve with blue cheese dressing.

6. Store extras in an airtight container in the refrigerator for up to 4 days. Reheat on a rimmed baking sheet in a preheated 400°F oven for 4 minutes or until the bacon is crisp and the mushrooms are warmed through.

nutritional info (per mushroom)				
calories	fat	protein	carbs	fiber
271	23g	13g	2g	0.2g

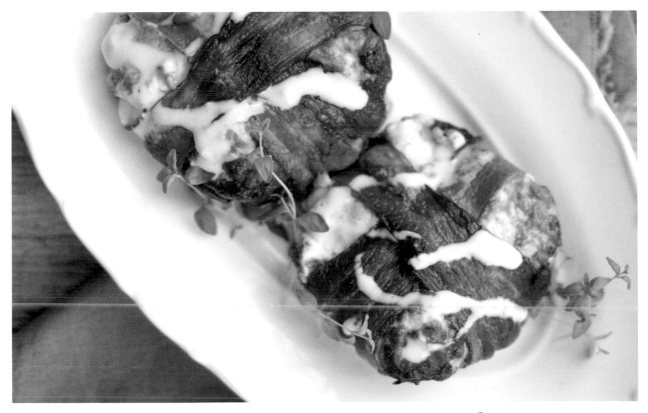

Loaded Chicken Nachos

L M H
KETO ✗ ✗

prep time: 10 minutes   *cook time:* 15 minutes   *yield:* 8 servings

chips

2 cups grated hard cheese, such as Parmesan, Asiago, or aged Gouda (about 8 ounces)

filling

3 teaspoons avocado oil, divided

1 green bell pepper, diced

1 red bell pepper, diced

2 cups diced leftover chicken or turkey

4 teaspoons lime juice

¼ teaspoon ground cumin

⅛ teaspoon fine sea salt

⅛ teaspoon ground black pepper

1 cup shredded sharp cheddar cheese

for garnish (optional)

Guacamole

Sour cream

Sliced jalapeño peppers

Finely diced onions

Lime wedges or slices

1. Preheat the oven to 375°F. Place a piece of parchment paper on a rimmed baking sheet.

2. Make the chips: Using a 2½-inch jar lid or round cookie cutter as a guide, drop 1 tablespoon of the cheese onto the parchment and use your fingers to spread the cheese to form a circle. Space the circles of cheese about 2 inches apart.

3. Bake the rounds for 5 minutes or until lightly browned and bubbly. Allow to cool on the pan; they will crisp up as they cool. Remove the chips from the parchment paper and place on a serving platter.

4. Meanwhile, make the filling: Heat 1½ teaspoons of the oil in a large skillet over medium-high heat. Add the bell peppers and sauté for 3 minutes or until crisp-tender; transfer the peppers to a small bowl.

5. While the peppers are cooking, combine the chicken, lime juice, cumin, salt, and pepper in a medium-sized bowl.

6. In a greased 13 by 9-inch baking dish, layer half of the peppers, half of the chicken, and then half of the cheddar cheese. Repeat the layers. Bake, uncovered, for 10 minutes or until heated through.

7. Use a spatula to transfer the nacho mixture from the baking dish onto the chips on the serving platter. Serve with guacamole, sour cream, sliced jalapeños, finely diced onions, and lime wedges or slices, if desired.

8. These nachos are best served fresh, but extra filling and chips can be stored in separate airtight containers in the refrigerator for up to 4 days. Reheat the filling in a baking dish in a preheated 375°F oven for 4 minutes or until warmed through.

nutritional info (per serving)				
calories	*fat*	*protein*	*carbs*	*fiber*
229	13g	24g	3g	1g

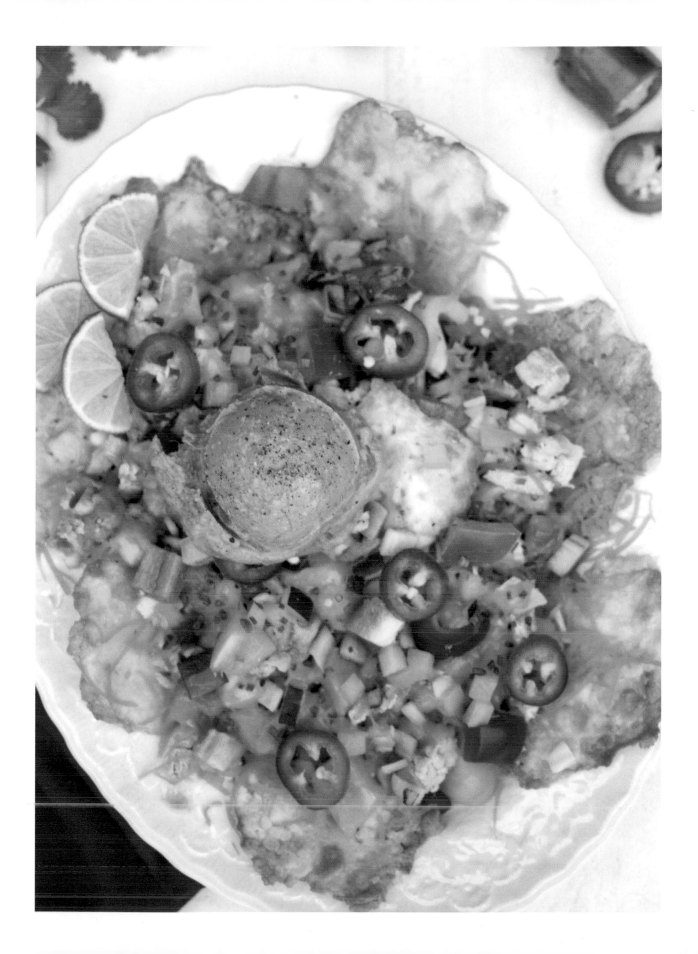

The Best Browned Butter Cheese Fondue

1 cup (2 sticks) unsalted butter

1 cup beef or chicken bone broth, homemade (page 356) or store-bought

2 ounces cream cheese (¼ cup)

4½ cups shredded extra-sharp cheddar cheese (about 1.2 pounds)

½ teaspoon fine sea salt

dipping ideas

1 batch cooked meatballs (from Meatballs with Brown Gravy, page 216)

3 cheddar sausages, homemade (page 266) or store-bought, cooked and cut into 1-inch rounds

Keto Buns (page 362), cut into ½-inch cubes and toasted

2 cups button mushrooms

2 cups black olives, pitted

1 cup celery sticks, about 3 inches long

½ cup cherry tomatoes

prep time: 10 minutes (not including time to prepare dipping options)
cook time: 7 minutes   *yield:* 12 servings

1. In a large saucepan over high heat, cook the butter for about 5 minutes, whisking constantly. The butter will start to sizzle and foam up. Watch for brown (but not black!) flecks; when you see them, remove the pan from the heat.

2. While whisking, slowly add the broth, cream cheese, and shredded cheese to the pan with the browned butter. Heat lightly, just until the cheese is pretty much melted. Add salt to taste.

3. Remove from the heat. Using an immersion blender or countertop blender, blend the fondue until very smooth. Pour into a fondue pot and enjoy with the dippers of your choice.

4. Store extra fondue in an airtight container in the refrigerator for up to 4 days. Reheat in the fondue pot over low heat until the cheese is loose and warmed through.

nutritional info (per serving)				
calories	*fat*	*protein*	*carbs*	*fiber*
316	30g	11g	2g	0g

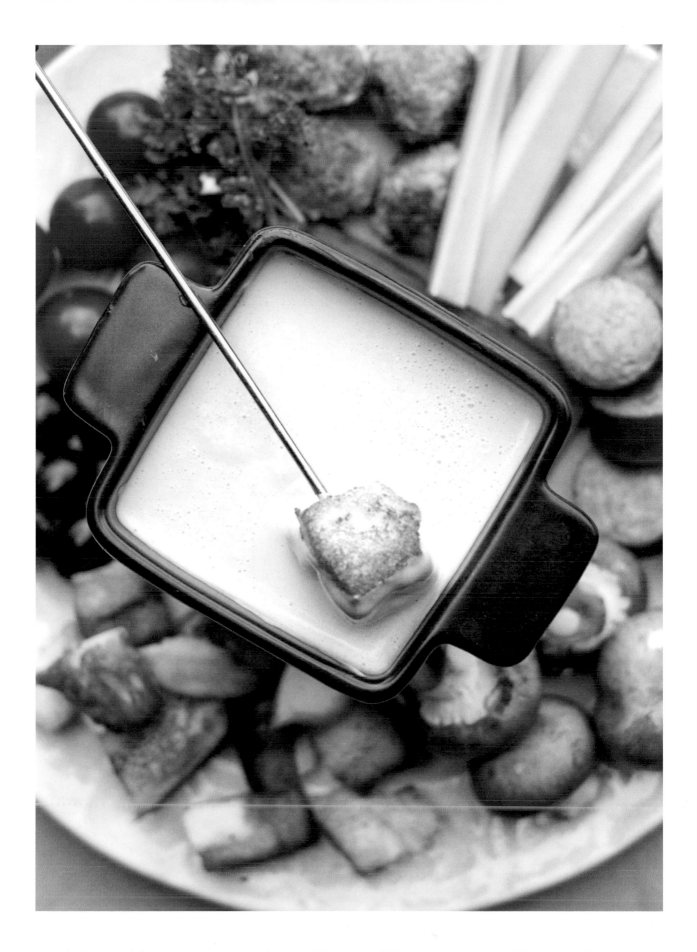

Parmesan Chips

2 cups grated Parmesan cheese (about 8 ounces)

prep time: 5 minutes   *cook time:* 25 minutes   *yield:* 32 chips (4 servings)

1. Preheat the oven to 375°F. Line a rimmed baking sheet with parchment paper.

2. Using a 2½-inch jar lid or round cookie cutter as a guide, drop 1 tablespoon of the cheese onto the parchment and use your fingers to spread the cheese to form a circle. Space the circles of cheese about 2 inches apart.

3. Bake the rounds for 5 minutes or until lightly browned and bubbly. Allow to cool on the pan; they will crisp up as they cool. Remove the chips from the parchment paper and serve with your favorite keto dip or toppings.

4. Store extras in an airtight container in the refrigerator for up to 4 days.

---

variation:

Pizza Chips. After forming the cheese circles in Step 2, scatter some mini pepperoni slices on each circle of cheese.

nutritional info (per serving of plain chips)				
calories	fat	protein	carbs	fiber
120	9g	12g	0g	0g

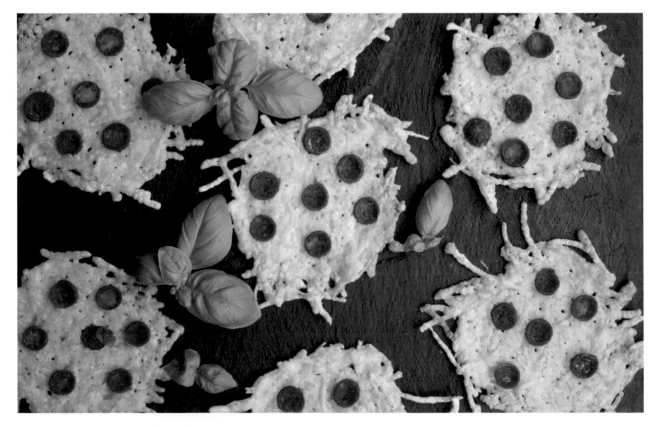

Buffalo Chicken Wings
with The Best Blue Cheese Dressing

L M H
KETO OPTION

prep time: 5 minutes (not including time to make dressing)
cook time: 35 minutes   yield: 6 servings

wings

2 pounds chicken wings and drumettes

3 tablespoons melted unsalted butter (or coconut oil if dairy-free)

1 teaspoon fine sea salt

½ teaspoon ground black pepper

1 tablespoon wing sauce or other medium-hot hot sauce, or to taste

for serving

½ batch The Best Blue Cheese Dressing (page 360) (omit for dairy-free)

Celery sticks

nutritional info (per serving)				
calories	fat	protein	carbs	fiber
585	43g	45g	1g	0.1g

1. Preheat the oven to 400°F.

2. Place the chicken wings and drumettes in a large bowl. Add the melted butter and toss to coat the chicken.

3. Place the buttered chicken on a rimmed baking sheet and season liberally with the salt and pepper.

4. Bake for 35 to 40 minutes, until the wings are crispy on the edges and cooked through.

5. Remove the chicken from the oven and brush it with the hot sauce. Serve with the blue cheese dressing and celery sticks.

6. Store extra wings in an airtight container in the refrigerator for up to 4 days. Reheat the wings on a baking sheet in a preheated 350°F oven for 5 minutes or until warmed through.

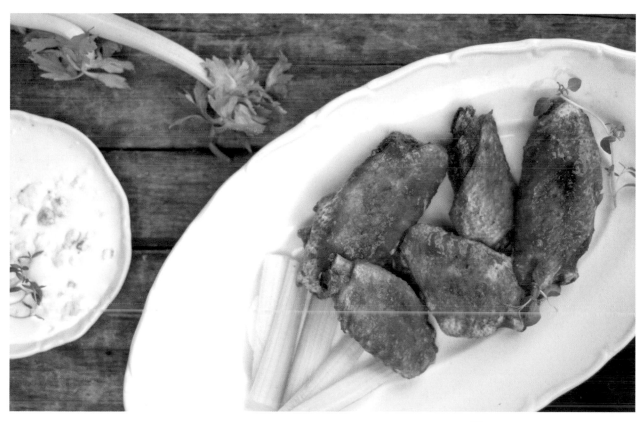

Baked Brie
with Keto Cherry Jelly

L **M** H
KETO

prep time: 15 minutes, plus at least 2 hours for jelly to cool and 1 hour to chill dough, if needed   *cook time:* 10 minutes   *yield:* 8 servings

jelly

1 cherry tea bag

2 teaspoons grass-fed powdered gelatin

⅓ cup Swerve confectioners'-style sweetener or equivalent amount of liquid or powdered sweetener (see page 24)

2 teaspoons cherry extract

⅛ teaspoon citric acid (for natural preservation and sour taste)

A few drops of natural red food coloring (optional)

dough

1¾ cups shredded mozzarella cheese

2 tablespoons unsalted butter

1 large egg

¾ cup blanched almond flour

⅛ teaspoon fine sea salt

1 (8-ounce) wheel Brie cheese

for garnish (optional)

2 tablespoons chopped pecans

2 tablespoons chopped fresh parsley

1. To make the jelly, bring 1 cup of water to a boil in a teakettle. Place the tea bag in a cup and pour the hot water into the cup. Let it steep for a few minutes, then remove the tea bag.

2. Place 2 tablespoons of cool water in a bowl. Sift the gelatin over the water and allow it to soften for a few minutes. Add the brewed tea to the softened gelatin.

3. Add the sweetener to the tea mixture and stir to combine. Taste and add more sweetener, if desired.

4. Add the extract, citric acid, and food coloring, if using, and stir to combine. Let cool on the counter for at least 2 hours before using.

5. To make the dough, place the mozzarella and butter in a microwave-safe bowl and microwave for 1 to 2 minutes, until the cheese is entirely melted. Stir well.

6. Add the egg and, using a hand mixer, combine well. Add the almond flour and salt and mix to combine. Using your hands, work it like a traditional dough, kneading for about 3 minutes. (*Note:* If the dough is too sticky, chill it in the refrigerator for an hour or overnight.)

7. Place a pizza stone (or a baking sheet, but a pizza stone will bake the bottom better) in the cold oven and preheat the oven to 400°F.

8. Place the dough on a greased sheet of parchment paper and pat it out with your hands to form a large circle, about 10 inches in diameter, or a rectangle, about 8 by 10 inches. This dough may be hard to roll out, but it is very forgiving. Shape the dough around the Brie.

9. Transfer the wrapped Brie on the parchment paper to the hot stone in the oven. Bake for 10 to 12 minutes, until the crust is golden brown.

10. Spread the cherry jelly all over the top of the baked Brie. Garnish with chopped pecans and parsley, if desired.

11. This dish is best served fresh, but any extras can be stored in an airtight container in the refrigerator for up to 3 days. Reheat in a preheated 350°F oven or toaster oven for 5 minutes or until the cheese is melted.

note: You can find citric acid in natural food stores. It is a natural preservative with a great sour taste.

nutritional info (per serving)				
calories	fat	protein	carbs	fiber
262	23g	13g	3g	1g

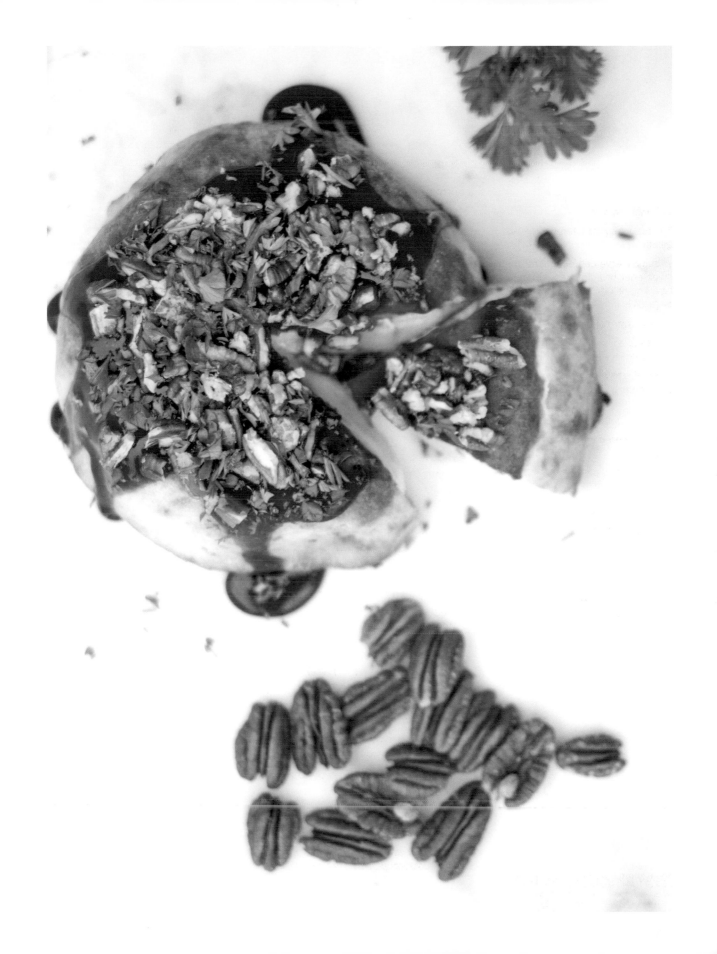

Spanakopita Flatbread

L M H
KETO

prep time: 10 minutes, plus 1 hour to chill dough, if needed

cook time: 12 minutes   *yield:* 4 servings

dough

1¾ cups shredded mozzarella cheese

2 tablespoons unsalted butter

¾ cup blanched almond flour

1 large egg

⅛ teaspoon fine sea salt

toppings

¼ cup Greek dressing, homemade (page 361) or store-bought, plus extra for serving

½ cup shredded mozzarella cheese

½ cup crumbled feta cheese

¼ cup diced green bell peppers

¼ cup chopped red onions

for garnish

¼ cup sliced black olives

2 tablespoons sliced cherry tomatoes

Handful of fresh spinach leaves

Fresh oregano leaves

1. Preheat the oven to 425°F.

2. To make the dough, place the mozzarella and butter in a microwave-safe bowl and microwave for 1 to 2 minutes, until the cheese is entirely melted. Stir well.

3. Add the egg and, using a hand mixer, combine well. Add the almond flour and salt and mix to combine. Using your hands, work it like a traditional dough, kneading for about 3 minutes. (*Note:* If the dough is too sticky, chill it in the refrigerator for an hour or overnight.)

4. Place a pizza stone (or a baking sheet, but a pizza stone will bake the bottom better) in the cold oven and preheat the oven to 400°F.

5. Place the dough on a greased sheet of parchment paper and pat it out with your hands to form a large circle, about 10 inches in diameter, or a rectangle, about 8 by 10 inches.

6. Spread the Greek dressing over the pizza crust. Sprinkle with the cheeses and top with the bell peppers and onions.

7. Bake until the cheese is melted, about 10 minutes. Remove from the oven and garnish with black olives, tomatoes, spinach leaves, and oregano leaves. Serve with extra Greek dressing on the side.

8. This flatbread is best consumed fresh, but any extras can be stored in an airtight container in the refrigerator for up to 3 days. Reheat in a preheated 350°F oven or toaster oven for 5 minutes or until the cheese is melted.

nutritional info (per serving)				
calories	fat	protein	carbs	fiber
419	35g	23g	8g	3g

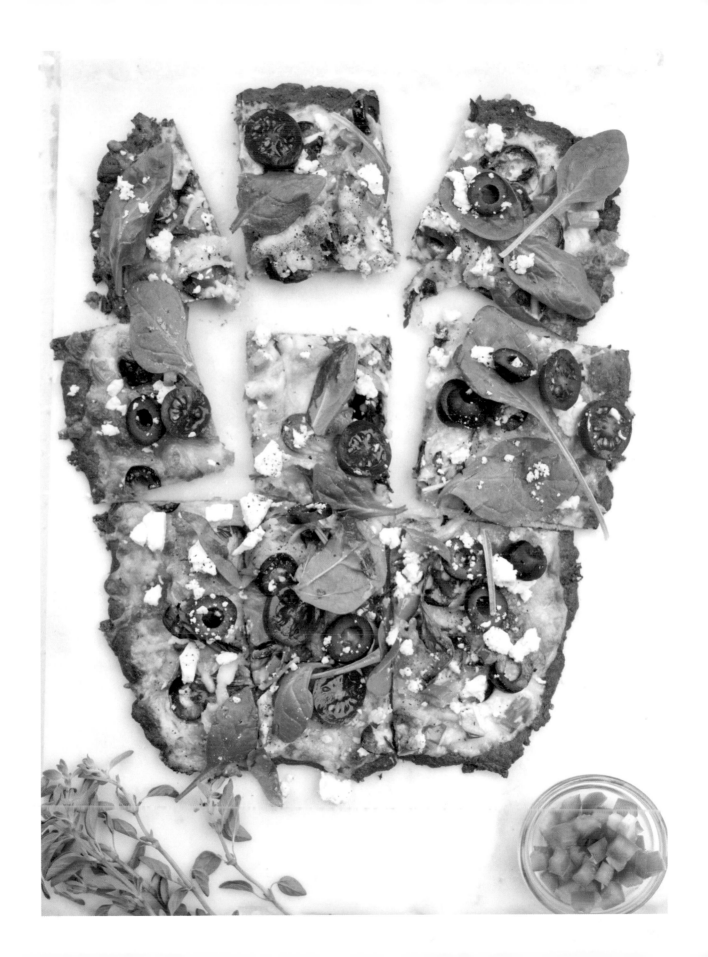

Bacon-Wrapped Stuffed Meatballs

L M H
KETO   OPTION

These meatballs are so amazing that I often make a triple batch and store unbaked meatballs in the freezer for easy appetizers or meals. If you can't find large cheese curds, about ½ inch in size, you can use a few smaller cheese curds per meatball instead, or substitute cubed cheese.

1 tablespoon ghee or unsalted butter (or coconut oil if dairy-free)

¼ cup chopped onions

½ teaspoon fine sea salt

1 pound ground beef

½ cup finely chopped mushrooms

½ cup powdered Parmesan cheese (see page 13; omit for dairy-free)

1 large egg

12 large cheese curds or ½-inch cubes of fontina or cheddar cheese (omit for dairy-free)

12 strips bacon, cut in half lengthwise

serving options

Ranch dressing, homemade (page 359) or store-bought

Cilantro Lime Ranch Dressing (page 360)

Stone-ground mustard

prep time: 5 minutes (not including time to make dressing)
cook time: 17 minutes
yield: 12 meatballs (2 per serving as an appetizer, 3 as a meal)

1. Preheat the oven to 400°F.

2. Heat the ghee in a heavy-bottomed skillet (such as cast iron). Add the onions, sprinkle with the salt, and cook for about 5 minutes, until the onions are translucent. Remove the onions to a bowl to cool.

3. Put the ground beef, chopped mushrooms, Parmesan cheese, and egg in a bowl. When the onions are no longer hot to the touch, add them to the bowl with the meat mixture and work everything together with your hands.

4. Shape the meat mixture into a 2-inch ball around a large cheese curd or cheese cube. Wrap a half strip of bacon around the entire meatball, then place another half strip, making an X, and wrap it around the meatball. Place the wrapped meatball on a rimmed baking sheet and secure the bacon to the meatball with a toothpick. Repeat with the rest of the meat mixture, cheese, and bacon.

5. Bake for 12 minutes or until the bacon is cooked and golden brown. Serve with ranch dressing or mustard, if desired.

6. Store extras in an airtight container in the refrigerator for up to 3 days. Reheat in a baking dish in a preheated 375°F oven for 5 minutes or until warmed through.

tip : To make this recipe even more keto, substitute ground pork for the ground beef.

nutritional info (per appetizer serving)				
calories	fat	protein	carbs	fiber
512	42g	33g	1g	0.2g

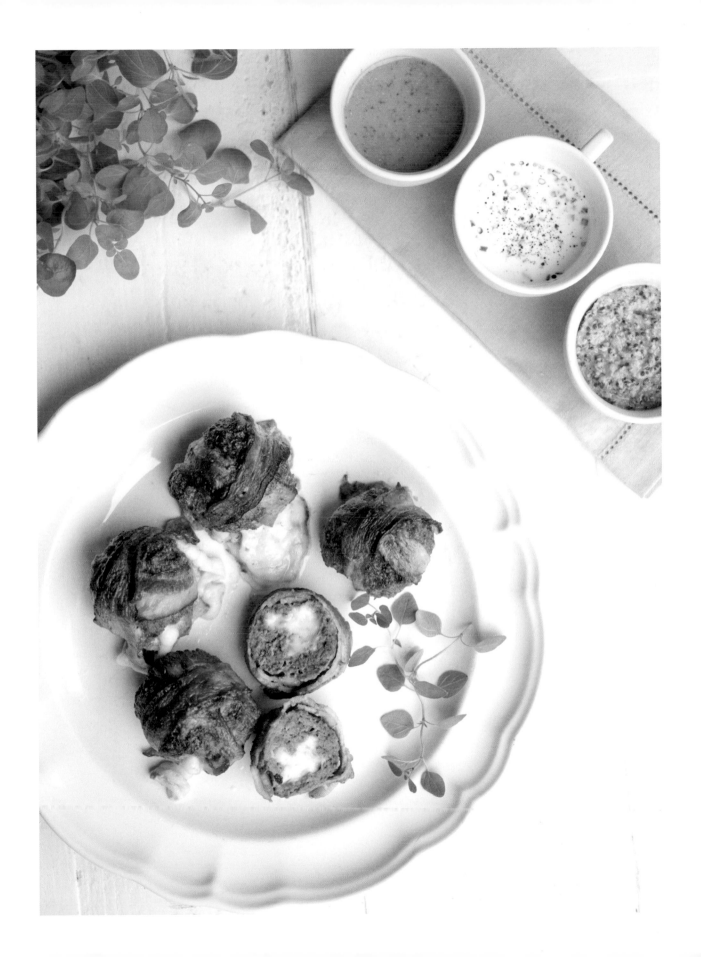

Hush Puppies
with Pimiento Mayo

pimiento mayo

½ cup mayonnaise, homemade (page 359) or store-bought

2 tablespoons jarred pimientos, drained

1 tablespoon lemon juice

1 teaspoon paprika

hush puppies

1 cup powdered Parmesan cheese (see page 13), plus more if needed

1 teaspoon baking powder

1 ounce cream cheese (2 tablespoons), softened

1 large egg, beaten

2 tablespoons minced onions

2 tablespoons jarred pimientos, drained

⅓ cup finely shredded sharp cheddar cheese

½ to 1 cup lard or coconut oil, for frying

1. To make the pimiento mayo, combine all the ingredients in a small bowl and whisk until well blended. Taste and adjust the balance of flavor as desired. (*Note:* The mayo can be made up to 2 days ahead and stored in an airtight container in the refrigerator.)

2. To make the hush puppies, combine the powdered Parmesan and baking powder in a medium-sized bowl. Add the softened cream cheese, beaten egg, and onions. Stir in the pimientos and cheddar cheese. If the mixture is too soft to shape into a ball, cover and place in the refrigerator; it will firm up as it chills. If the dough is still too soft after chilling, stir in an additional ¼ cup of powdered Parmesan.

3. When ready to fry the hush puppies, place ½ cup of lard in the tallest, skinniest pot you have. Heat the lard to 375°F over medium-high heat. The hot fat should be at least 1½ inches deep; add more lard to the pot if needed.

4. Take 2 tablespoons of the hush puppy dough and form it into a 1-inch ball. Use a spoon to drop a few balls at a time into the hot fat. Fry until golden brown, about 4 minutes. Remove from the heat and place on a plate lined with paper towel. Repeat with the remaining hush puppies.

5. Transfer the hush puppies to a serving platter and serve with the pimiento mayo.

6. Store extra hush puppies and mayo in separate airtight containers in the refrigerator for up to 3 days. To reheat the hush puppies, either place them in a preheated 350°F oven or fry them in a greased skillet on all sides until warmed through, about 5 minutes.

nutritional info (per serving)				
calories	fat	protein	carbs	fiber
127	12g	5g	1g	0.1g

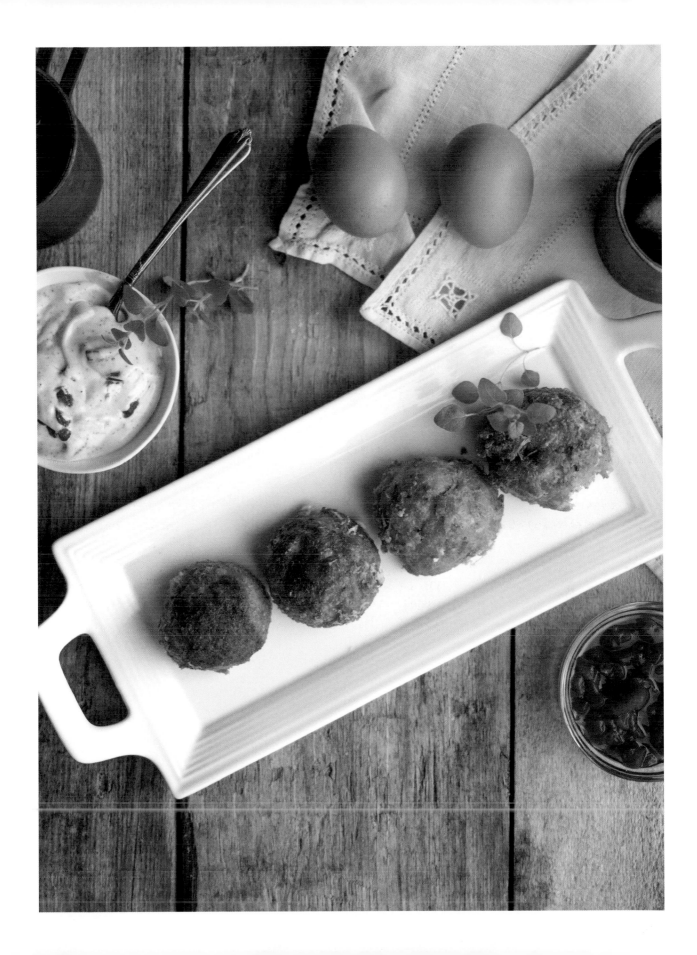

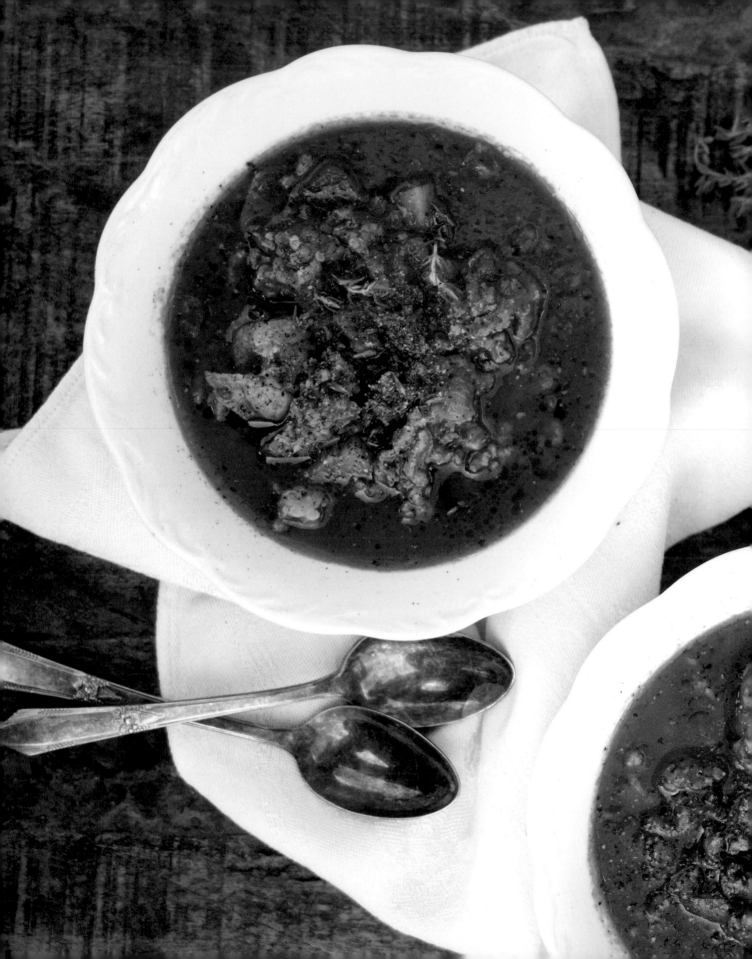

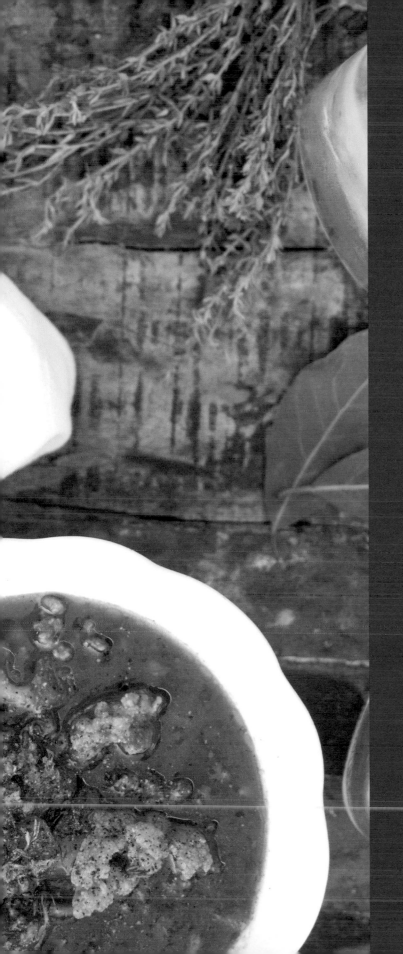

Soups, Salads, and Sides

Seafood Bisque

prep time: 10 minutes *cook time:* 40 minutes *yield:* 4 servings

3 tablespoons ghee or unsalted butter (or butter-flavored coconut oil if dairy-free)

2 cups cauliflower florets and chunked cauliflower stem, about ½ inch in size

1 leek, halved lengthwise, thoroughly rinsed and chopped

½ cup diced onions

1 stalk celery, cut into ½-inch chunks

Leaves from 3 sprigs fresh thyme

2 strips orange zest

2 drops orange oil (optional)

1 (8-ounce) package cream cheese (Kite Hill brand cream cheese style spread if dairy-free), softened

3 cups chicken bone broth, homemade (page 356) or store-bought, divided

Fine sea salt and ground black pepper

1½ cups chopped cooked baby langostino or shrimp

Oregano leaves, for garnish

Melted ghee or extra-virgin olive oil, for drizzling

1. Heat the 3 tablespoons of ghee in a saucepan over medium heat. Add the cauliflower, leek, onions, celery, thyme, orange zest, and orange oil, if using. Cook for 10 to 15 minutes, until the cauliflower is soft. Scoop out half of the cauliflower and place it in a food processor or blender with the cream cheese and 1 cup of the broth; puree until smooth. Return the pureed cauliflower to the pot, pour in the rest of the broth, and bring to a boil.

2. Immediately decrease the heat and gently simmer until the soup is reduced and thickened, about 20 minutes.

3. Strain the soup into a clean pot and season with salt and pepper to taste. Add the langostino to the strained bisque. Cook over low heat for 6 more minutes or until heated through.

4. To serve, ladle the bisque into warmed soup bowls. Garnish with oregano leaves and a drizzle of melted ghee. Store extras in an airtight container in the refrigerator for up to 3 days. Reheat in a saucepan over medium heat for a few minutes or until warmed through.

nutritional info (per serving)				
calories	fat	protein	carbs	fiber
521	39g	29g	8g	1g

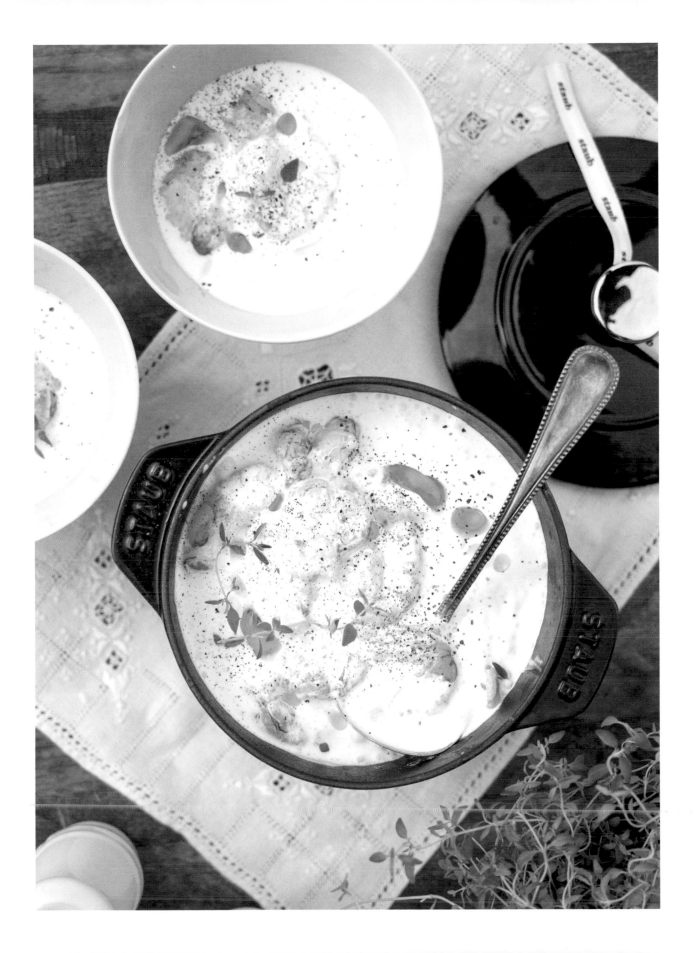

Clam Chowder

When I was in high school, I worked at a restaurant called High View, which was on an adorable fishing lake. We always served clam chowder on Friday nights. I still love clam chowder, so I made a ketogenic clam chowder with browned butter and bacon!

L M H
KETO OPTION

prep time: 10 minutes   *cook time:* 20 minutes   *yield:* 6 servings

4 strips bacon, chopped

¼ cup (½ stick) unsalted butter (or butter-flavored coconut oil if dairy-free)

2 cups cauliflower florets, cut into 1-inch pieces

½ cup minced onions

½ cup diced celery

1 (8-ounce) package cream cheese (Kite Hill brand cream cheese style spread if dairy-free), softened

2 cups chicken bone broth, homemade (page 356) or store-bought, divided

3 (6½-ounce) cans minced clams, with juices

1½ teaspoons fine sea salt

½ teaspoon ground black pepper

1. In a large skillet over medium-high heat, fry the bacon until crisp, about 4 minutes. Set the skillet aside.

2. Place the butter in a large pot over medium-high heat, whisking, until the butter froths and brown (but not black!) flecks appear, about 6 minutes. Reduce the heat to low. Add the cauliflower, onions, and celery to the browned butter and sauté for 2 minutes. Add the cream cheese and ¼ cup of the broth and whisk until well combined.

3. Add the rest of the broth to the pot and cook over medium heat until the veggies are tender, about 7 minutes. Do not allow the soup to boil. Stir in the clams with the juices just before serving. If they cook too long, they will get tough. Season with the salt and pepper and serve.

4. Store extras in an airtight container in the refrigerator for up to 3 days. Reheat in a saucepan over medium heat for a few minutes or until warmed through.

nutritional info (per serving)				
calories	fat	protein	carbs	fiber
371	26g	22g	8g	1g

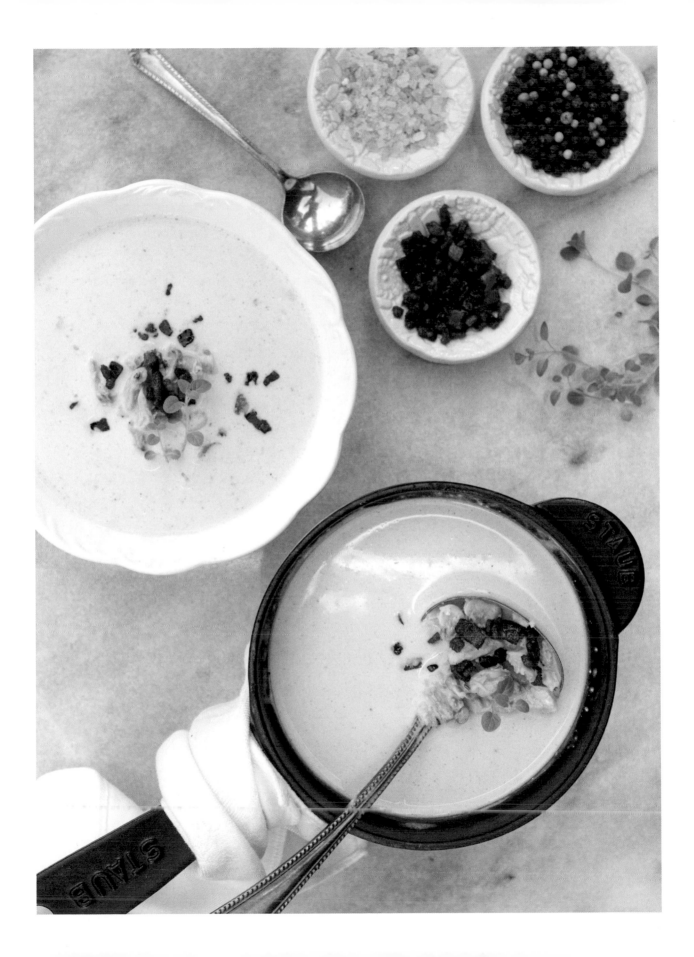

Chicken "Wild Rice" Soup

In this recipe, I've replaced the toothsome texture of wild rice, a classic component of chicken soup, with chicken cracklings and fried bacon bits. They provide great flavor and add a satisfying texture: I call them "crunchy rice." I often use the leftover meat from my Herb Roasted Chicken (page 184) to make this soup.

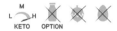

prep time: 20 minutes *cook time:* 1½ hours *yield:* 10 servings

½ cup (1 stick) unsalted butter (or lard or butter-flavored coconut oil if dairy-free)

½ cup diced onions

½ cup diced celery

8 ounces mushrooms, sliced

6 cups chicken bone broth, home-made (page 356) or store-bought

1 (8-ounce) package cream cheese (Kite Hill brand cream cheese style spread if dairy-free), softened

2 cups cooked cubed chicken

1 teaspoon fresh thyme, finely chopped

½ teaspoon fine sea salt

½ teaspoon curry powder

½ teaspoon dry mustard

½ teaspoon dried parsley

½ teaspoon ground black pepper

chicken cracklings (for crunchy "rice")

(Makes about 2 cups)

½ pound chicken skin and fat

½ teaspoon ghee (or lard if dairy-free)

2 tablespoons finely diced onions

1 small clove garlic, smashed to a paste or minced

½ tablespoon fresh sage leaves or other herb of choice, such as thyme

½ teaspoon fine sea salt

½ teaspoon ground black pepper

1 pound bacon, diced, for crunchy "rice"

1. In a stockpot, melt the butter over medium heat. Stir in the onions and celery and sauté for 5 minutes or until soft. Add the mushrooms and sauté for 2 more minutes. Pour in the chicken broth and stir. Bring to a boil, then reduce the heat to low.

2. Add the softened cream cheese and whisk until it is fully incorporated and heated through.

3. Add the chicken and seasonings and simmer, covered, for 1 hour.

4. While the soup is simmering, make the crunchy "rice," starting with the cracklings: Chop the chicken skin into ¼-inch pieces and pat them completely dry with paper towels. Heat the ghee in a medium-sized cast-iron skillet over medium heat. Add the chicken skin pieces, cover, and reduce the heat to low. Cook for 12 to 15 minutes, until there is a layer of liquid fat in the pan.

5. Meanwhile, fry the bacon in a large cast-iron skillet until crispy, about 8 minutes. Remove the bacon from the skillet and set aside until you're ready to serve the soup; reserve the bacon fat for another use.

6. After the chicken fat has cooked on low for 12 to 15 minutes, bring the heat back up to medium and uncover the skillet. Cook the chicken skin pieces for an additional 15 minutes, stirring often, until they start to curl up and there is a lot of fat in the pan. Carefully pour the chicken skin pieces and liquid fat through a colander into a jar. Save the chicken fat for later use—it's a great ketogenic fat—and put the drained chicken skin pieces back in the skillet.

7. To the skillet, add the onions, garlic, and sage and cook over medium heat for another 15 minutes, stirring, until the cracklings are golden brown and crispy. Remove the skillet from the heat. Season the cracklings with the salt and pepper.

8. Ladle the soup into bowls and stir most of the crunchy "rice"—the prepared cracklings and crispy bacon—into the soup. Sprinkle the remaining "rice" on top as a garnish.

busy family tip:

The cracklings can be made up to 3 days ahead. Once cool, store in an airtight container in the fridge. When ready to add them to the soup, reheat the cracklings in a skillet over medium heat for a few minutes or until warmed through.

nutritional info (per serving)				
calories	fat	protein	carbs	fiber
642	54g	33g	4g	1g

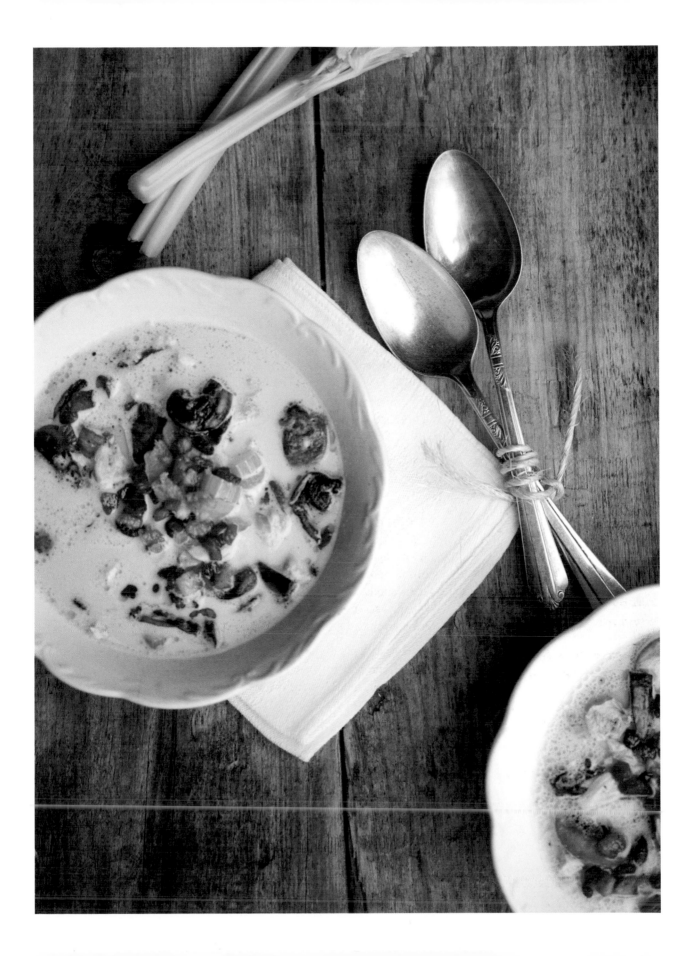

Cream of Chicken Soup

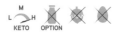
KETO OPTION

2 cups chicken bone broth, home-made (page 356) or store-bought

½ cup diced celery

4 ounces cream cheese (½ cup) (Kite Hill brand cream cheese style spread if dairy-free), softened

1 tablespoon ghee or unsalted butter (or coconut oil or bacon fat if dairy-free)

2 tablespoons minced shallots

2 cloves garlic, smashed to a paste

2 boneless, skinless chicken thighs, chopped into ¼-inch pieces

1 teaspoon dried thyme leaves

1 teaspoon fine sea salt

½ teaspoon ground black pepper

½ bay leaf

1 tablespoon lemon juice, or more to taste

Fresh herbs of choice, such as oregano or thyme, for garnish

Avocado oil or extra-virgin olive oil, for drizzling

1. In a food processor, puree the broth, celery, and softened cream cheese. Set aside.

2. Melt the ghee in a saucepan over medium heat. Add the shallots and garlic and lightly sauté for 2 minutes, until fragrant. Add the chopped chicken and sauté for 6 minutes or until the chicken is cooked through and no longer pink.

3. Add the celery puree, thyme, salt, pepper, and bay leaf to the soup and cook over medium heat for 25 minutes. Remove the bay leaf. Stir in the lemon juice. Taste and add more salt, pepper, or lemon juice, if desired. Serve garnished with fresh herbs and a drizzle of oil.

4. Store extras in an airtight container in the refrigerator for up to 3 days. Reheat in a saucepan over medium heat for a few minutes or until warmed through.

nutritional info (per serving)				
calories	fat	protein	carbs	fiber
268	21g	15g	4g	1g

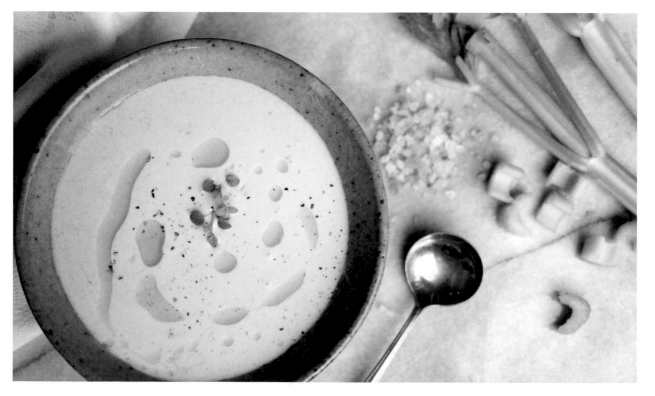

Mushroom Truffle Bisque

LongHorn Steakhouse serves amazing steaks, but the soup that inspired this recipe is also a hit at its restaurants. This bisque is rich, creamy, and flavorful and tastes fantastic paired with a juicy steak!

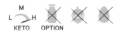

L M H
KETO OPTION

prep time: 5 minutes (not including time to cook bacon)
cook time: 10 minutes   *yield:* 4 servings

2 tablespoons unsalted butter or ghee (or coconut oil if dairy-free)

4 ounces button mushrooms, sliced

4 ounces baby portobello mushrooms, sliced

¼ cup chopped white onions

½ teaspoon fine sea salt

1 clove garlic, minced

2 cups chicken bone broth, homemade (page 356) or store-bought

1 (8-ounce) package cream cheese (Kite Hill brand cream cheese style spread if dairy-free), softened

Diced cooked bacon, for garnish (optional)

1 teaspoon truffle oil, for drizzling (optional)

1. Melt the butter in a stockpot or large saucepan over medium heat. Add the mushrooms and onions and sauté until the onions are translucent, about 4 minutes. Season with the salt. Add the garlic and sauté for another minute. Remove some of the mushrooms and reserve for garnish.

2. Add the broth and cream cheese to the pot and heat through. Use an immersion blender to puree the soup. Ladle into serving bowls and garnish each bowl with a few of the reserved mushrooms, some diced cooked bacon, and a drizzle of truffle oil, if desired.

3. Store extras in an airtight container in the refrigerator for up to 3 days. Reheat in a saucepan over medium heat for a few minutes or until warmed through.

nutritional info (per serving)				
calories	fat	protein	carbs	fiber
304	27g	8g	6g	1g

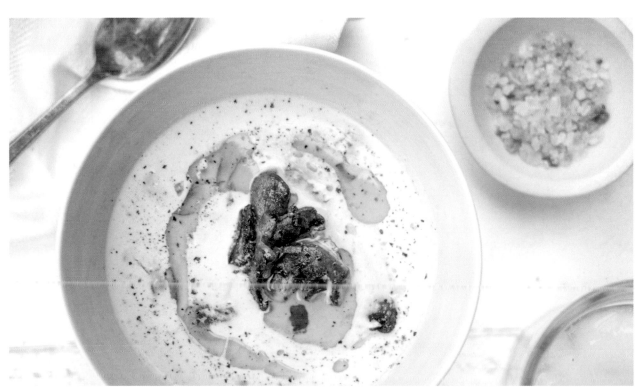

Fauxtato Leek Soup

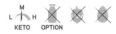

KETO   OPTION

4 strips bacon, diced

½ cup chopped leeks

½ cup diced celery

2 cups cauliflower florets and chunked cauliflower stem, about ½ inch in size

2 cups chicken bone broth, homemade (page 356) or store-bought

1 (8-ounce) package cream cheese (Kite Hill brand cream cheese style spread if dairy-free), softened

½ teaspoon fish sauce (optional)

1½ teaspoons fine sea salt

½ teaspoon ground black pepper

Avocado oil or extra-virgin olive oil, for drizzling

Fresh thyme leaves, for garnish

Here's a secret when you want to make faux-potato anything using cauliflower: use the stem! When cut into chunks, cauliflower stem resembles potatoes, and instead of throwing out the core when you use the florets for another recipe, you've put it to great use.

prep time: 5 minutes   *cook time:* 25 minutes   *yield:* 6 servings

1. In a large saucepan or Dutch oven, fry the bacon over medium-high heat until crisp, about 4 minutes. Remove the bacon and set aside, leaving the drippings in the pan. Add the leeks, celery, and cauliflower pieces to the pan. Sauté for 5 minutes or until the leeks are soft.

2. Pour in the chicken broth and cook over medium heat until the veggies are tender, about 10 minutes. Place ½ cup of the cooked cauliflower mixture and the cream cheese in a food processor and puree until smooth. (This will help thicken the soup.)

3. Return the puree to the pan with the vegetables. Stir in the fish sauce (if using), salt, and pepper. Taste and adjust the seasoning as desired. Heat through, but do not allow the soup to boil. Serve the soup drizzled with oil and garnished with thyme and the reserved bacon.

4. Store extras in an airtight container in the refrigerator for up to 3 days. Reheat in a saucepan over medium heat for a few minutes or until warmed through.

nutritional info (per serving)				
calories	fat	protein	carbs	fiber
195	16g	6g	4g	1g

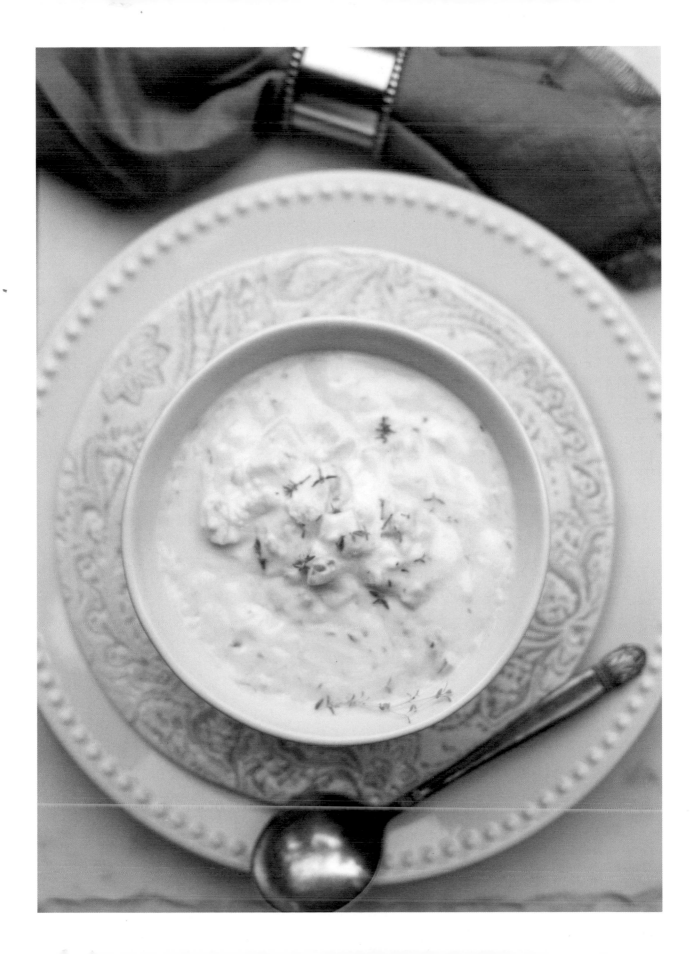

Beef Stew

L M H KETO ✗ ✗ ✗

1 (1-pound) boneless beef roast

Fine sea salt and ground black pepper

3 tablespoons MCT oil or bacon fat

½ head (2 cups) cauliflower, cut into 1-inch pieces

2 cups button mushrooms, sliced in half

1 cup diced onions

2 large stalks celery, cut into ¼-inch pieces

3 cloves garlic, minced, or 1 head roasted garlic, cloves squeezed from the head

4 cups beef bone broth, homemade (page 356) or store-bought

1 (28-ounce) can diced tomatoes, or 2 fresh tomatoes, diced

½ teaspoon dried rosemary, or 1 teaspoon fresh rosemary, finely chopped

½ teaspoon dried thyme, or 1 teaspoon fresh thyme, finely chopped

1. Pat the roast dry with a paper towel and cut it into 1-inch pieces. Season the meat on all sides with salt and pepper. Place the MCT oil in a Dutch oven over medium-high heat. When hot, sear the beef chunks in the oil until they are golden brown on all sides, about 3 minutes.

2. Add the cauliflower, mushrooms, onions, celery, and garlic to the pot with the beef. Sauté for 3 minutes.

3. Add the broth, tomatoes, rosemary, and thyme to the pot. Cover and cook for 1 hour, stirring every 20 minutes or so.

4. Uncover and cook for another 30 minutes to thicken the stew. Remove from the heat and serve.

5. Store extras in an airtight container in the refrigerator for up to 4 days or in the freezer for up to 1 month. Reheat in a saucepan over medium heat for 5 minutes or until warmed through.

nutritional info (per serving)				
calories	*fat*	*protein*	*carbs*	*fiber*
245	17g	13g	7g	2g

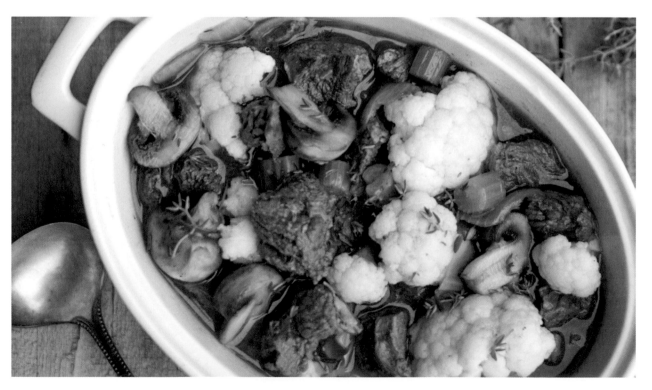

Slow Cooker Chipotle Lime Steak Soup

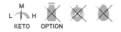

prep time: 10 minutes   *cook time:* 4 to 8 hours   *yield:* 8 servings

8 cups beef bone broth, homemade (page 356) or store-bought

1 cup diced onions

1 green bell pepper, thinly sliced

1 (16-ounce) jar salsa

¼ cup diced pickled jalapeños

1 chipotle chile pepper in adobo sauce, chopped

2½ teaspoons fine sea salt

2 teaspoons chili powder

1 teaspoon ground cumin

1 teaspoon paprika

½ teaspoon ground black pepper

1 pound boneless beef roast, cut into 2-inch cubes

2 limes, halved

for garnish (optional)

Fresh cilantro

Shredded sharp cheddar cheese

Sour cream

Lime wedges

1. Combine the broth, onions, bell pepper, salsa, jalapeños, chipotle pepper, salt, and spices in a slow cooker. Place the cubed beef on top of the other ingredients.

2. Cover and cook on low for 8 hours or on high for 4 hours. When the beef is tender, shred the meat with 2 forks. Stir well. Squeeze the lime juice into the slow cooker. Taste and add more salt, if desired.

3. Serve topped with fresh cilantro, cheddar cheese, sour cream, and a lime wedge, if desired. Store extras in an airtight container in the refrigerator for up to 3 days. Reheat in a saucepan over medium heat for a few minutes or until warmed through.

nutritional info (per serving)				
calories	fat	protein	carbs	fiber
204	13g	13g	7g	2g

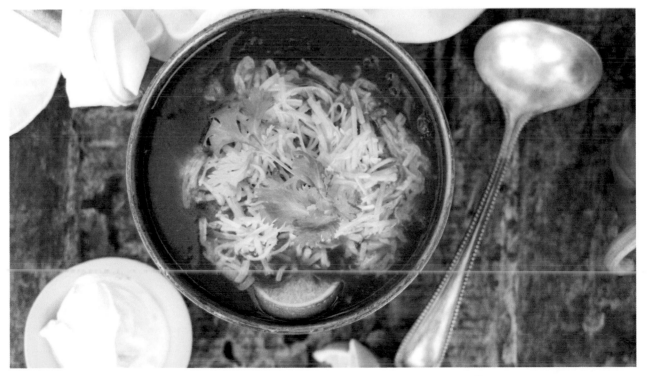

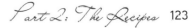

Italian Sausage Soup

1 tablespoon ghee (or avocado oil if dairy-free)

1 pound hot Italian sausages, casings removed

6 cups chicken bone broth, homemade (page 356) or store-bought, divided

3 celery stalks, diced

½ cup diced onions

2 large cloves garlic, minced

2 cups cauliflower florets, cut into ½-inch pieces

1 cup diced zucchini

1 red bell pepper, diced

1 teaspoon minced fresh rosemary

1 teaspoon minced fresh sage

1 teaspoon minced fresh thyme

½ teaspoon fine sea salt

½ teaspoon ground black pepper

½ cup pizza sauce, homemade (page 358), or store-bought pizza or marinara sauce

1 bay leaf

Chopped fresh parsley, for garnish (optional)

1. Heat the ghee in a Dutch oven or stockpot over medium heat. Add the sausage and cook for about 6 minutes, breaking it up into small chunks as it browns. When the sausage is fully cooked, remove it from the pot with a slotted spoon. Put it in a bowl and set aside.

2. Add ¼ cup of the chicken broth to the pot and scrape the bottom to deglaze. Add the celery, onions, and garlic and cook, stirring frequently, until the onions are translucent, about 5 minutes.

3. Add the cauliflower, zucchini, bell pepper, herbs, salt, and pepper. Cook, stirring, for another 3 minutes. Add the remaining broth, pizza sauce, and bay leaf. Simmer over medium heat for 8 minutes. Add the cooked sausage and simmer for another 10 minutes. Taste and adjust the seasoning, if desired.

4. Remove and discard the bay leaf. Serve the soup garnished with chopped parsley, if desired.

5. Store extras in an airtight container in the refrigerator for up to 3 days. Reheat in a saucepan over medium heat for a few minutes or until warmed through.

nutritional info (per serving)				
calories	fat	protein	carbs	fiber
340	26g	18g	8g	2g

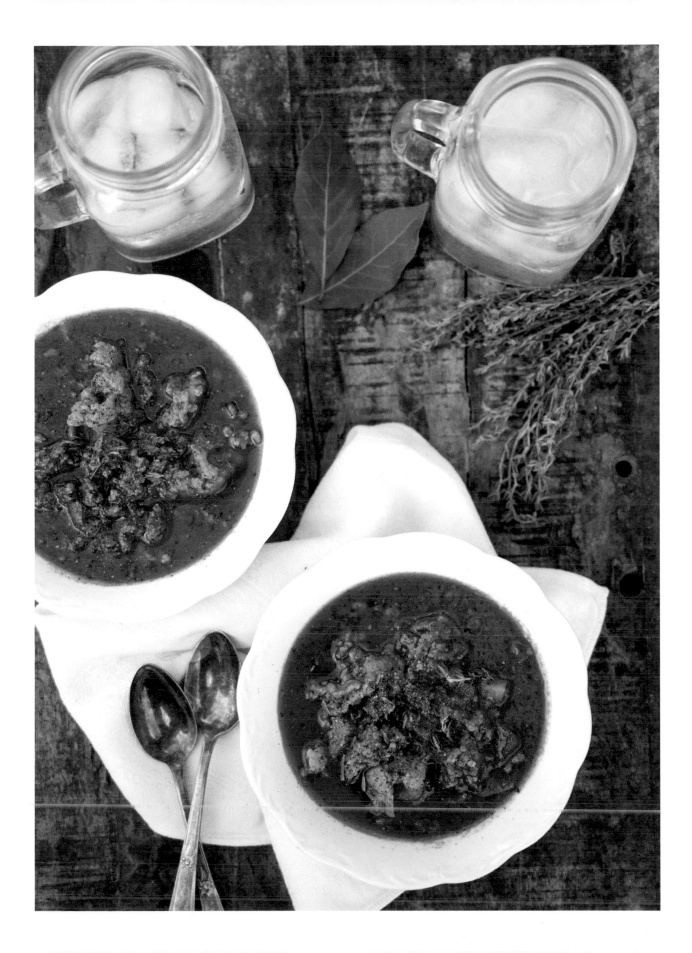

Philly Cheesesteak Soup

L M H
KETO OPTION

2 pounds boneless sirloin steak, cubed

Fine sea salt and ground black pepper

¼ cup (½ stick) unsalted butter (or coconut oil if dairy-free), divided

1 cup chopped onions

3 cloves garlic, minced

6 cups beef bone broth, homemade (page 356) or store-bought, divided

1 green bell pepper, thinly sliced

¼ teaspoon cayenne pepper

1 (8-ounce) package cream cheese (Kite Hill brand cream cheese style spread if dairy-free), softened

1 cup shredded provolone cheese, for garnish (omit for dairy-free)

prep time: 15 minutes *cook time:* 6 to 8 hours *yield:* 8 servings

1. Season the steak generously on all sides with salt and pepper.

2. Heat 2 tablespoons of the butter in a large skillet over medium-high heat. Add the onions and garlic and cook until soft, 3 to 5 minutes. Transfer the mixture to a slow cooker.

3. Add the cubed steak to the skillet and sear on all sides until the meat is dark golden brown, adding more butter if needed to keep the meat from sticking to the pan. Then transfer the meat to the slow cooker with the onions and garlic.

4. Add 5 cups of the beef broth, the bell pepper, and the cayenne pepper to the slow cooker. Cover and cook on low for 6 to 8 hours, until the meat is cooked through and fork-tender. Shred the meat with 2 forks.

5. A few minutes before serving, place the softened cream cheese and remaining 1 cup of broth in a blender, puree until smooth, and then add the puree to the slow cooker. Stir to combine and turn the heat up to high. Continue to cook, covered, just until warmed through.

6. Ladle the soup into bowls and top with shredded provolone cheese.

7. Store extras in an airtight container in the refrigerator for up to 3 days. Reheat in a saucepan over medium heat for a few minutes or until warmed through.

nutritional info (per serving)				
calories	fat	protein	carbs	fiber
409	31g	25g	4g	1g

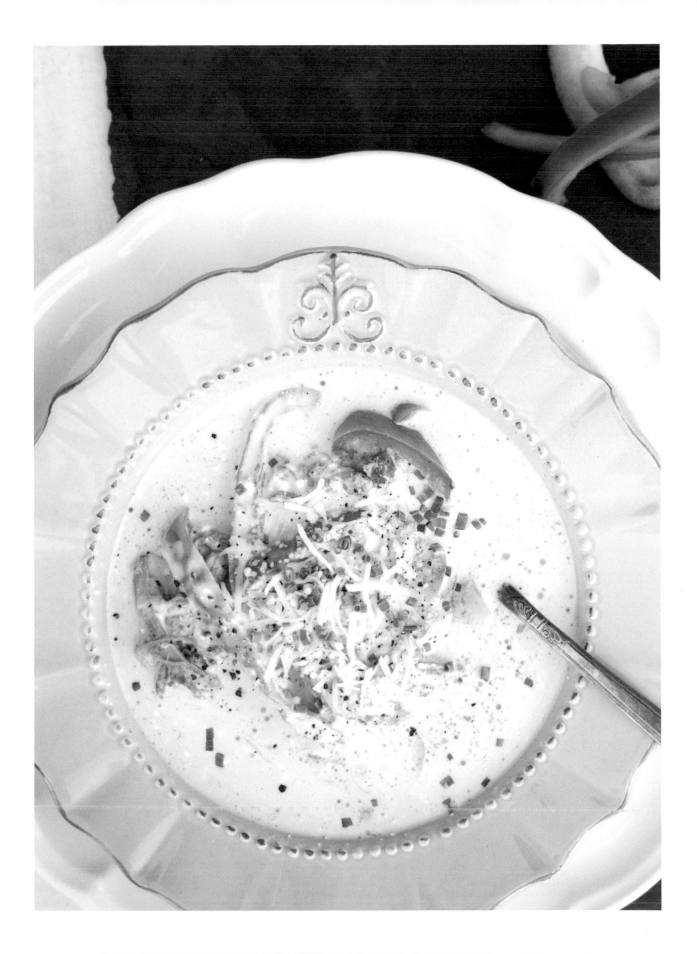

Warm Goat Cheese Salad
with Bacon Vinaigrette

½ pound bacon, diced

1 (8-ounce) log fresh goat cheese

½ cup pork dust (or pork rinds crushed into a powder)

3 tablespoons plus 2 teaspoons coconut vinegar or red wine vinegar

3 tablespoons avocado oil, MCT oil, or extra-virgin olive oil

1 teaspoon Dijon mustard

½ teaspoon fine sea salt

¼ teaspoon ground black pepper

2 drops stevia glycerite (optional)

4 cups leafy greens

½ avocado, sliced (optional)

½ cup raw walnuts, for garnish (optional; omit for nut-free)

nutritional info (per serving)				
calories	fat	protein	carbs	fiber
766	67g	36g	8g	4g

Nothing says fall like a warm goat cheese salad with a warm bacon vinaigrette! I've always enjoyed flavorful salads, even before I started eating keto. But in my pre-keto life, I often made my salads too high in carbs by adding dried cranberries or sun-dried tomatoes. This warm salad needs nothing like that. It is delicious and creamy without the carbs!

prep time: 5 minutes   *cook time:* 10 minutes   *yield:* 4 servings

1. Sauté the diced bacon in a skillet over medium heat until crisp, about 5 minutes. Using a slotted spoon, remove the bacon to a bowl, leaving the drippings in the pan.

2. Meanwhile, cut the goat cheese log into 8 medallions that are about ¼ inch thick.

3. Place the pork dust in a shallow bowl. Gently roll each goat cheese medallion in the pork dust to cover the medallions.

4. In batches, fry the medallions in the hot skillet with the bacon drippings over medium heat for 1 minute or until golden brown, then flip and fry for another minute. Remove the medallions from the skillet and set aside on a plate.

5. Add the vinegar, oil, mustard, salt, pepper, and stevia, if using, to the skillet and stir well to combine. Stir in the cooked bacon.

6. Plate the greens and avocado slices, if using, on a serving platter and top with the fried goat cheese medallions. Drizzle the bacon vinaigrette over the greens and garnish with walnuts and freshly ground pepper, if desired.

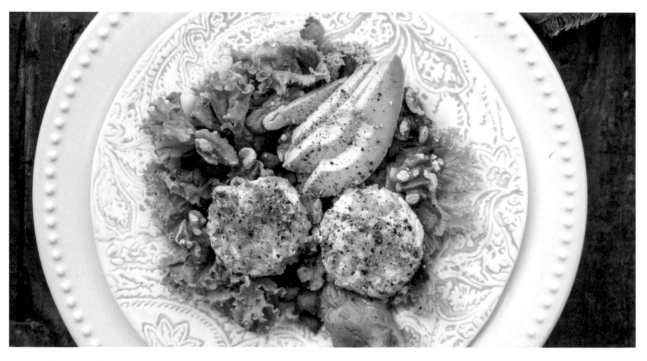

Mashed Fauxtatoes

If you are a visual learner like me, check out the video about how to make this recipe on my site, MariaMindBodyHealth.com (type the word *video* in the search field).

L M H
KETO ✕ ✕

2 cups chicken bone broth, homemade (page 356) or store-bought

Florets from 1 medium head cauliflower, cut into bite-sized pieces

1 tablespoon dried chives, plus extra for garnish

1 clove garlic, minced

2 ounces cream cheese (¼ cup), softened

½ cup shredded sharp cheddar or grated Parmesan cheese

Fine sea salt and ground black pepper

Unsalted butter, for serving

prep time: 5 minutes *cook time:* 8 minutes
yield: 4 servings (1 cup per serving)

1. Pour the broth into a large saucepan. Use enough that you have about ½ inch of broth in the pan. Bring the broth to a boil, then add the cauliflower, chives, and garlic and cover the pan with a tight-fitting lid. Steam the cauliflower until tender, 6 to 8 minutes. Drain well. Pat it very dry between several layers of paper towels.

2. Place the cauliflower in a high-powered blender or food processor. Add the cheeses and puree until very smooth. Season to taste with salt and pepper. Transfer the mixture to a serving dish and garnish with pats of butter and chopped chives.

3. Store extras in an airtight container in the refrigerator for up to 3 days. Reheat in a saucepan over medium heat for a few minutes or until warmed through.

nutritional info (per serving)				
calories	fat	protein	carbs	fiber
178	12g	9g	9g	4g

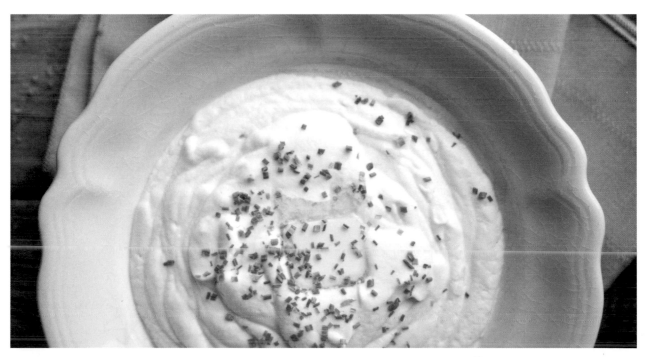

Roasted Cauliflower
with Béarnaise Sauce

prep time: 5 minutes (not including time to make béarnaise sauce)
cook time: about 20 minutes *yield:* 6 servings

¼ cup (½ stick) melted unsalted butter, coconut oil, lard, or avocado oil

2 teaspoons minced garlic

1 medium head cauliflower, cored and separated into medium to large florets

2 teaspoons fine sea salt

1 batch Béarnaise Sauce (page 357)

Fresh thyme leaves, for garnish (optional)

nutritional info (per serving)				
calories	fat	protein	carbs	fiber
147	13g	3g	6g	2g

1. Preheat the oven to 450°F.

2. Place the melted butter and garlic in a small bowl and stir to combine. Drizzle the melted garlic butter over the cauliflower and toss to coat. Spread out the cauliflower on one or two rimmed baking sheets (don't overcrowd or they won't roast) and sprinkle with the salt. Roast for 18 to 22 minutes, until dark golden brown (I like mine a little charred).

3. Place the roasted cauliflower on a serving platter, drizzle with the béarnaise sauce, and garnish with thyme leaves, if desired.

4. Store the roasted cauliflower and béarnaise sauce in separate airtight containers in the refrigerator for up to 3 days. To reheat the cauliflower, place on a baking sheet in a preheated 350°F oven for a few minutes or until warmed through. To reheat the sauce, see page 357.

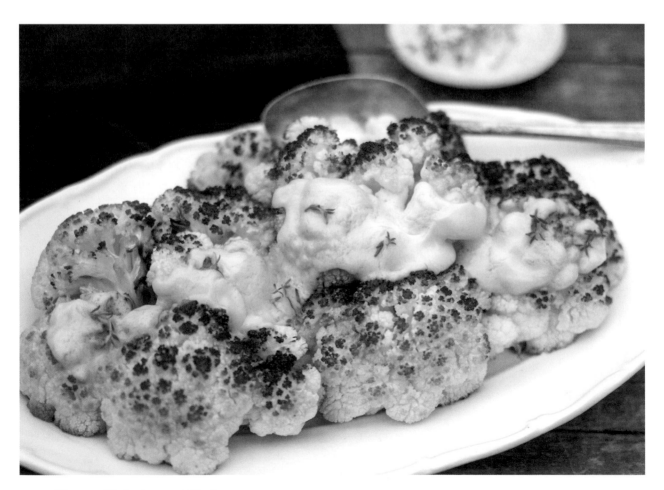

Steak Fries

KETO
L — M — H

2 large eggs

1 cup powdered Parmesan cheese
(see page 13)

2 large portobello mushrooms,
sliced into ¼-inch-thick fries

Coconut oil, for frying

Cilantro Lime Ranch Dressing
(page 360), The Best Blue Cheese
Dressing (page 360), or pizza
sauce, homemade (page 358) or
store-bought, for serving

nutritional info (per serving)				
calories	fat	protein	carbs	fiber
171	12g	17g	2g	1g

prep time: 5 minutes (not including time to make dressing)

cook time: 10 minutes yield: 4 servings

1. In a shallow bowl, beat the eggs.

2. Place the Parmesan cheese in another shallow bowl.

3. Dip the portobello fries into the eggs, then dredge in the Parmesan, using your hands to coat each fry well.

4. Put enough coconut oil in a 4-inch-deep (or deeper) cast-iron skillet so that it is about 1½ inches deep. Heat the oil to 350°F. Fry the steak fries in 2 batches for about 5 minutes per batch, until golden brown. Remove from the skillet and place on paper towels to drain.

5. Arrange the fries on a serving platter. Serve with the keto dipping sauce of your choice.

6. These fries are best served fresh, but any extras can be stored in an airtight container in the refrigerator for up to 3 days. To reheat, place the fries on a rimmed baking sheet and broil for 3 minutes or until crispy.

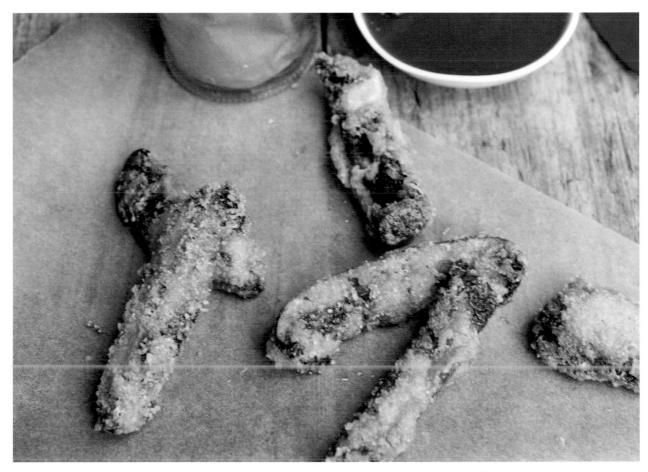

Brussels Sprouts with Soft-Boiled Eggs and Avocado

If you had told me when I was a child that someday I would love Brussels sprouts, I would have laughed. But you know what? I do! Especially when you use my method for making the *best* Brussels sprouts!

My technique requires two steps, but it's worth it: first I blanch them and then I sauté them. Blanching Brussels preserves their bright color and cuts down the cooking time to retain more nutrients and a fresh flavor.

Why are these the best Brussels sprouts? Well, it isn't just the way they're prepared. The garnish of soft-boiled egg and avocado really steps it up! I love anything with a soft-boiled egg added to it. If you are a keto-vegetarian (or if, like my son Kai, you do not like bacon), feel free to leave the bacon out.

KETO   OPTION OPTION OPTION

1½ pounds Brussels sprouts, trimmed

1 cup chopped radicchio or kale

2 strips bacon, diced (optional)

2 tablespoons unsalted butter (or coconut oil if dairy-free)

1 shallot, finely chopped, or 2 tablespoons diced onions

½ teaspoon fine sea salt (1 teaspoon if not using bacon)

for garnish

3 soft-boiled eggs (see below; omit for egg-free)

2 tablespoons chopped walnuts (omit for nut-free)

½ avocado, sliced

prep time: 10 minutes   *cook time:* 8 minutes   *yield:* 6 servings

1. Bring a large pot of water to a boil. Add the Brussels sprouts and radicchio or kale (I used radicchio for a contrasting purple color) and blanch for about 15 seconds. Quickly drain and rinse the vegetables in cold water. Cut the large sprouts in half lengthwise.

2. If using bacon, cook the bacon in a medium-sized skillet over medium heat for about 3 minutes, until browned. Remove the bacon to a bowl and set aside; leave the drippings in the pan.

3. Add the butter and shallot to the skillet and sauté for about 2 minutes, until the shallot is soft. Add the blanched Brussels sprouts and radicchio and toss to coat in the butter. Sauté the vegetables for about 3 minutes, until they begin to soften, then season with the salt and cook until crisp-tender, another 2 minutes.

4. With a slotted spoon, transfer the vegetables to a serving dish. Top with the cooked bacon, if using, and soft-boiled eggs sliced in half. Sprinkle with chopped walnuts, if using, and serve with sliced avocado.

5. This dish is best served fresh, but any extras can be stored in an airtight container in the refrigerator for up to 3 days. Reheat in a baking dish in a preheated 350°F oven for 5 minutes or until warmed through.

how to cook perfect soft-boiled eggs:

Fill a medium saucepan halfway with water and bring to a simmer, but not quite a boil. Gently place the eggs in the simmering water and cook for 5 minutes, holding the water at a simmer, not a boil. Remove the eggs and run under cool water. Once cool, carefully peel the eggs.

nutritional info (per serving)				
calories	fat	protein	carbs	fiber
204	14g	9g	13g	6g

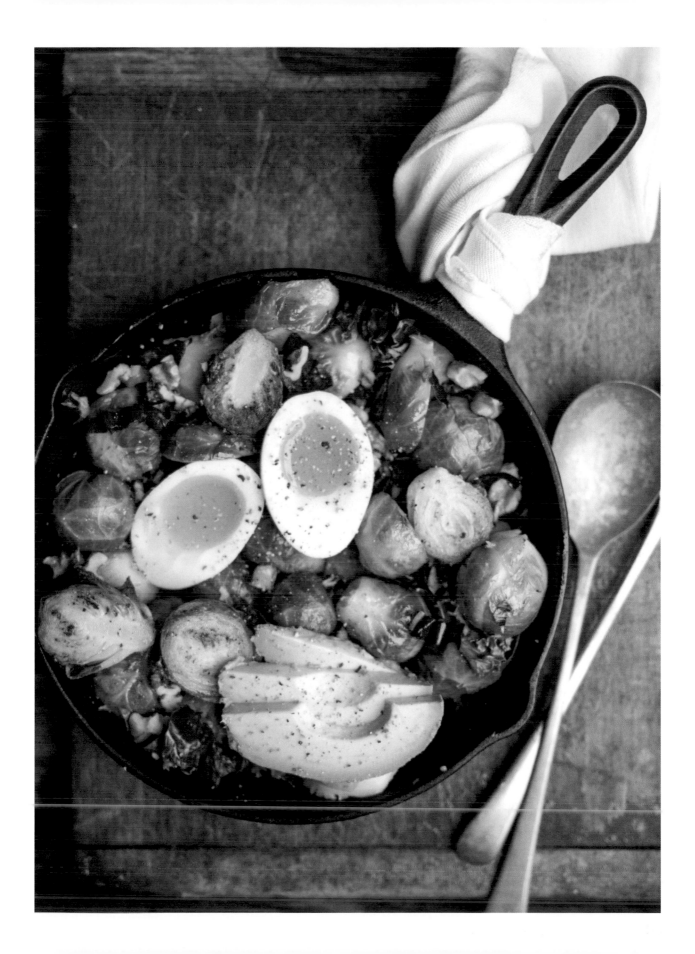

Yorkshire Pudding

KETO · OPTION

When making this side dish, I like to use a vintage cast-iron muffin pan to make individual puddings. But a regular muffin pan works just fine, or you can use a pie pan to make one large pudding.

½ cup pan drippings from a roast prime rib of beef (see page 220) (see note)

3 large eggs, separated

¾ cup unsweetened almond milk (or full-fat coconut milk if nut-free)

½ teaspoon fine sea salt

¾ cup unflavored egg white protein powder

prep time: 5 minutes *cook time:* 20 minutes *yield:* 12 servings

1. Preheat the oven to 375°F.

2. Pour the beef drippings into a standard-size 12-well muffin pan (or a 9-inch metal pie pan). Place the pan in the oven and get the drippings very hot.

3. In the bowl of a stand mixer or in a large bowl with a hand mixer, beat the egg whites until very stiff. Set aside.

4. In a separate bowl, using a hand mixer, beat together the egg yolks, almond milk, and salt until light and foamy.

5. With the mixer on low speed, slowly add the protein powder to the beaten egg whites and mix just until incorporated. Add the egg yolk mixture to the egg white mixture and gently fold to combine.

6. Carefully take the hot pan out of the oven and pour the drippings into the batter. Give the batter a quick stir and pour the batter into the pan (if using a muffin pan, fill each well about two-thirds full). Put the pan back in the oven and cook until the pudding is puffed and dry, 15 to 20 minutes (or 30 minutes if using a pie pan). Allow to rest for a few minutes before removing from the pan.

7. This dish is best served fresh, but any extras can be stored in an airtight container in the refrigerator for up to 3 days. Reheat on a baking sheet in a preheated 350°F oven for 5 minutes or until warmed through.

tip : If you are a vegetarian, you can use coconut oil rather than beef drippings to grease the pan.

nutritional info (per serving)				
calories	fat	protein	carbs	fiber
42	1g	7g	0.4g	0g

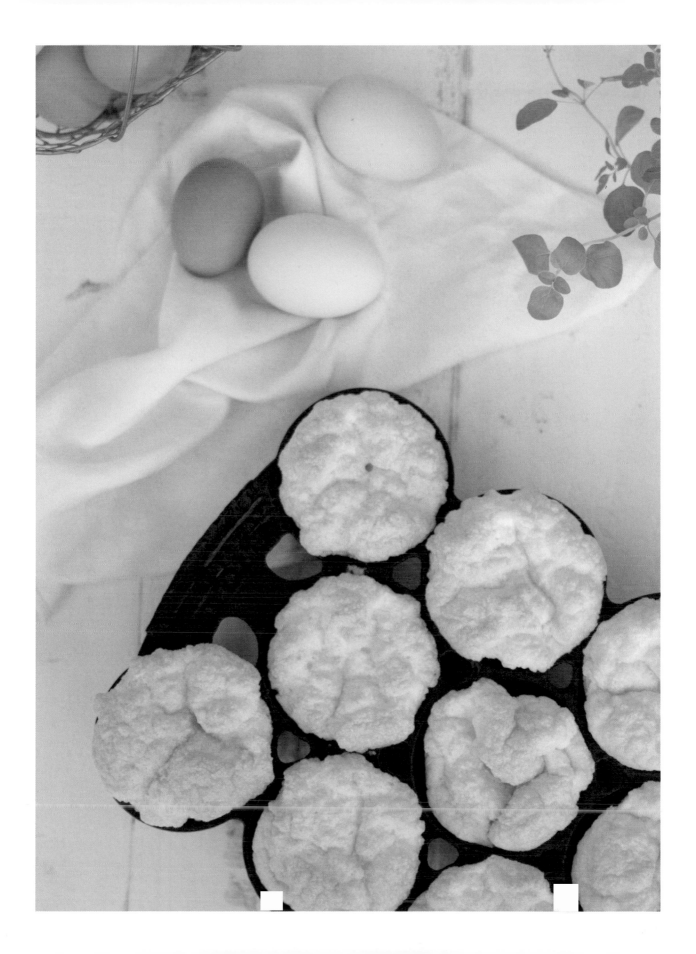

Roasted Asparagus
with Poached Eggs and Hollandaise

KETO   OPTION

1 pound medium-thick asparagus

1 tablespoon melted ghee or unsalted butter (or avocado oil if dairy-free)

¼ teaspoon fine sea salt

¼ teaspoon ground black pepper

4 large eggs

Coconut vinegar

½ batch Hollandaise (page 358), for serving

Purple salt, for garnish

prep time: 5 minutes (not including time to make hollandaise)
cook time: 15 minutes *yield:* 4 servings

1. Preheat the oven to 450°F.

2. Trim the tough ends off the asparagus and place the asparagus in a single layer on a rimmed baking sheet. Pour the melted ghee over the asparagus and roll them around to coat. Sprinkle with the salt and pepper. Roast for 10 minutes or until slightly browned. Meanwhile, poach the eggs.

3. To poach the eggs, fill a large saucepan halfway full with water and add a tablespoon of coconut vinegar per quart of water. Bring to a simmer, then gently add the eggs and poach until cooked to a soft stage, about 3 minutes. Set the poached eggs aside.

4. Divide the roasted asparagus among 4 plates. Top each plate with 2 tablespoons of hollandaise and a poached egg. Sprinkle with purple salt and serve.

5. This dish is best served fresh, but any extras can be stored in an airtight container in the refrigerator for up to 3 days. Reheat the asparagus on a rimmed baking sheet in a preheated 350°F oven for 5 minutes or until warmed through. Reheat leftover poached eggs in a pan of gently simmering water for a minute. To reheat the hollandaise, see page 358.

nutritional info (per serving)				
calories	fat	protein	carbs	fiber
291	26g	9g	5g	2g

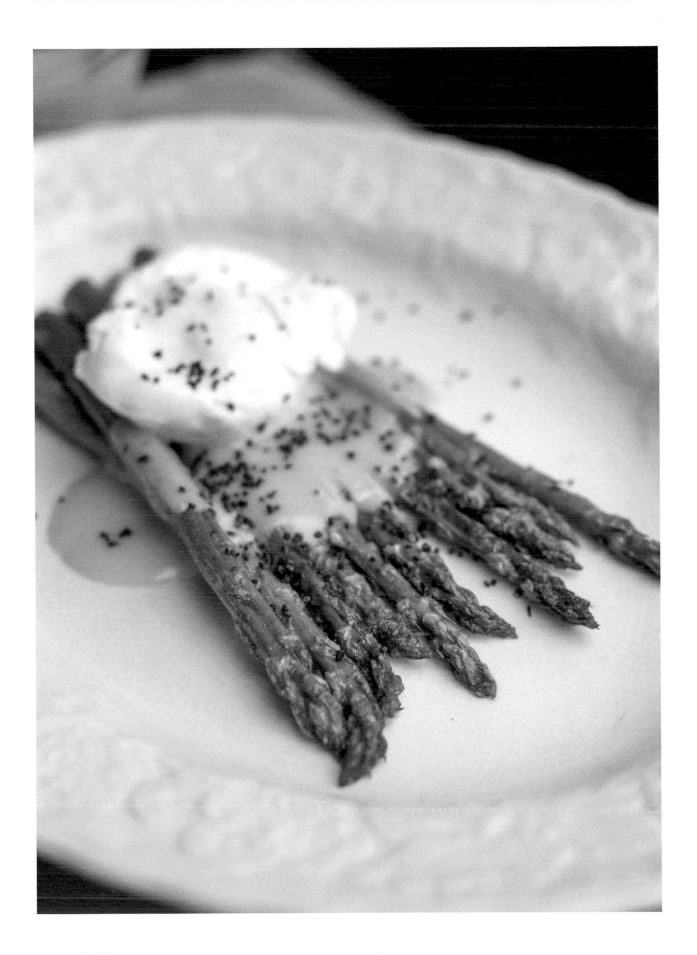

Zucchini and Bacon Gratin

KETO
L M H ✖ ✖

2 strips bacon, diced

¼ cup sliced onions

1 medium zucchini

½ cup grated Parmesan cheese, divided

¼ cup chopped leeks, divided (optional)

¼ cup small cherry tomatoes, cut in half

Fresh dill or thyme, for garnish

prep time: 10 minutes *cook time:* 15 minutes *yield:* 4 servings

1. Preheat the oven to 425°F.

2. Place the diced bacon in a cast-iron skillet over medium heat. Add the onions and sauté until the bacon is cooked through and the onions are caramelized a little, about 5 minutes.

3. Meanwhile, cut the zucchini into ⅛-inch-thick rounds.

4. Place a layer of zucchini over the onions and bacon in the skillet. (Reserve a few pieces of bacon for garnish, if desired.) Sprinkle half of the Parmesan cheese and half of the leeks, if using, over the zucchini layer. Add another layer of zucchini and top with the remaining Parmesan, remaining leeks, and the tomatoes.

5. Transfer the skillet to the oven and bake for 10 minutes or until the zucchini is tender and crispy around the edges and the tomatoes shrivel and get caramelized. You could even place the pan under the broiler at the end to crisp up the cheese. Serve hot, garnished with fresh dill or thyme.

6. Store extras in an airtight container in the refrigerator for up to 3 days. Reheat in a greased skillet over medium heat for a few minutes or until warmed through.

nutritional info (per serving)				
calories	fat	protein	carbs	fiber
112	8g	9g	4g	1g

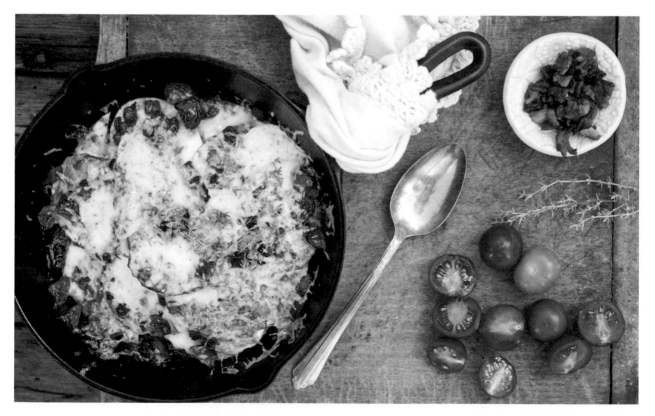

"Cornbread" Muffins

The pecan meal in this recipe creates the perfect texture of cornbread—without the corn! You can either purchase pecan meal or make your own by pulsing raw pecans in a food processor or blender until a rough powder forms. (Do not process the nuts too much or you will end up with pecan butter.) These muffins taste great with keto soups!

½ cup pecan meal

¼ cup coconut flour

2 tablespoons Swerve confectioners'-style sweetener or equivalent amount of liquid or powdered sweetener (see page 24)

½ teaspoon baking powder

½ teaspoon fine sea salt

3 large eggs, beaten

½ cup unsweetened cashew milk or almond milk (or heavy cream if not dairy-sensitive)

¼ cup (½ stick) unsalted butter or ghee (or butter-flavored coconut oil if dairy-free), melted but not hot, plus extra for serving

1 teaspoon maple extract (optional)

prep time: 5 minutes *cook time:* 15 minutes
yield: 6 jumbo or 12 regular-size muffins (1 jumbo or 2 regular-size per serving)

1. Preheat the oven to 325°F. Grease a jumbo 6-well muffin pan or standard-size 12-well muffin pan.

2. Place the pecan meal, coconut flour, powdered sweetener (if using powdered), baking powder, and salt in a medium-sized bowl and mix well to combine. Add the eggs, cashew milk, melted butter, liquid sweetener (if using liquid), and maple extract, if using, and blend well.

3. Pour the batter into the greased muffin pan, filling each well about two-thirds full, and bake for 15 to 20 minutes if using a jumbo muffin pan or 12 to 15 minutes if using a regular-size muffin pan, until a toothpick inserted in the center of a muffin comes out clean. Allow to cool to room temperature before removing from the pan. Serve with additional butter or ghee.

4. Store extras in an airtight container in the refrigerator for up to 3 days, or freeze for up to 1 month.

nutritional info (per serving)				
calories	fat	protein	carbs	fiber
192	17g	5g	4g	2g

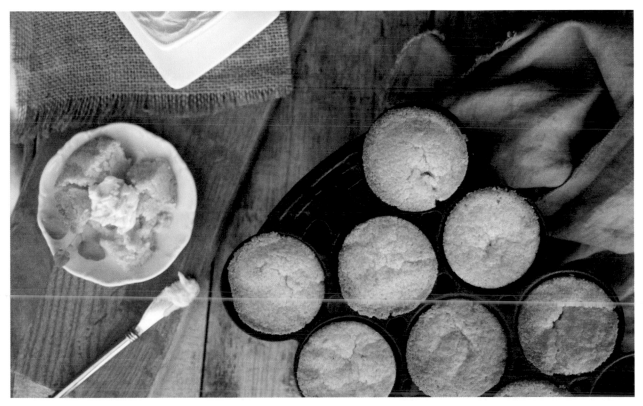

Stuffing Cupcakes

KETO OPTION

½ cup (1 stick) unsalted butter (or bacon fat or lard if dairy-free)

8 ounces white mushrooms, sliced

3 stalks celery, chopped

¼ cup chopped onions

½ teaspoon dried ground sage

½ teaspoon poultry seasoning

1 pound bulk pork sausage

1 batch Keto Buns (page 362)

1 cup beef or chicken bone broth, homemade (page 356) or store-bought

1 teaspoon fine sea salt

½ teaspoon ground black pepper

2 large eggs, beaten

prep time: 5 minutes (not including time to make buns) *cook time:* 30 minutes
yield: 12 cupcakes (1 per serving)

1. Preheat the oven to 325°F. Grease a standard-size 12-well muffin pan.

2. Place the butter in a large cast-iron skillet over medium-high heat. Cook, whisking, until brown (but not black!) flecks appear—this is browned butter. Reserve ¼ cup for drizzling over the top of the cupcakes before serving. (*Note:* If using bacon fat or lard, simply heat the fat in the skillet before continuing with Step 3.)

3. Add the mushrooms, celery, onions, sage, and poultry seasoning to the skillet with the browned butter and sauté until tender and translucent, about 5 minutes.

4. Add the sausage and sauté, using a wooden spoon to break up the pieces, until the meat is cooked through and no longer pink, about 4 minutes. While the meat is cooking, cut the buns into ½-inch cubes.

5. Add the bread cubes to the pan with the sausage mixture. Pour in the broth and mix well. Season with the salt and pepper. Slide the pan off the heat and stir in the beaten eggs.

6. Pour the mixture into the greased muffin pan, filling each well about three-quarters full. Bake, covered, for 15 to 20 minutes, until cooked through. Uncover and bake for 5 more minutes, until the cupcakes are golden brown on the top.

7. Drizzle the reserved ¼ cup of browned butter over the tops of the cupcakes and serve.

nutritional info (per cupcake)				
calories	fat	protein	carbs	fiber
221	19g	10g	2g	0.5g

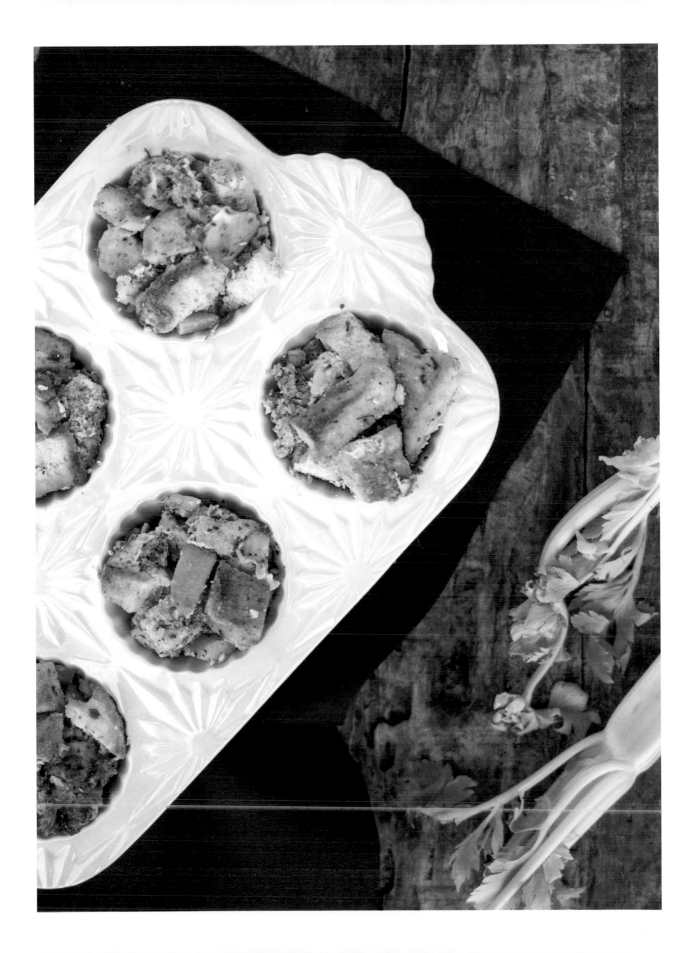

Creamed Collards
with Browned Butter and Bacon

Are you superstitious? Have you ever heard that eating collard greens on New Year's Day brings good fortune for the new year? Here is a perfect recipe to celebrate!

KETO   OPTION

prep time: 10 minutes   *cook time:* 25 minutes   *yield:* 8 servings

4 strips thick-cut bacon, diced

½ cup (1 stick) unsalted butter (or coconut oil if dairy-free)

2 cups chicken or beef bone broth, homemade (page 356) or store-bought

1 cup finely chopped onions

1 bay leaf

3 pounds (2 small bunches) collard greens

½ cup heavy cream (or full-fat coconut milk if dairy-free)

2 cloves garlic, smashed to a paste

1 tablespoon coconut vinegar or apple cider vinegar

¾ teaspoon fine sea salt

½ teaspoon ground black pepper

1. In a large saucepan, cook the diced bacon over medium heat until slightly crisp, about 5 minutes. Remove the bacon and drippings to a bowl and set aside.

2. Place the butter in the same saucepan and cook over high heat for about 5 minutes, whisking. The butter will start to sizzle and foam up. Watch for brown (but not black!) flecks; when they begin to appear, lower the heat. While whisking, slowly add the broth, then add the onions and bay leaf. Bring to a boil and allow to boil for 5 minutes. (*Note:* If using coconut oil instead of butter, put the oil, broth, onions, and bay leaf in the pan at the same time and boil for 5 minutes.)

3. Meanwhile, prepare the collards: Remove and discard the ribs and stems. Coarsely chop the collard leaves.

4. Stir the greens, cream, garlic, vinegar, salt, and pepper into the broth mixture. Boil for 10 minutes or until the greens are tender. Stir in the reserved bacon and drippings and serve.

5. Store extras in an airtight container in the refrigerator for up to 3 days. Reheat in a saucepan over medium heat for a few minutes or until warmed through.

nutritional info (per serving)				
calories	fat	protein	carbs	fiber
284	25g	7g	11g	5g

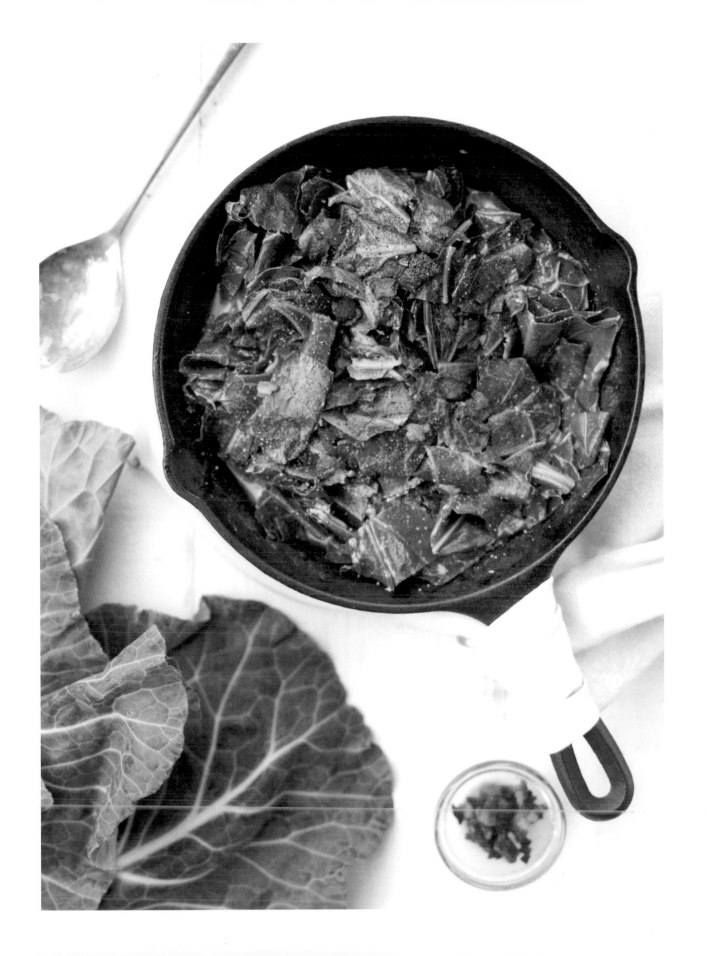

Scalloped Fauxtatoes
with Bacon, Leeks, and Gruyère

4 strips bacon, diced

3 leeks, thinly sliced

¾ teaspoon fine sea salt, divided

⅜ teaspoon ground black pepper, divided

4 cauliflower stems or 1 medium head cauliflower

2½ cups heavy cream, divided

6 ounces Gruyère cheese, shredded

2 teaspoons chopped fresh thyme

¼ teaspoon ground nutmeg

¼ cup grated Parmesan cheese

In this amazing recipe, you can use cauliflower florets if you like, but if you really want to fool your dinner guests, use only the stem and save the florets for Fauxtato Leek Soup (page 120), Roasted Cauliflower with Béarnaise Sauce (page 357), Mashed Fauxtatoes (page 129), or any other recipe that uses florets. Cauliflower stem makes this dish look and taste just like traditional scalloped potatoes! Not only that, but using cauliflower instead of potatoes reduces the cooking time by half.

prep time: 10 minutes, plus 10 minutes to rest *cook time:* 40 minutes
yield: 8 servings

1. Preheat the oven to 400°F and grease an 8-inch square or similar-sized casserole dish.

2. Cook the diced bacon in a cast-iron skillet over medium heat for about 4 minutes, stirring occasionally, until browned and crispy. Remove the bacon from the skillet with a slotted spoon, leaving the drippings in the pan.

3. Add the leeks to the bacon drippings and sauté over medium heat until they're soft and starting to turn golden brown, about 3 minutes. Sprinkle the leeks with ¼ teaspoon of the salt and ⅛ teaspoon of the pepper.

4. Using a mandoline on the thinnest setting, cut the cauliflower stems into very thin slices to resemble scalloped potatoes. Place half of the cauliflower and half of the cream in the greased casserole dish. Sprinkle with ¼ teaspoon of the salt and ⅛ teaspoon of the pepper.

5. Top the cauliflower with the leeks, bacon, Gruyère, thyme, and nutmeg, then add the remaining cauliflower and cream. Sprinkle with the Parmesan, remaining ¼ teaspoon of salt, and remaining ⅛ teaspoon of pepper.

6. Bake the gratin until it's bubbly, the top is brown, and the cauliflower is soft, about 30 minutes. Remove from the oven and allow to rest for 10 to 15 minutes before serving; otherwise it will be too soupy. Store extras in an airtight container in the refrigerator for up to 3 days. Reheat in a baking dish in a preheated 350°F oven for about 10 minutes.

nutritional info (per serving)				
calories	*fat*	*protein*	*carbs*	*fiber*
415	41g	12g	6g	3g

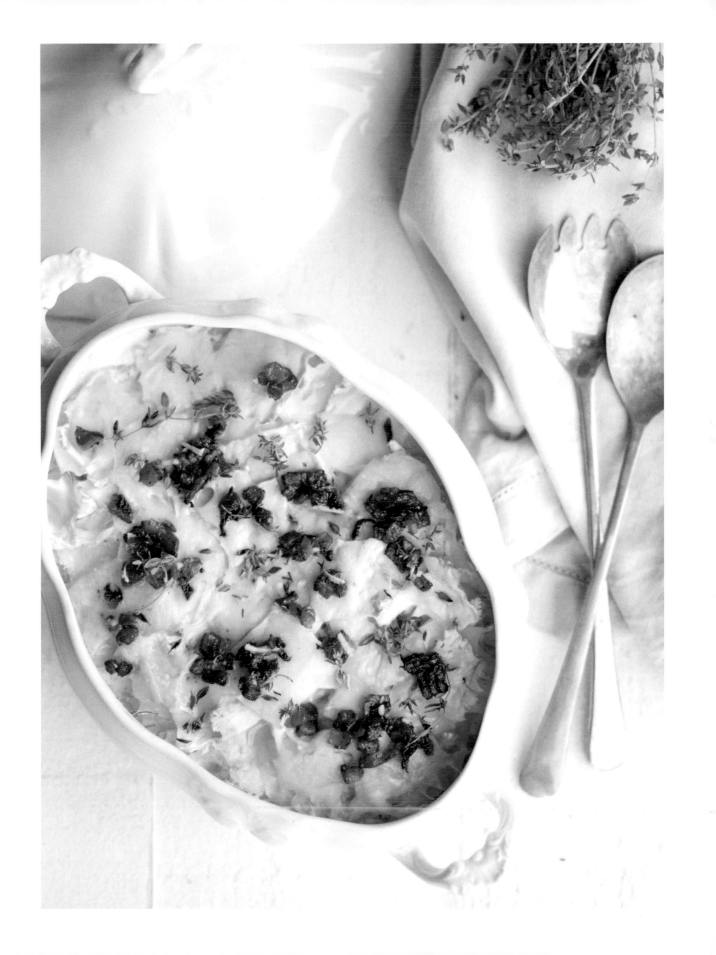

Pimiento Cheese Muffins

L↑H
M
KETO

prep time: 5 minutes   *cook time:* 15 minutes   *yield:* 6 jumbo or 12 regular-size muffins (1 jumbo or 2 regular-size per serving)

½ cup blanched almond flour

¼ cup coconut flour

½ teaspoon baking powder

½ teaspoon fine sea salt

3 large eggs, beaten

½ cup unsweetened cashew milk, almond milk, or heavy cream

¼ cup (½ stick) unsalted butter or ghee, melted but not hot

¾ cup shredded extra-sharp cheddar cheese

¼ cup drained jarred pimientos, chopped

¼ cup minced onions

3 tablespoons sliced green onions

3 tablespoons minced fresh parsley

2 tablespoons finely chopped fresh chives

½ batch Homemade Pimiento Cheese (recipe below), for serving

1. Preheat the oven to 325°F. Grease a jumbo 6-well muffin pan or a standard-size 12-well muffin pan.

2. Place the almond flour, coconut flour, baking powder, and salt in a medium-sized bowl and mix well to combine. Add the beaten eggs, cashew milk, and melted butter and blend well. Stir in the cheddar cheese, pimientos, onions, green onions, parsley, and chives.

3. Pour the batter into the greased muffin pan, filling each well two-thirds full, and bake for 15 to 20 minutes if using a jumbo muffin pan or 12 to 15 minutes if using a regular-size muffin pan, until a toothpick inserted in the center of a muffin comes out clean. Allow to cool to room temperature before removing from the pan. Serve with pimiento cheese.

4. Store extras in an airtight container in the refrigerator for up to 3 days.

nutritional info (per serving)				
calories	*fat*	*protein*	*carbs*	*fiber*
341	29g	13g	8g	3g

Homemade Pimiento Cheese

L↑H
M
KETO ✕

prep time: 5 minutes   *yield:* 2 cups (12 servings)

1 cup shredded extra-sharp cheddar cheese

4 ounces cream cheese (½ cup), softened

¼ cup mayonnaise, homemade (page 359) or store-bought

¼ teaspoon onion powder

⅛ teaspoon garlic powder

1 (2-ounce) jar diced pimientos, drained

Fine sea salt and ground black pepper

1. Place the cheddar cheese, softened cream cheese, mayonnaise, onion powder, garlic powder, and pimientos in a large bowl and mix well. Season to taste with salt and pepper.

2. Place in the fridge to firm up a bit before serving. Store extras in an airtight container in the refrigerator for up to 3 days.

nutritional info (per serving)				
calories	*fat*	*protein*	*carbs*	*fiber*
101	9g	3g	1g	0.1g

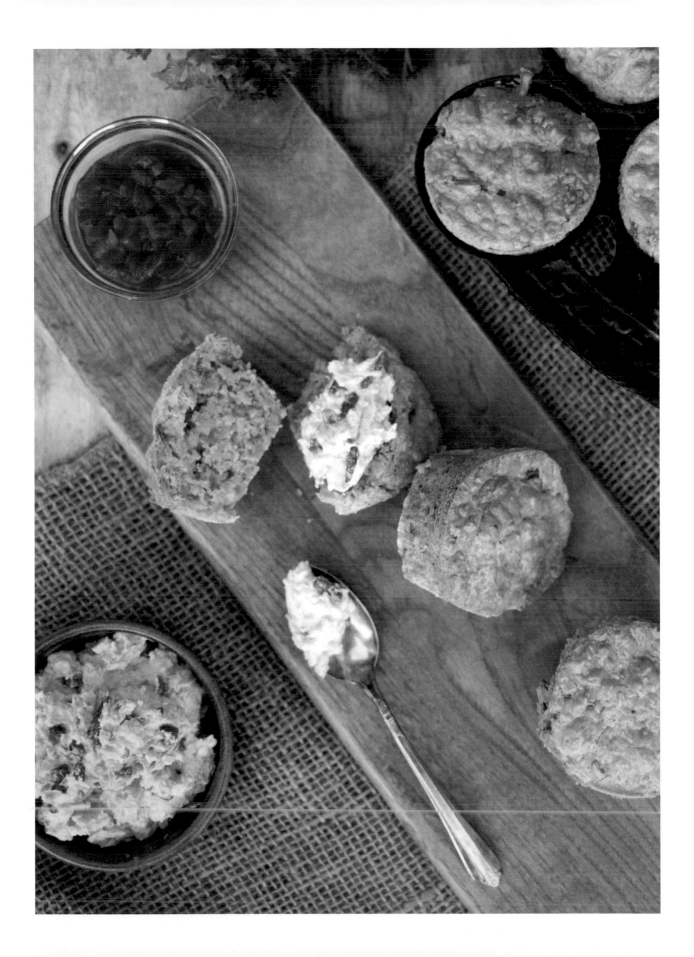

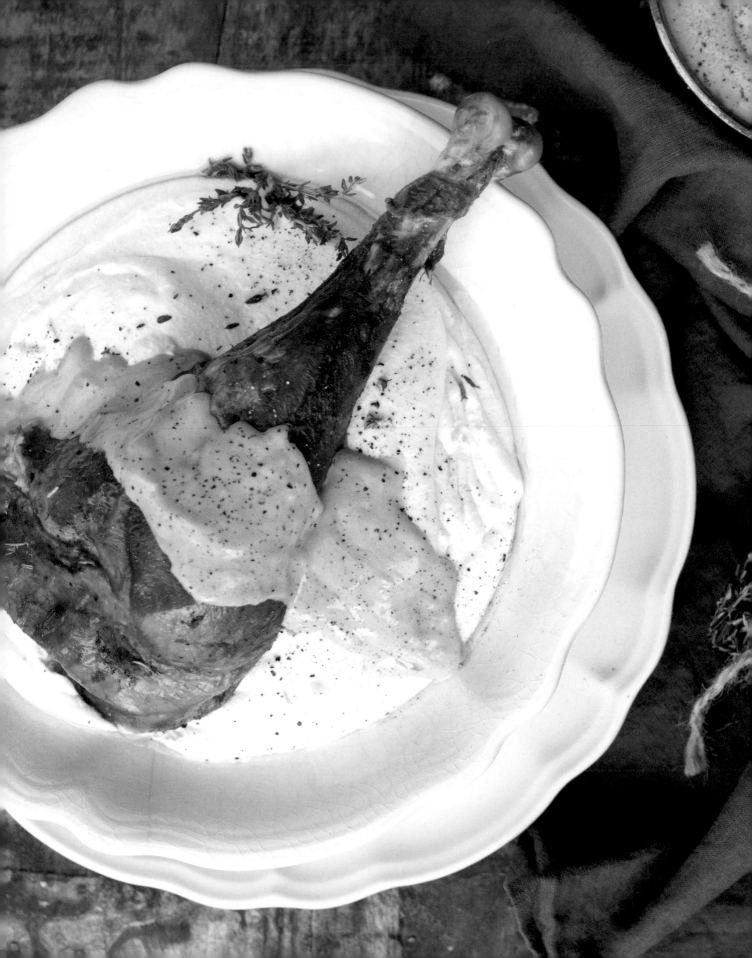

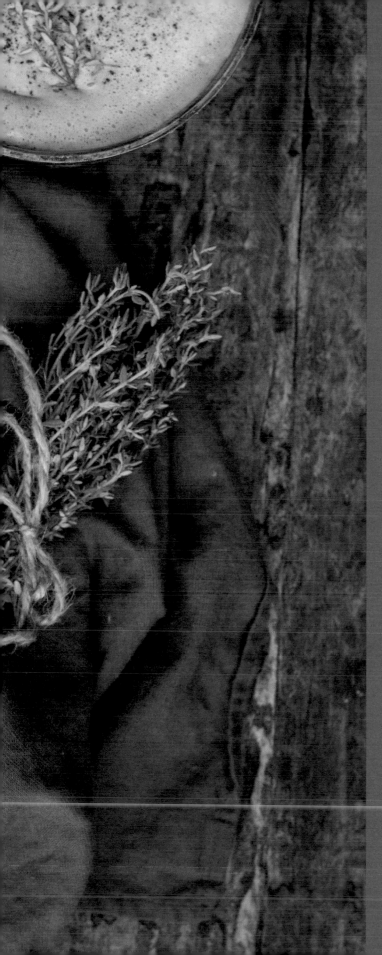

main dishes
Poultry

Cordon Bleu Lasagna

L M H
KETO ✕ ✕

I ate my first bite of Chicken Cordon Bleu when I was seventeen, and it was love at first forkful. It was creamy and ever so flavorful. I thought that turning classic Chicken Cordon Bleu into a lasagna would make it an extra-comforting recipe!

prep time: 12 minutes *cook time:* 1 hour 40 minutes (see tip for shortcut)
yield: 10 servings

chicken

3 tablespoons bacon fat, lard, or ghee

4 chicken leg quarters (about 3 pounds)

1½ teaspoons fine sea salt

½ teaspoon ground black pepper

¼ cup diced onions

1 teaspoon minced garlic

1 cup chicken bone broth, homemade (page 356) or store-bought

sauce

¼ cup (½ stick) unsalted butter

1½ ounces cream cheese (3 tablespoons)

¼ cup beef or chicken bone broth, homemade (page 356) or store-bought

1 cup shredded Swiss cheese

Fine sea salt and ground black pepper

casserole

1 large zucchini (about 10 inches long), trimmed and sliced lengthwise into ¼-inch planks

1 (4-ounce) package sliced Swiss cheese

1 (4-ounce) package thin-sliced ham

1. To cook the chicken: Heat the bacon fat in a deep sauté pan over medium-high heat. Season the chicken leg quarters with the salt and pepper. Place the chicken in the hot fat and cook until golden brown on all sides, about 8 minutes total.

2. Add the onions and garlic to the pan, reduce the heat to medium, and cook for about 8 minutes, stirring occasionally, until the onions are golden brown.

3. Add the broth and simmer, covered, for about 1 hour, until the chicken is almost falling off the bone.

4. Remove the chicken legs from the pan and allow them to cool until you can handle them. Remove the skin (see note), then shred the meat and set it aside.

5. To make the sauce: In a saucepan, melt the butter over medium heat. Stir in the cream cheese and broth and cook, stirring, for 2 minutes or until thickened. Reduce the heat. Add the Swiss cheese and stir until the cheese is melted. Season with salt and pepper to taste, then remove from the heat.

6. Preheat the oven to 350°F. Layer the zucchini "noodles" in an 8-inch square casserole dish (you should have two stacked layers of noodles), then drizzle ½ cup of the sauce over the zucchini. Top the sauced zucchini with a layer of Swiss cheese slices, then a layer of ham slices. Layer the shredded chicken on top of the ham. Drizzle the rest of the sauce into the casserole dish. Top this with another layer of ham, then the rest of the cheese slices.

7. Bake the lasagna for 20 minutes or until the zucchini is soft and the cheese is melted. Store extras in an airtight container in the refrigerator for up to 3 days. Reheat in a baking dish in a preheated 350°F oven for 5 minutes or until warmed through.

note: After removing the skin from the cooked chicken, don't discard it! Save it to make the "crunchy rice" for Chicken "Wild Rice" Soup (page 116). You can always freeze chicken skin for later use.

busy family tip:

To skip Steps 1 through 3 and shave about 1¼ hours off of the cooking time, replace the chicken leg quarters with a precooked clean-ingredient rotisserie chicken from the supermarket or leftover cooked chicken.

nutritional info (per serving)				
calories	fat	protein	carbs	fiber
314	26g	16g	3g	1g

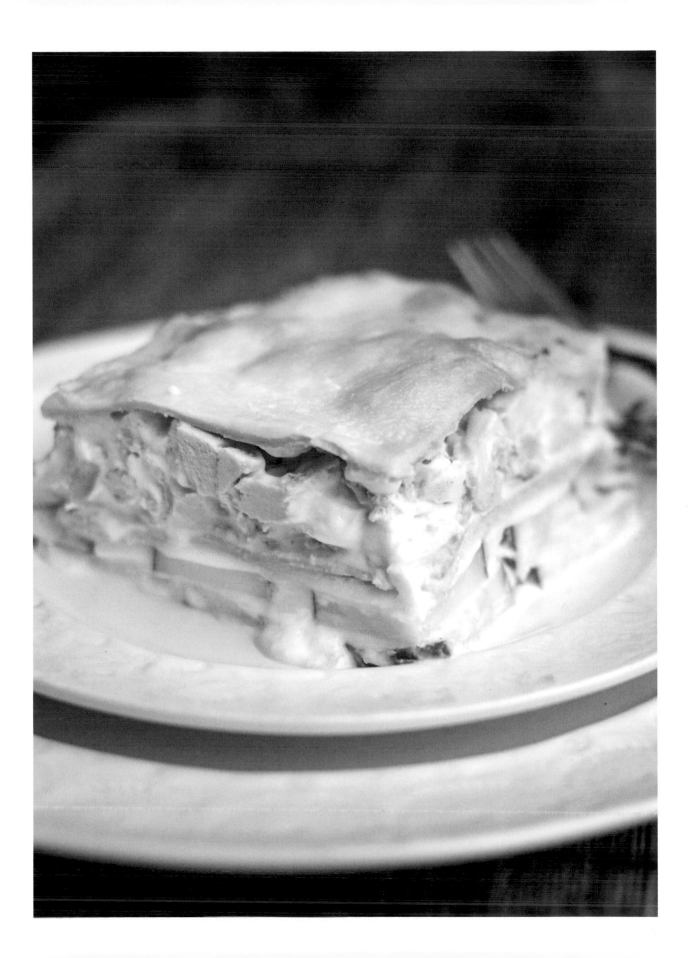

Poulet Grand-Mère

4 bone-in, skin-on chicken thighs

1 teaspoon fine sea salt, divided

¼ cup ghee (or coconut oil if dairy-free)

4 sprigs fresh thyme, plus extra for garnish

4 strips thick-cut bacon, diced

¼ cup sliced onions

1 cup sliced mushrooms

Ground black pepper

2 cups chicken bone broth, homemade (page 356) or store-bought

2 tablespoons melted ghee or unsalted butter (or avocado oil if dairy-free) (optional)

prep time: 15 minutes   *cook time:* 30 minutes   *yield:* 4 servings

1. Preheat the oven to 350°F.

2. Sprinkle the chicken thighs with ½ teaspoon of the salt. In a large cast-iron skillet, heat the ghee (enough to coat the bottom of the pan) over medium-high heat. Add the thyme. Place the seasoned chicken thighs skin side down in the pan and sear until golden brown, using a spoon to baste the flesh side with the melted ghee from the pan as they cook. Flip the thighs and cook for another 2 minutes or until the chicken is golden brown. Remove the chicken from the skillet and place on a rimmed baking sheet; leave the drippings in the skillet.

3. Bake the chicken for 7 minutes or until it is cooked through and no longer pink inside.

4. Meanwhile, cook the bacon: Place the diced bacon in the skillet with the chicken drippings. Cook over medium heat for 4 minutes or until the bacon is crisp and cooked through. Use a slotted spoon to scoop out the bacon pieces and set them aside.

5. Place the onions in the hot skillet and cook until soft and translucent, about 5 minutes. Add the mushrooms and cook until the mushrooms are golden brown on all sides, 3 to 5 minutes. Season with the remaining ½ teaspoon of salt and a couple pinches of pepper.

6. Add the broth and scrape up all the browned bits that have collected on the bottom of the pan. Cook down until the gravy has reduced a bit. Taste and add more seasoning, if desired. Serve the chicken with the mushroom gravy from the pan. Garnish with the reserved bacon pieces and fresh thyme. Drizzle with 2 tablespoons of melted ghee, if desired.

7. Store extras in an airtight container in the refrigerator for up to 3 days. Reheat on a rimmed baking sheet in a preheated 350°F oven for a few minutes, until warmed through.

nutritional info (per serving)				
calories	fat	protein	carbs	fiber
489	42g	23g	3g	1g

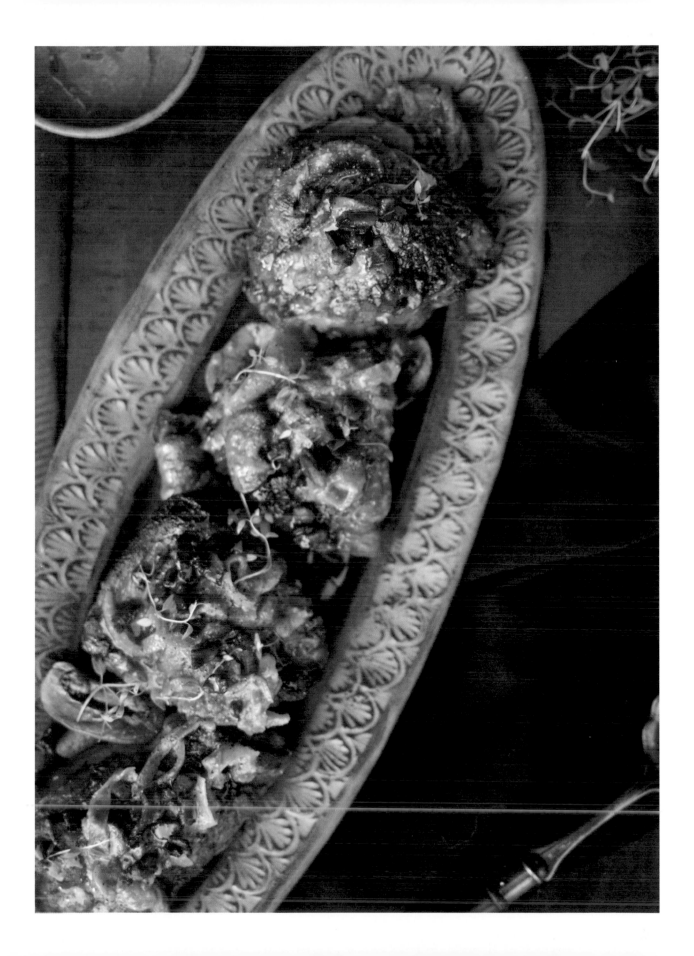

Chicken and Gravy Cobbler

KETO OPTION

prep time: 20 minutes *cook time:* 25 minutes *yield:* 8 servings

filling

2 tablespoons ghee or unsalted butter (or coconut oil if dairy-free)

1½ cups sliced mushrooms

¼ cup diced onions

2 stalks celery, finely chopped

1 cup chopped asparagus

1½ pounds boneless, skinless chicken thighs, chopped into ¼-inch pieces

1 teaspoon fine sea salt

½ teaspoon ground black pepper

4 ounces cream cheese (½ cup) (Kite Hill brand cream cheese style spread if dairy-free)

¾ cup chicken bone broth, homemade (page 356) or store-bought

biscuits

4 large egg whites

1 cup blanched almond flour

1 teaspoon baking powder

¼ teaspoon fine sea salt

3 tablespoons very cold butter (or lard if dairy-free), cut into pieces

Fresh thyme, for garnish

Melted ghee, butter, or extra-virgin olive oil, for drizzling

1. Preheat the oven to 400°F.

2. In a cast-iron skillet, melt the ghee over medium heat. Add the mushrooms and onions and sauté for 4 minutes or until the mushrooms are golden brown. Add the celery and asparagus and sauté for another 3 minutes.

3. Season the chopped chicken on all sides with the salt and pepper. Add the chicken to the skillet and sauté until it is seared on all sides. It doesn't need to be cooked through.

4. Add the cream cheese to the skillet and use a whisk to combine well until no lumps are present. Slowly whisk in the broth. Set aside and make the biscuits for the topping.

5. To make the biscuits, place the egg whites in a mixing bowl or the bowl of a stand mixer and whip until very firm and stiff. In a separate medium-sized bowl, whisk together the almond flour, baking powder, and salt, then cut in the butter. (If the butter isn't chilled, the biscuits won't turn out.) Gently fold the flour mixture into the egg whites. Use a large spoon or ice cream scooper to scoop out and form the dough into 2-inch-round biscuits, making sure the butter stays in separate clumps.

6. Place the biscuits on top of the chicken mixture in the skillet. Bake for 12 to 15 minutes, until the biscuits are golden brown. Serve garnished with thyme and a drizzle of melted ghee.

7. Store extras in an airtight container in the refrigerator for up to 3 days. Reheat in a baking dish in a preheated 350°F oven for 5 minutes or until warmed through.

nutritional info (per serving)				
calories	fat	protein	carbs	fiber
438	33g	28g	6g	2g

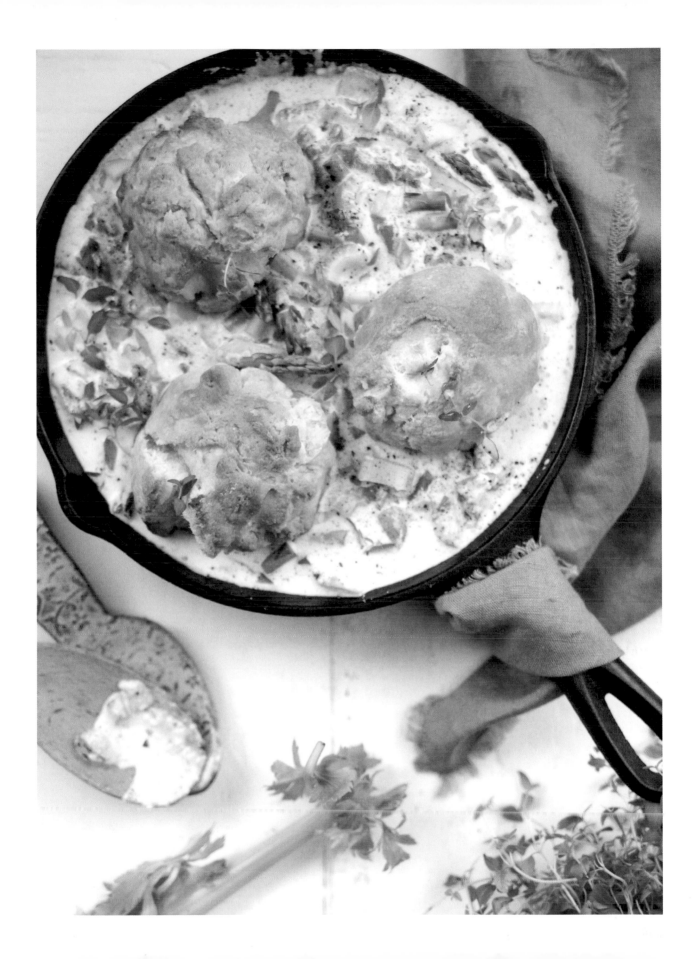

Lemon Pepper Roast Turkey with Bacon Gravy

1 (12-pound) turkey

3 lemons, plus extra for garnish

2 tablespoons ground black pepper

1 tablespoon fine sea salt

1 cup diced onions

2 cloves garlic, minced

1 large stalk celery, diced

4 small sprigs fresh thyme

10 strips bacon, diced

½ cup ghee or unsalted butter

⅛ teaspoon guar gum (a natural thickener), or 1 ounce cream cheese (2 tablespoons)

for serving (optional)

Mashed Fauxtatoes (page 129; see note)

A nice piece of freshly roasted turkey with a side of mashed fauxtatoes just screams comfort to me. It looks like you slaved all day in the kitchen for your loved ones, but both recipes are really quite simple, and there are lots of uses for the meat. If you find yourself with leftover turkey after making this dish, you can use it to make Turkey Tetrazzini (page 158) or Turkey Goulash (page 180), for example. And you can use the carcass to make a rich turkey bone broth (page 356) for use in Braised Turkey Legs with Creamy Gravy (page 166) or the goulash.

prep time: 15 minutes (not including time to make fauxtatoes)
cook time: 3 hours *yield:* 14 servings

1. Preheat the oven to 350°F.

2. Remove the neck and giblets from the turkey.

3. Grate the zest of the lemons into a small bowl. Add the pepper and salt. Using paper towels, pat the turkey dry. Season the turkey cavity with a bit of the zest mixture, then rub the rest all over the outside of the turkey. Cut the lemons in half. Place 1 lemon inside the cavity along with the onions, garlic, celery, and thyme sprigs.

4. Tie the turkey legs together using kitchen twine or a small string. Place the turkey on a rack set inside a large roasting pan. Tuck the wings under the body to prevent burning.

5. Cook the diced bacon in a large skillet over medium heat until crisp, about 5 minutes. Transfer to paper towels to drain, keeping the drippings in the skillet.

6. Add the ghee to the skillet with the drippings and stir until melted, then pour into a bowl and stir in the juice of the remaining 2 lemons. Rub this mixture all over the turkey. Place the turkey in the oven and roast for 30 minutes. After 30 minutes, baste the turkey with the drippings. Continue to roast for a total of about 3 hours, basting every half hour, until a meat thermometer inserted into the thigh registers 165°F. Remove the turkey to a serving tray to rest for at least 25 minutes before carving.

7. Meanwhile, pour the drippings from the roasting pan into a saucepan and place over medium heat. Whisk in the guar gum or cream cheese until well combined and no clumps are present. Cook for 5 minutes, stirring, until the gravy is thick. Then add the reserved bacon for an amazing gravy. Serve with extra lemon halves or quarters.

8. Store extras in an airtight container in the refrigerator for up to 3 days. Reheat on a baking sheet in a preheated 350°F oven for 5 minutes or until warmed through.

note: One batch of mashed fauxtatoes serves four people. Double or triple the recipe as needed depending on how many people you are serving.

nutritional info (per serving)				
calories	fat	protein	carbs	fiber
349	19g	39g	3g	1g

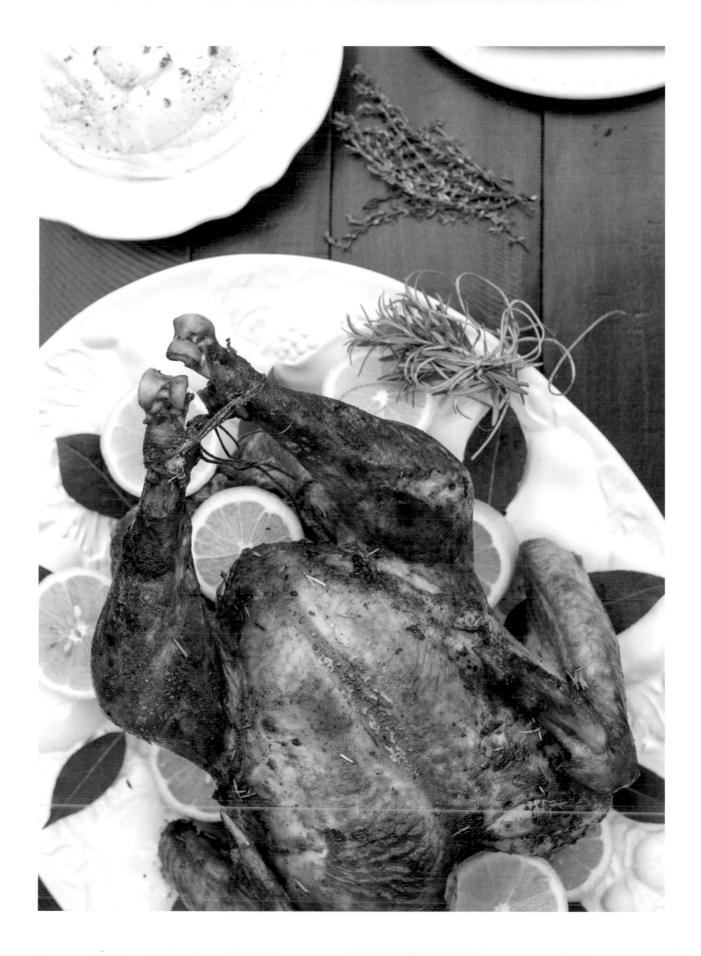

Turkey Tetrazzini

prep time: 5 minutes   *cook time:* 45 minutes   *yield:* 8 servings

noodles

2 tablespoons unsalted butter or ghee (for cabbage noodles)

4 cups very thinly sliced green cabbage or raw spiral-sliced zucchini noodles

2 teaspoons fine sea salt (for zucchini noodles)

1 tablespoon unsalted butter or ghee

1 cup sliced mushrooms

¼ cup diced leeks or onions

6 spears asparagus, cut into 1-inch pieces (tough ends trimmed)

1 clove garlic, smashed to a paste

4 ounces cream cheese (½ cup), softened

½ cup turkey or chicken bone broth, homemade (page 356) or store-bought

1 large egg, beaten

2 cups shredded cheddar cheese, divided

½ cup grated Parmesan cheese

1 teaspoon poultry seasoning

½ teaspoon fine sea salt

¼ teaspoon ground black pepper

3 cups diced leftover cooked turkey

Chopped fresh parsley, for garnish (optional)

1. Preheat the oven to 400°F. Grease a 13 by 9-inch casserole dish.

2. If making cabbage noodles, place 2 tablespoons of butter and the cabbage in a large cast-iron skillet over medium-low heat. Cover and cook, stirring often, for 15 minutes or until the cabbage is very tender.

   If making zucchini noodles, place them in a colander over the sink and sprinkle with 2 teaspoons of salt. Allow to drain for 5 minutes, then squeeze out the excess liquid and salt. Place the noodles in a large cast-iron skillet.

3. Meanwhile, place 1 tablespoon of butter in a medium-sized skillet over medium heat. Add the mushrooms, leeks, and asparagus and sauté for 4 minutes or until the asparagus is crisp-tender. Add the garlic and sauté for another minute. Slide the pan off the heat.

4. In a medium-sized bowl, whisk together the cream cheese, broth, and egg. Stir this mixture into the cabbage or zucchini noodles. Add 1½ cups of the cheddar cheese, along with the Parmesan cheese, poultry seasoning, salt, and pepper. Stir until melted; do not allow the mixture to boil.

5. Stir in the turkey and asparagus mixture and remove from the heat. Transfer the mixture to the prepared casserole dish. Sprinkle with the remaining ½ cup of cheddar cheese.

6. Bake for 12 minutes or until hot and bubbly. Serve garnished with parsley, if desired.

7. Store extras in an airtight container in the refrigerator for up to 3 days. Reheat in a baking dish in a preheated 350°F oven for 5 minutes or until warmed through.

tip: You can make extra cabbage "pasta" and store it in the freezer or fridge for easy additions to meals. Zucchini noodles, however, do not freeze well.

nutritional info (per serving)				
calories	fat	protein	carbs	fiber
372	24g	33g	6g	1g

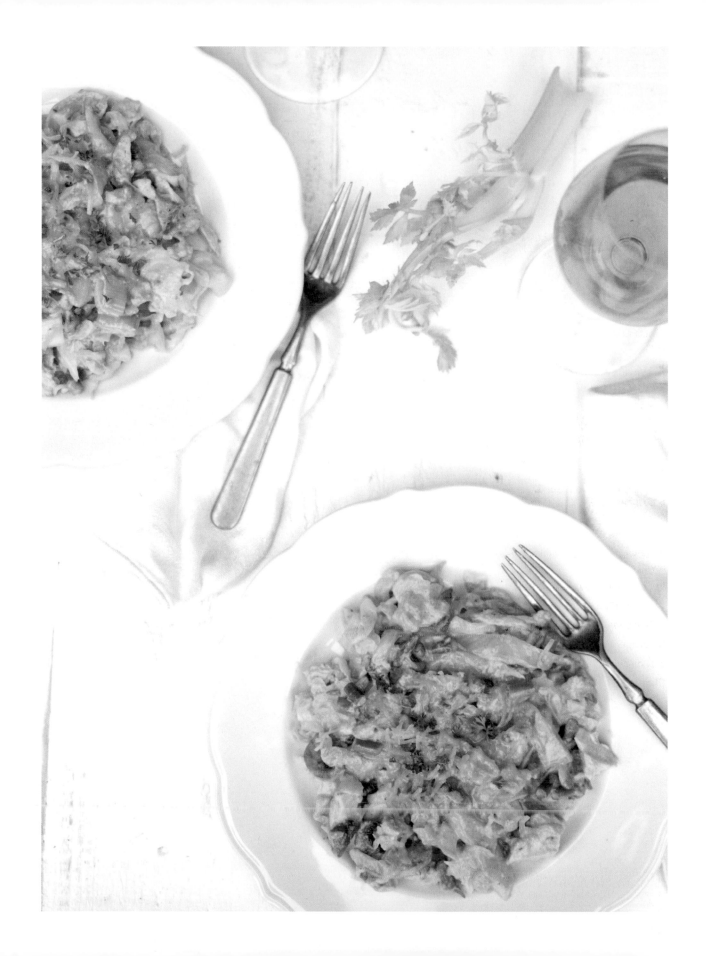

Skillet Enchilada Casserole

This amazing casserole will warm your soul and fill your kitchen with amazing smells! This dish also makes fantastic leftovers for the week!

L **M** H KETO ✗ ✗

prep time: 10 minutes   *cook time:* 55 minutes   *yield:* 8 servings

3 tablespoons ghee or coconut oil, divided

1 onion, roughly chopped

4 cloves garlic, roughly chopped

2½ tablespoons chili powder, divided

3 teaspoons ground cumin, divided

2½ teaspoons fine sea salt, divided

1½ cups chicken bone broth, homemade (page 356) or store-bought

2 (28-ounce) cans diced tomatoes

2 pounds boneless, skinless chicken thighs

2 teaspoons paprika

1 teaspoon dried ground oregano

10 slices deli chicken breast

3 cups shredded Monterey Jack cheese

for garnish

Sliced avocado

Chopped fresh cilantro and/or sprigs

Crumbled Cotija cheese

Lime wedges

1. Heat 2 tablespoons of the ghee in a cast-iron skillet over medium-high heat. Add the onion and sauté for 4 minutes. Reduce the heat to medium and add the garlic, 1 tablespoon of the chili powder, 2 teaspoons of the cumin, and 1½ teaspoons of the salt. Sauté for 2 more minutes.

2. Add the chicken broth and tomatoes and simmer for 8 minutes. Transfer the mixture to a blender and blend until smooth, then set the sauce aside.

3. Season the chicken thighs on all sides with the remaining 1½ tablespoons of chili powder, the remaining teaspoon of cumin, the remaining teaspoon of salt, the paprika, and the oregano. Add the remaining tablespoon of ghee to the skillet, still over medium-high heat. Add the chicken and cook for a few minutes on each side until browned on both sides. Add the reserved sauce, cover, and reduce the heat to medium. Cook for 12 minutes or until the chicken is cooked through and no longer pink. Remove the chicken from the sauce and shred the meat with 2 forks. Set the shredded chicken and sauce aside.

4. Preheat the oven to 350°F.

5. Place 5 slices of the deli chicken in a 9-inch cast-iron skillet or casserole dish. Top with half of the shredded chicken, half of the sauce, and half of the Monterey Jack cheese. Top with the remaining deli chicken slices, shredded chicken, sauce, and cheese. Bake for 20 minutes or until the casserole is heated through and the cheese is melted.

6. Garnish the casserole with slices of avocado, chopped cilantro, and crumbled Cotija cheese. Store extras in an airtight container in the refrigerator for up to 3 days. Reheat in a baking dish in a preheated 350°F oven for 5 minutes or until warmed through.

nutritional info (per serving)				
calories	fat	protein	carbs	fiber
442	30g	36g	6g	2g

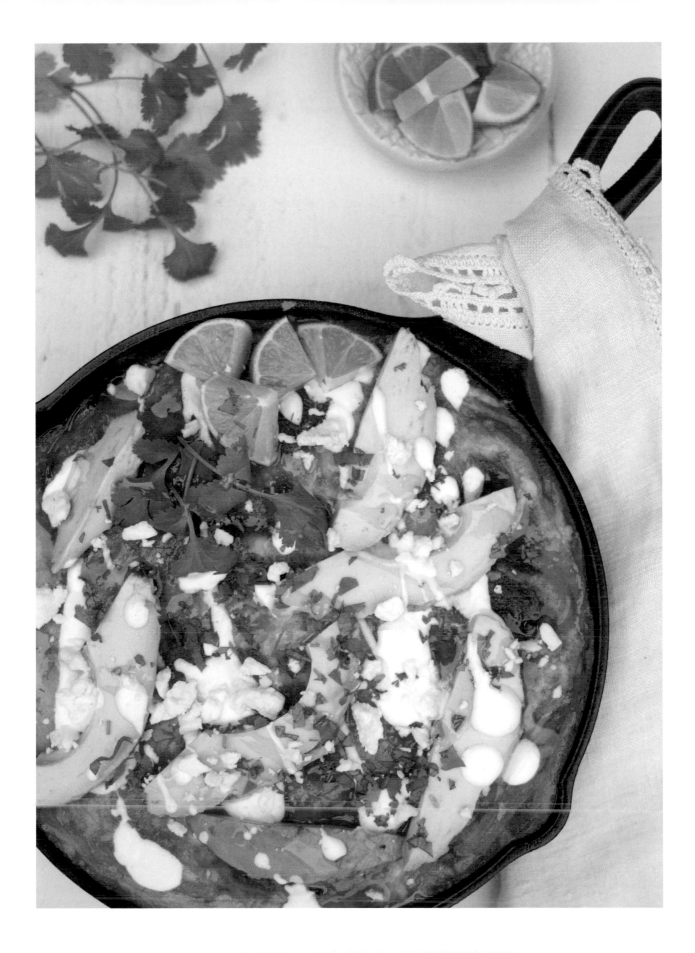

Turkey Meatloaf Cupcakes

Instead of using breadcrumbs or cracker crumbs, I use an egg as a binder for the meatloaf in this recipe, along with grated Parmesan cheese and finely chopped mushrooms. (Don't worry, you won't taste the mushrooms, but they make the meatloaf very moist!) Mushrooms and aged cheeses have something called umami, a pleasant savory taste produced by glutamate and ribonucleotides, which are chemicals that occur naturally in many foods. Umami is subtle and not generally identifiable, but it blends well with other tastes to intensify and enhance flavors. Umami plays an important role in making food taste delicious.

L M H
KETO

prep time: 6 minutes (not including time to make fauxtatoes)

cook time: 15 minutes   *yield:* 12 cupcakes (2 per serving)

meatloaf

2 pounds ground turkey

¾ cup finely chopped mushrooms

½ cup grated Parmesan cheese

½ cup tomato sauce

1 large egg, beaten

2 teaspoons poultry seasoning

1 teaspoon dried thyme leaves

1 clove garlic, smashed to a paste

glaze

1 cup tomato sauce

2 teaspoons prepared yellow mustard

2 tablespoons Swerve confectioners'-style sweetener or equivalent amount of liquid or powdered sweetener (see page 24)

1 teaspoon onion powder

1 cup tomato sauce, warmed

3 cups Mashed Fauxtatoes (page 129)

Fresh parsley or oregano, for garnish

1. Preheat the oven to 350°F.

2. In a large bowl, mix together the ground turkey, mushrooms, Parmesan cheese, ½ cup of tomato sauce, and beaten egg. Season with the poultry seasoning, thyme, and garlic and mix to combine.

3. Make the glaze by mixing together the 1 cup of tomato sauce, mustard, sweetener, and onion powder in a small bowl.

4. Press the meat mixture into a standard-size 12-well muffin pan, filling each well about three-quarters full. Top each "cupcake" with glaze. Bake for 15 minutes or until the internal temperature reaches 160°F.

5. Remove the cupcakes from the pan onto a serving tray. Top each cupcake with a spoonful of tomato sauce, then a dollop of mashed fauxtatoes. (I use a piping bag with a tip for a pretty presentation.) Garnish with fresh parsley or oregano.

6. Store extras in an airtight container in the refrigerator for up to 3 days. Reheat on a rimmed baking sheet in a preheated 350°F oven for 5 minutes or until warmed through.

nutritional info (per serving)				
calories	fat	protein	carbs	fiber
329	13g	42g	10g	2g

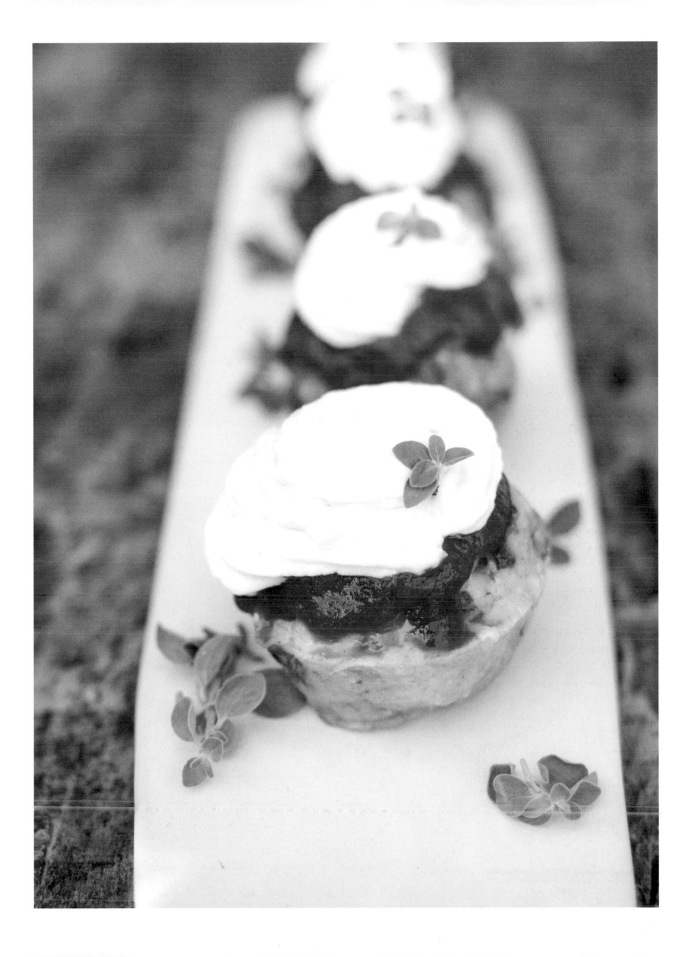

Saucy Crispy Chicken

This recipe has been a big hit with everyone who tries it. It has an amazing crispy crust and a flavorful sauce that can't be beat!

prep time: 7 minutes, plus 1 hour to marinate *cook time:* 12 minutes
yield: 4 servings

marinade

½ cup avocado oil

½ cup ranch dressing, homemade (page 359) or store-bought

3 tablespoons coconut aminos

1 tablespoon minced garlic

1 teaspoon coconut vinegar

1 teaspoon lemon juice

1 teaspoon ground black pepper

4 boneless, skinless chicken thighs, pounded to ¾-inch thickness

Fine sea salt and ground black pepper

2 teaspoons coconut oil or avocado oil, for frying

parmesan sauce

½ cup ranch dressing, homemade (page 359) or store-bought

¼ cup grated Parmesan cheese

parmesan topping

½ cup pork dust (or blanched almond flour if not nut-sensitive)

⅓ cup grated Parmesan cheese

2 tablespoons unsalted butter, melted

1 teaspoon garlic salt

1 cup shredded provolone cheese

1. Combine the ingredients for the marinade in a shallow dish. Add the chicken thighs and stir well to coat. Cover and let marinate in the refrigerator for 1 hour or overnight.

2. Preheat the broiler. Remove the chicken from the marinade, pat dry, and season on all sides with salt and pepper; discard the marinade. Heat the coconut oil in a large cast-iron skillet over medium-high heat, then add the chicken and sauté for 3 minutes. Flip and cook for another 3 to 5 minutes, until the chicken is cooked through and no longer pink.

3. Meanwhile, make the Parmesan sauce: Place ½ cup of ranch dressing and ¼ cup of Parmesan cheese in a small bowl and stir well to combine.

4. Prepare the Parmesan topping by placing the pork dust, ⅓ cup of Parmesan cheese, melted butter, and garlic salt in another small bowl. Stir well to combine.

5. Cover the chicken in the skillet with the Parmesan sauce, top with the provolone cheese, and then sprinkle on the Parmesan topping. Place in the oven and broil for 4 minutes or until the cheese is melted and the topping is starting to brown.

6. Store extras in an airtight container in the refrigerator for up to 3 days. Reheat in a baking dish in a preheated 350°F oven for 5 minutes or until warmed through.

nutritional info (per serving)				
calories	*fat*	*protein*	*carbs*	*fiber*
544	42g	40g	0.2g	0g

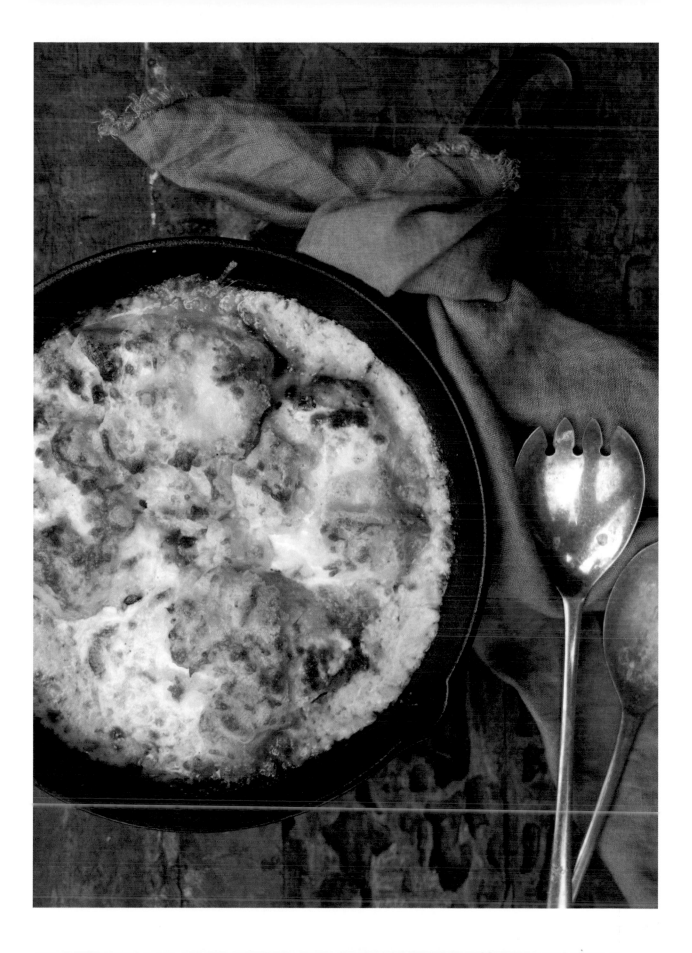

Braised Turkey Legs
with Creamy Gravy

This tasty meal reminds me of Thanksgiving dinner, but without the hassle! Braising turkey legs seems daunting, but it creates one amazing meal without much daunting work.

L M↑ H
KETO ✕ ✕

2 tablespoons ghee or coconut oil

4 turkey legs

Fine sea salt and ground black pepper

¼ cup diced onions

¼ cup diced celery

2 sprigs thyme, plus extra for garnish

1½ cups turkey or chicken bone broth, homemade (page 356) or store-bought, or water, or more as needed

½ batch Mashed Fauxtatoes (page 129), for serving

1 ounce mascarpone or cream cheese (2 tablespoons), softened

Chopped fresh herbs, such as thyme, for garnish

Melted ghee or extra-virgin olive oil, for drizzling

prep time: 15 minutes (not including time to make fauxtatoes)
cook time: about 2 hours   *yield:* 4 servings

1. Preheat the oven to 300°F.

2. Heat the ghee in a cast-iron skillet over medium-high heat. Season the turkey legs on all sides with salt and pepper. Place the legs in the skillet and sear on all sides until golden brown, about 3 minutes per side. Remove from the skillet and place in a roasting pan.

3. Place the onions, celery, and thyme sprigs in the skillet and fry for 8 minutes or until the onions are translucent. Transfer the veggies to the roasting pan, tucking them under the turkey legs so they don't burn. Pour the broth into the pan. Place the pan in the oven and roast, uncovered, for about 1 hour 40 minutes, until the turkey is cooked through and no longer pink inside when pierced with a knife.

4. To serve, divide the fauxtatoes among 4 plates. Place a turkey leg on top of the mash on each plate.

5. Pour the sauce and veggies from the roasting pan into a blender. Add the mascarpone and puree until smooth. Cover each turkey leg with the creamy gravy. Garnish with herbs and a drizzle of melted ghee.

6. Store extras in an airtight container in the refrigerator for up to 3 days. Reheat on a rimmed baking sheet in a preheated 350°F oven for 5 minutes or until warmed through.

nutritional info (per serving)				
calories	fat	protein	carbs	fiber
650	30g	80g	10g	4g

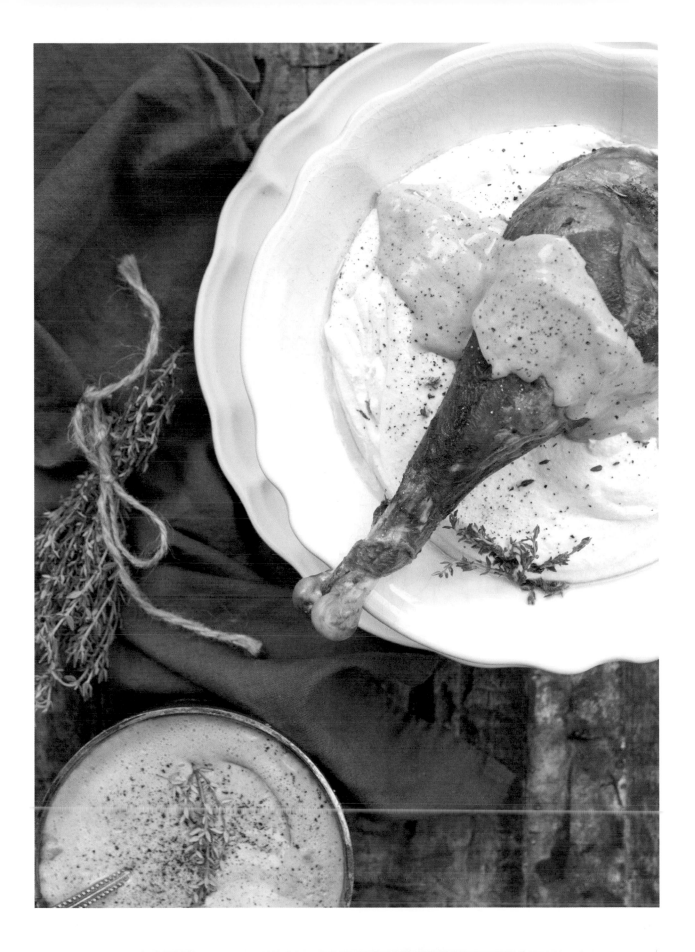

Chicken Club Hand Pies

These hand pies are super-tasty and really cute to serve. If you love them as much as we do, I highly suggest making a quadruple batch and storing unbaked pies in the freezer for easy meals: all you have to do is pop one in the toaster oven or oven!

L ⟩ M H
KETO

prep time: 10 minutes, plus 1 hour to chill dough, if needed
cook time: 15 minutes   *yield:* 4 servings

dough

1¾ cups shredded mozzarella cheese

2 tablespoons unsalted butter

1 large egg, beaten

¾ cup blanched almond flour

⅛ teaspoon fine sea salt

filling

2 strips bacon, diced

2 tablespoons diced onions

⅛ teaspoon minced fresh thyme

1 boneless, skinless chicken thigh, cut into ¼-inch pieces (about ½ cup)

¼ cup mayonnaise, homemade (page 359) or store-bought

Fresh oregano, for garnish

Ranch dressing, homemade (page 359) or store-bought, for serving

1. Place a pizza stone in the cold oven, then turn the oven on to 425°F. (You can use a baking sheet, but a pizza stone will bake the bottoms better.)

2. To make the dough, place the mozzarella cheese and butter in a microwave-safe bowl and microwave for 1 to 2 minutes, until the cheese is entirely melted. Stir well.

3. Add the egg and, using a hand mixer, combine well. Add the almond flour and salt and combine well with the mixer. Use your hands and work it like a traditional dough, kneading for about 3 minutes. Set the dough aside. (*Note:* If the dough is too sticky, chill it in the refrigerator for an hour or overnight.)

4. To make the filling, place the diced bacon and onions in a skillet over medium heat. Cook until the bacon is crispy and the onions are soft, about 3 minutes. Add the thyme and chicken and sauté until the chicken is cooked through. Remove from the heat. Add the mayo and stir well to combine. Set aside.

5. Place a greased piece of parchment paper on a rimless baking sheet. Place one-quarter of the dough on the greased parchment and pat it out with your hands to form a small circle, about 4 inches in diameter. Repeat with the remaining dough, making a total of 4 circles. Divide the cooked filling among the pies. Seal each pie closed by folding it in half and crimping the edges with your fingers.

6. Transfer the pies to the hot stone in the oven by sliding the parchment with the pies off of the baking sheet and onto the stone. Bake for 10 minutes or until the pies are golden brown. Garnish with oregano and serve with ranch dressing.

7. Store extras in an airtight container in the refrigerator for up to 3 days. Reheat on a baking sheet in a preheated 350°F oven or toaster oven for 5 minutes or until warmed through.

nutritional info (per hand pie)				
calories	fat	protein	carbs	fiber
513	43g	27g	7g	2g

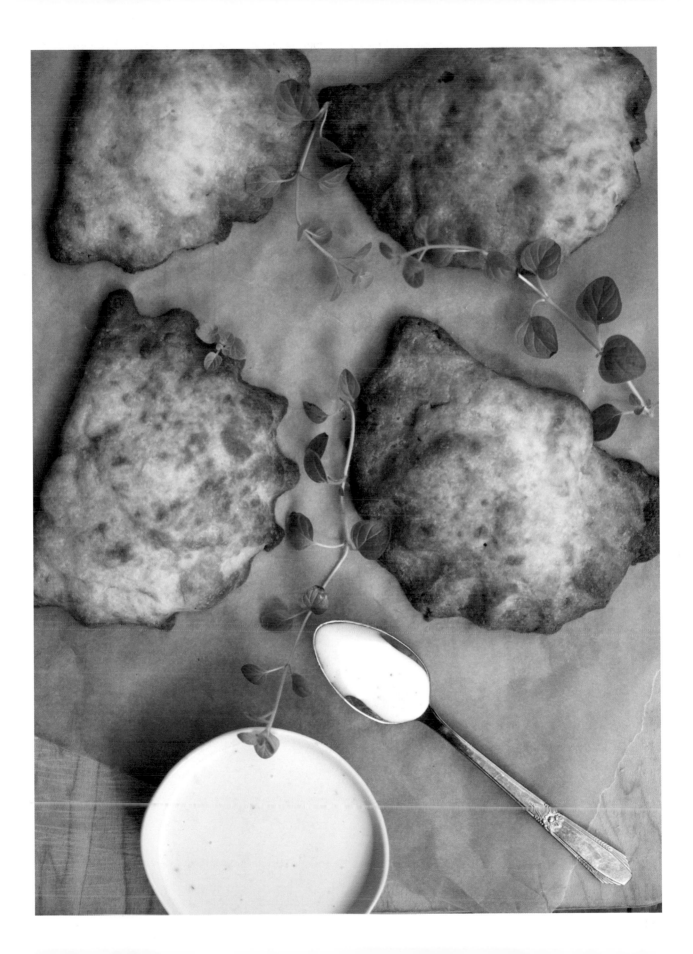

Fried Chicken
with Cheesy Grits

Nothing screams "comfort food" louder than fried chicken and grits! This keto remake will have you asking for more just to make sure the dish is keto—it tastes that good!

2 cups coconut oil or rendered keto fat, such as lard, for frying (see note)

1 large egg

½ cup powdered Parmesan cheese (see page 13) or pork dust

¼ teaspoon ground black pepper

4 chicken legs

Double batch Keto Grits (page 361), for serving

Chopped fresh herbs of choice, for garnish (optional)

Kale chips (recipe below), for serving (optional)

prep time: 8 minutes (not including time to make grits or kale chips)
cook time: 13 minutes *yield:* 4 servings

1. Heat the oil in a 4-inch-deep (or deeper) cast-iron skillet over medium heat to 375°F.

2. While the oil is heating, place the egg in a shallow bowl and beat it lightly with a fork. Combine the Parmesan cheese and pepper in a separate shallow bowl. Dip the chicken legs into the egg, then into the Parmesan mixture. Using your hands, press the cheese onto the chicken to form a nice crust.

3. Fry the chicken legs in the hot oil until the chicken is cooked through, about 10 minutes, rotating the legs as needed. Remove from the oil and set aside.

4. Divide the grits among 4 plates and top each plate with a chicken leg. Sprinkle with chopped herbs and serve with kale chips, if desired.

5. Store extras in an airtight container in the refrigerator for up to 3 days. Reheat the chicken on a rimmed baking sheet in a preheated 350°F oven for 5 minutes or until warmed through. Reheat the grits in a saucepan over low heat.

---

note: This may seem like a lot of oil, but I strain it after use and save it in a large mason jar in the refrigerator for future frying.

how to make kale chips:

To make kale chips, preheat the oven to 250°F. For this recipe, have on hand about 2 bunches of kale leaves. Wash the leaves, then dry them very well. Using a sharp knife, carve out the thick inner stems. Place the destemmed kale leaves on a rimmed baking sheet. Lightly mist with coconut oil spray and sprinkle with salt. Bake for 40 minutes to 1 hour, until the chips are crisp. Remove from the oven and set aside to cool. Kale chips can be stored in an airtight container for up to 1 week but are best eaten within 3 days. Makes 8 cups of chips (½ cup per serving).

nutritional info (per serving)				
calories	*fat*	*protein*	*carbs*	*fiber*
592	46g	45g	1g	0g

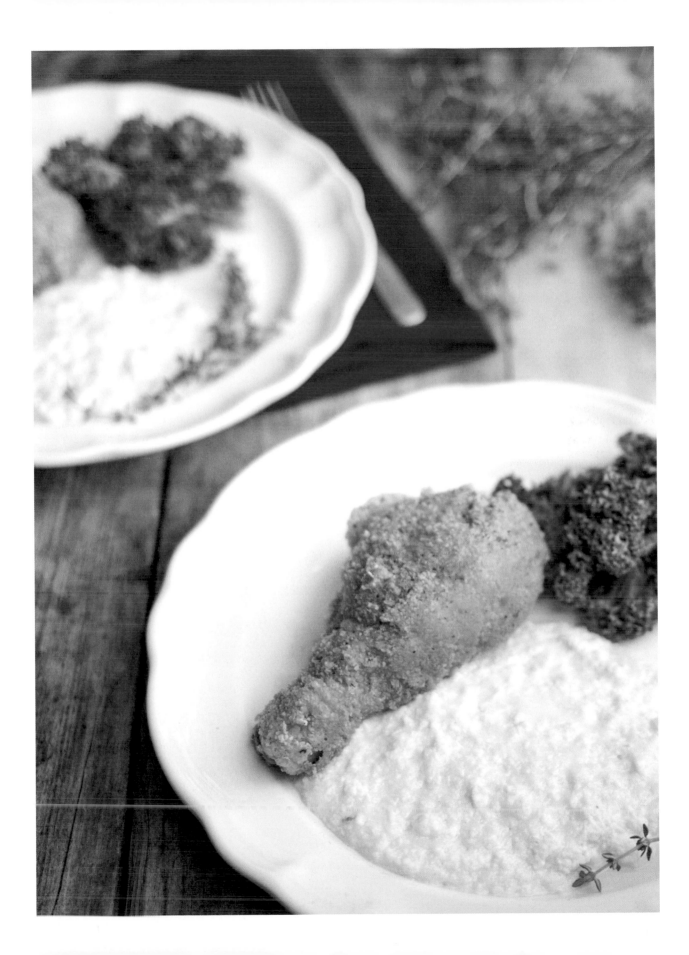

Chicken Divan

This diner classic is typically made with multiple types of "cream of" soups. I find it interesting that those canned soups don't even have cream in them! This dish is way better than what you'd get at a diner. The casserole mixture can be prepared ahead, covered, and stored in the refrigerator until ready to bake.

L M H
KETO

1 cup mayonnaise, homemade (page 359) or store-bought

1 cup chicken bone broth, homemade (page 356) or store-bought

1 cup shredded cheddar cheese

1 teaspoon chopped fresh chives

1 teaspoon fine sea salt, divided

1 (12-ounce) package broccoli florets

1 tablespoon ghee or coconut oil

4 (4-ounce) boneless, skinless chicken thighs, cut into 1-inch strips

prep time: 5 minutes *cook time:* 30 minutes *yield:* 4 servings

1. Preheat the oven to 350°F. Grease an 8-inch square casserole dish.

2. Place the mayo, broth, cheese, chives, and ½ teaspoon of the salt in a large mixing bowl and stir to combine well.

3. Bring about 1 inch of water to a boil in a pot. Add the broccoli, cover, and steam for 3 to 5 minutes, until crisp-tender. Drain and transfer to the mixing bowl with the mayo mixture.

4. Heat the ghee in a skillet over medium heat. Sprinkle the chicken strips with the remaining ½ teaspoon of salt and place in the skillet. Sauté the chicken until cooked through, about 4 minutes per side. Add the chicken to the mixing bowl with the mayo mixture. Stir until well combined.

5. Place the chicken mixture in the prepared casserole dish. Bake for 15 to 20 minutes, until the casserole is melted and gooey. Remove from the oven and enjoy! Store extras in an airtight container in the refrigerator for up to 3 days. Reheat in a baking dish in a preheated 350°F oven for 5 minutes or until warmed through.

nutritional info (per serving)				
calories	fat	protein	carbs	fiber
691	63g	29g	4g	1g

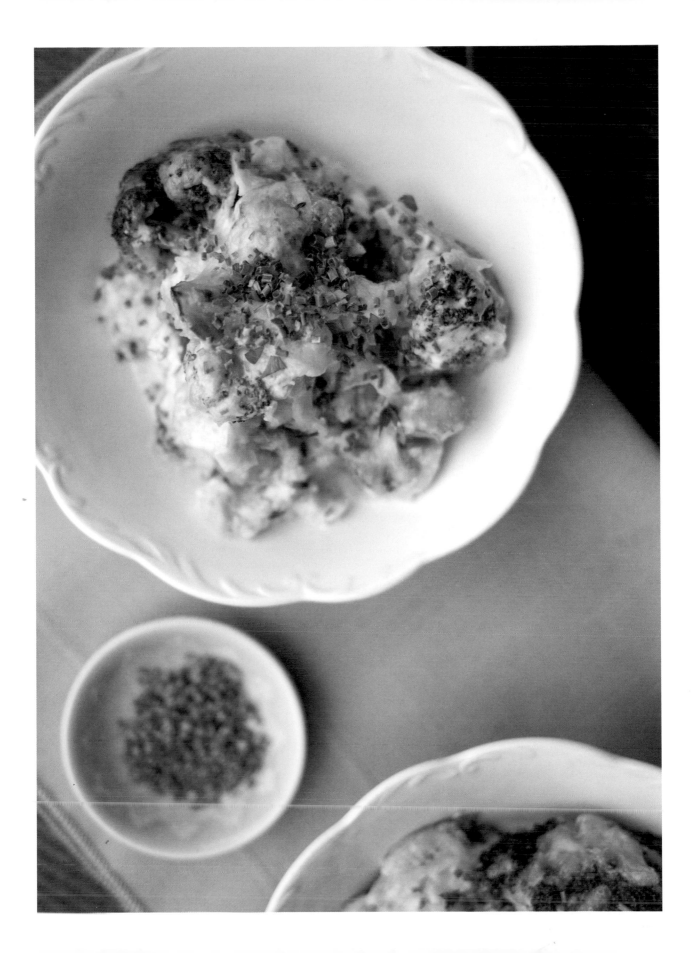

Smothered Fried Cabin Chicken

prep time: 10 minutes   *cook time*: about 10 minutes   *yield*: 4 servings

L →H M KETO OPTION

4 boneless, skinless chicken thighs

Fine sea salt and ground black pepper

2 large eggs

½ cup pork dust or powdered pork rinds

½ cup powdered Parmesan cheese (see page 13) (or more pork dust if dairy-free)

2 strips bacon, diced

1 cup shredded sharp cheddar cheese (omit for dairy-free)

¼ cup diced tomatoes

2 cups leafy salad greens mix, such as mesclun

1 lemon, quartered

¼ cup ranch dressing, homemade (page 359) or store-bought

Sliced green onions, for garnish

1. Preheat the oven to 400°F.

2. Place the chicken thighs between 2 pieces of parchment paper and, using a rolling pin or meat tenderizer, pound gently until the chicken is about ¼ inch thick. Season well on both sides with salt and pepper.

3. Beat the eggs in a shallow bowl. Beat in 1 tablespoon of water and season with a pinch of salt and pepper. In another shallow bowl, combine the pork dust and Parmesan cheese.

4. Dredge each chicken thigh in the beaten eggs and let the excess drip off, then press both sides of the chicken into the pork dust mixture.

5. In a large cast-iron skillet over medium-high heat, fry the diced bacon for about 4 minutes, stirring, until crisp. Remove from the skillet and set aside. Leave the bacon drippings in the skillet.

6. If needed, add a tablespoon or two of avocado oil or coconut oil to the bacon drippings in the skillet for frying. Once hot, sear the breaded chicken thighs until golden brown on one side, about 2 minutes. Flip and sear until golden brown on the other side, about another 2 minutes. Remove the skillet from the heat. Top the fried chicken with the shredded cheese, fried bacon, and diced tomatoes. Place in the oven for 3 minutes or until the cheese is melted.

7. Meanwhile, make the salad by cleaning and roughly chopping the salad greens.

8. Divide the smothered chicken and salad among 4 plates. Squirt a lemon quarter over each portion of chicken and salad. Then drizzle with ranch dressing and garnish with sliced green onions.

9. Store extra chicken and salad in separate airtight containers in the refrigerator for up to 3 days. Reheat the chicken on a rimmed baking sheet in a preheated 350°F oven for 5 minutes or until warmed through.

nutritional info (per serving)				
calories	fat	protein	carbs	fiber
517	36g	45g	4g	1g

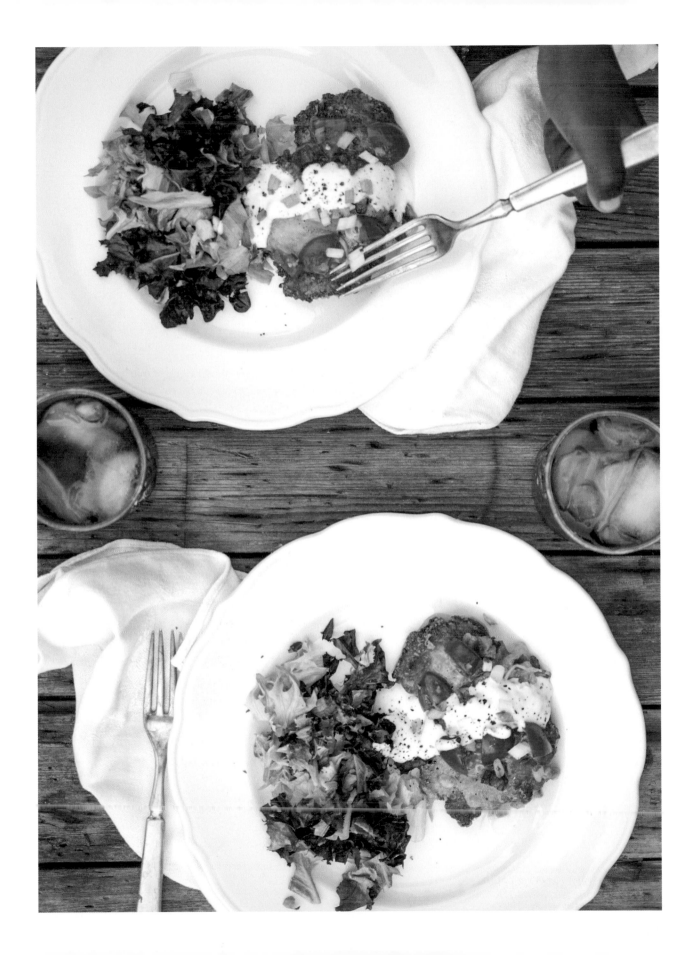

Shredded Amish Chicken and Gravy

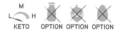

KETO   OPTION OPTION OPTION

6 boneless, skinless chicken thighs

1 cup chicken bone broth, homemade (page 356) or store-bought

1 (8-ounce) package cream cheese (Kite Hill brand cream cheese style spread if dairy-free), softened

1 tablespoon poultry seasoning

1 teaspoon ground black pepper

Fresh herbs of choice, such as thyme, for garnish (optional)

Melted ghee or unsalted butter, for drizzling (optional; omit for dairy-free)

serving suggestions

1 batch Mashed Fauxtatoes (page 129)

6 Garlicky Cheddar Biscuits, split in half (page 42)

1 batch Cauliflower Rice (page 362)

I grew up in a small town in north-central Wisconsin, where Amish chicken and gravy is a traditional meal served at everything from graduation parties to weddings. You often find this dish made with turkey instead of chicken.

prep time: 5 minutes (not including time to make fauxtatoes, biscuits, or rice)
cook time: 6 hours   *yield:* 6 servings

1. Place the chicken thighs in a 4-quart slow cooker. Combine the broth, cream cheese, poultry seasoning, and pepper in a blender and puree until smooth. Add the blended mixture to the slow cooker. Cover and cook on low for 6 hours or until the chicken falls apart easily. Shred the meat with 2 forks and stir it into the gravy. Taste and add salt, if desired.

2. Serve the chicken over mashed fauxtatoes, biscuits, or cauliflower rice with lots of gravy from the slow cooker. Garnish with fresh herbs and a drizzle of melted ghee, if desired.

3. Store extras in an airtight container in the refrigerator for up to 3 days. Reheat in a baking dish in a preheated 350°F oven for 5 minutes or until warmed through.

note: If dairy-free, serve the chicken over cauliflower rice or make the dairy-free version of the biscuits. If nut-free or egg-free, serve it over fauxtatoes or cauliflower rice.

nutritional info (per serving, with fauxtatoes)				
calories	fat	protein	carbs	fiber
453	31g	32g	10g	3g

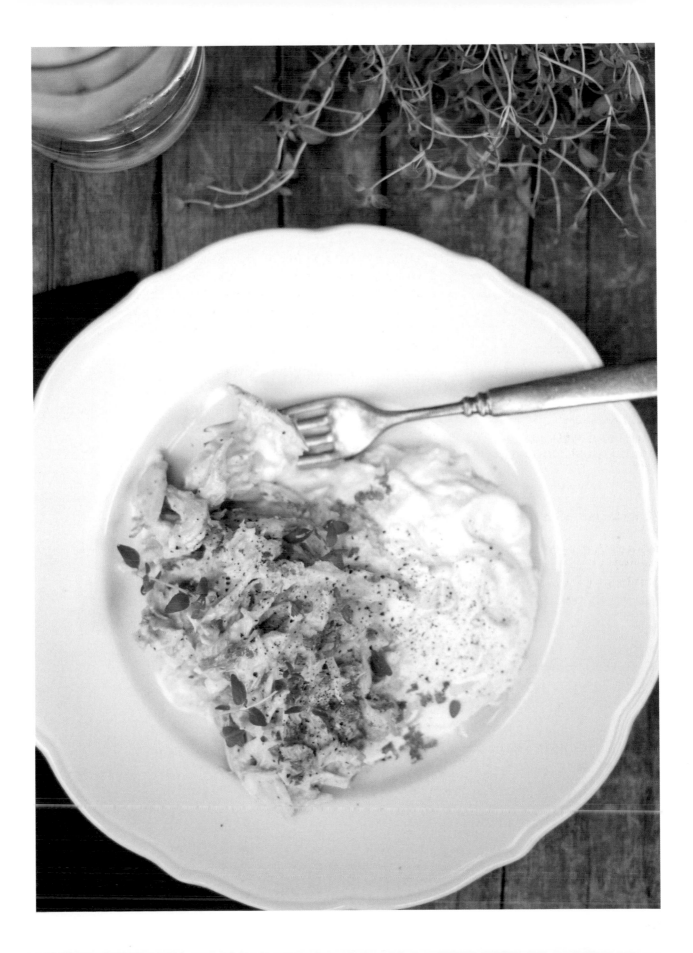

BBQ Chicken Lasagna

I made this recipe about five years ago for my brothers and sisters. Since I'm always trying new recipes, I had totally forgotten about this one until my sister-in-law reminded me of how much they loved the BBQ chicken lasagna I made for them. For her to remember this dish from years ago, it must have been good! And trust me, it is.

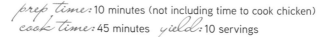

prep time: 10 minutes (not including time to cook chicken)
cook time: 45 minutes *yield:* 10 servings

1. Preheat the oven to 375°F. Grease a 13 by 9-inch baking dish.

2. Prepare the sauce: Place the tomato sauce in a large bowl. Add the liquid smoke and sweetener and mix to combine. Set aside.

3. Assemble the lasagna: Pour 1 cup of the sauce into the greased baking dish. Layer with half of the deli chicken "noodles," then half of the cheese, half of the shredded chicken, and half of any other fillings you like. (I love mushrooms sautéed in butter and seasoned with a touch of salt.) Layer with the remaining sauce, then noodles, then chicken (with any additional toppings). Top with the remaining cheese.

4. Bake the lasagna for 45 minutes or until the sauce is bubbly and the cheese is golden brown. Let it rest for 10 minutes before serving.

5. Store extras in an airtight container in the refrigerator for up to 3 days. Reheat in a baking dish in a preheated 350°F oven for 5 minutes or until warmed through.

sauce

4 cups tomato sauce

2 teaspoons liquid smoke

¼ cup Swerve confectioners'-style sweetener or equivalent amount of liquid or powdered sweetener (see page 24)

noodles

16 thin slices deli roasted chicken breast

filling

2 cups shredded cheddar cheese

3 cups shredded cooked chicken thighs (from about 2 pounds bone-in thighs; see below)

optional fillings

1 pound button mushrooms, sliced and sautéed in butter

1 green bell pepper, chopped and sautéed in butter

½ cup diced onions, sautéed in butter

how to make slow cooker shredded chicken thighs

2 pounds bone-in, skin-on chicken thighs

2 cups chicken bone broth, homemade (page 356) or store-bought

¼ cup diced onions

2 teaspoons minced garlic

1 teaspoon fine sea salt

½ teaspoon ground black pepper

Place all the ingredients in a 6-quart (or larger) slow cooker. Cover and cook on low until the chicken is fork-tender, about 6 hours. Remove the chicken from the slow cooker, then remove the skin (reserve the skin for making chicken cracklings, page 116). Pull the meat from the bones, discard the bones, and shred the meat using 2 forks. Store the chicken in an airtight container in the refrigerator for up to 5 days, or freeze for up to 1 month. (*Note:* If you're not using the chicken right away, store it with some of the juices from the slow cooker. It will help keep the meat moist until you use it.) *Makes 3 cups shredded chicken.*

nutritional info (per serving)				
calories	fat	protein	carbs	fiber
345	21g	31g	8g	2g

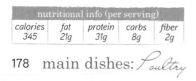

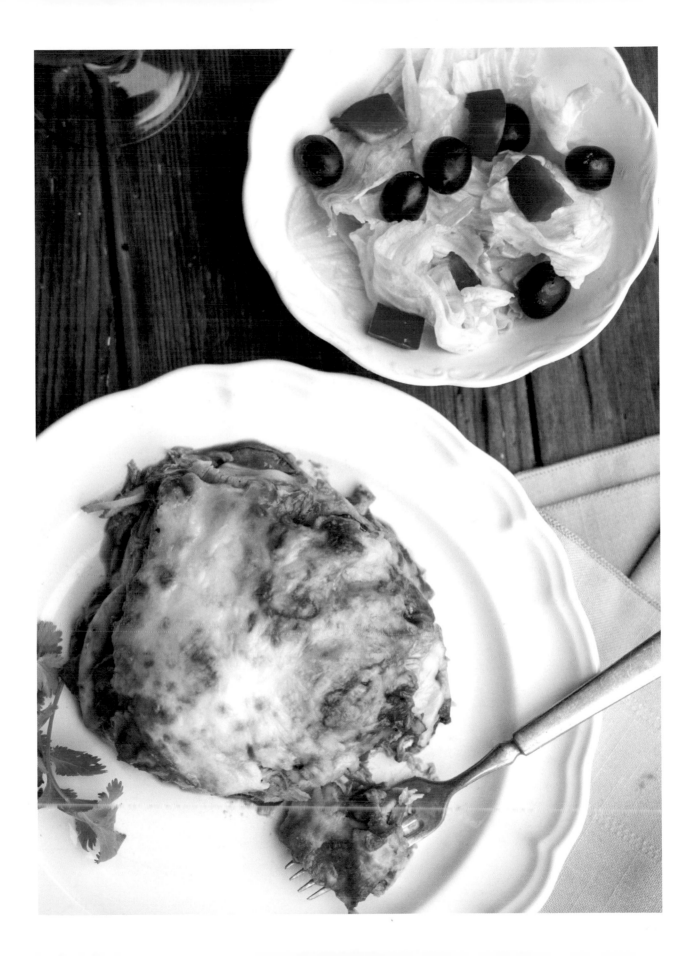

Turkey Goulash Over Mashed Fauxtatoes

I turn to this delicious recipe whenever I have leftover meat after roasting a whole turkey (see page 156) or turkey parts (see page 166).

prep time: 10 minutes (not including time to make fauxtatoes)
cook time: 1 hour *yield:* 8 servings

2 tablespoons ghee or coconut oil

1 green bell pepper, diced

½ cup diced onions

2 cloves garlic, smashed to a paste

8 ounces Mexican-style fresh (raw) chorizo, removed from casings

4 cups (¾-inch-cubed) leftover cooked turkey

3 tablespoons chili powder

1 tablespoon ground cumin

1 tablespoon dried oregano leaves

1 tablespoon paprika

½ teaspoon ground black pepper

1 teaspoon fine sea salt

1 (24-ounce) jar fire-roasted diced tomatoes

2 cups turkey or chicken bone broth, homemade (page 356) or store-bought

1 lime, halved

1 batch Mashed Fauxtatoes (page 129), for serving

Sour cream, for garnish

Chopped fresh chives, for garnish

1. Heat the ghee in a Dutch oven or soup pot over medium-high heat. Add the bell pepper and onions and cook, stirring often, until the onions are translucent, about 5 minutes. Add the garlic and cook for 1 more minute.

2. Add the chorizo and sauté, using a wooden spoon to crumble the sausage, until cooked through. Add the turkey, spices, and salt. Pour in the tomatoes and broth, bring to a simmer over medium heat, and cook, uncovered, until the liquid has reduced by a few inches and the stew has thickened, about 1 hour. Squeeze the lime juice into the pot and stir.

3. Taste and adjust the seasoning, if desired. Serve in bowls over fauxtatoes, garnished with a dollop of sour cream and a sprinkle of chopped chives.

4. Store extras in an airtight container in the refrigerator for up to 3 days. Reheat in a saucepan over medium heat for 5 minutes or until warmed through.

nutritional info (per serving)				
calories	*fat*	*protein*	*carbs*	*fiber*
342	18g	32g	12g	4g

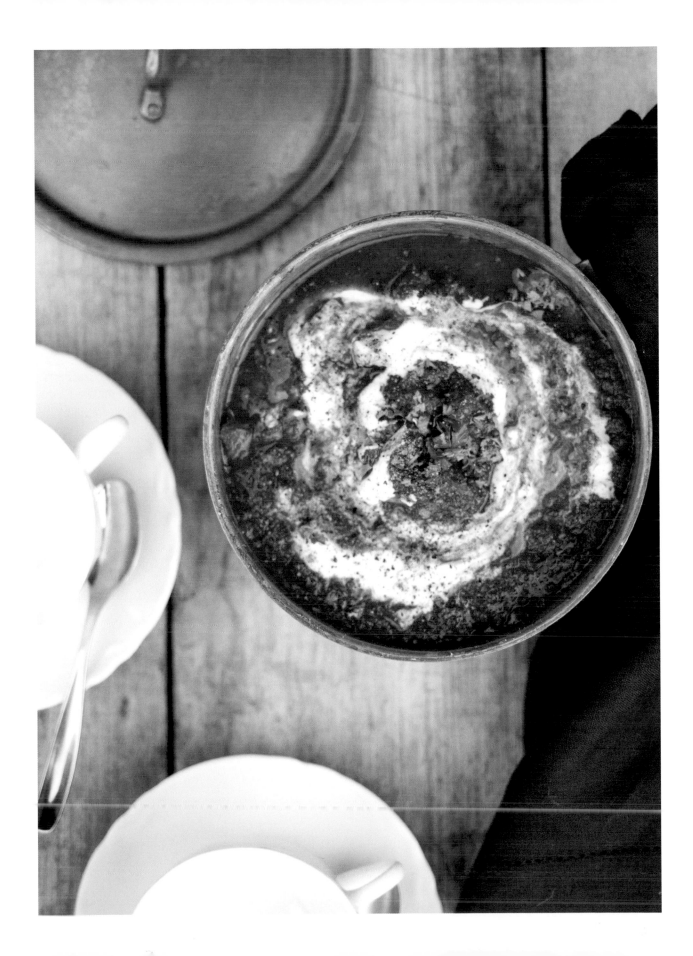

Red Curry Chicken Over Cauliflower Rice

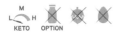

prep time: 5 minutes (not including time to make rice)

cook time: about 45 minutes *yield:* 4 servings

1 tablespoon ghee or unsalted butter (or avocado oil if dairy-free)

3 shallots, finely diced

1½ cups chicken bone broth, homemade (page 356) or store-bought

1 (14-ounce) can full-fat coconut milk

1½ tablespoons Thai red curry paste

2 boneless, skinless chicken thighs, cut into ½-inch chunks

¼ cup chopped fresh cilantro

1 to 2 green onions, sliced into ½-inch pieces (about ¼ cup)

¼ teaspoon fine sea salt

Juice of 1 lime

2 cups Cauliflower Rice (page 362), for serving

½ tablespoon melted ghee (or extra-virgin olive oil if dairy-free), for drizzling (optional)

½ teaspoon ground black pepper, for garnish (optional)

Lime or lemon wedges, for garnish (optional)

1. Place the ghee in a cast-iron skillet over medium heat. When hot, add the shallots and sauté until tender, about 2 minutes. Reduce the heat to low.

2. Whisk in the broth, coconut milk, and curry paste. Stir in the chunks of chicken. Simmer, uncovered, for 40 minutes or until the sauce has reduced a bit. The longer you simmer the sauce, the thicker it will be.

3. Add the cilantro, green onions, and salt. Cover and cook for about 5 minutes. Stir in the lime juice and immediately remove the pan from the heat.

4. Divide the cauliflower rice among 4 serving bowls and spoon the curry over the top. Serve drizzled with melted ghee and sprinkled with freshly ground pepper, with lime or lemon wedges on the side, if desired.

5. Store extras in an airtight container in the refrigerator for up to 3 days. Reheat in a saucepan over medium heat for a few minutes, until warmed through.

nutritional info (per serving)				
calories	*fat*	*protein*	*carbs*	*fiber*
355	27g	16g	10g	3g

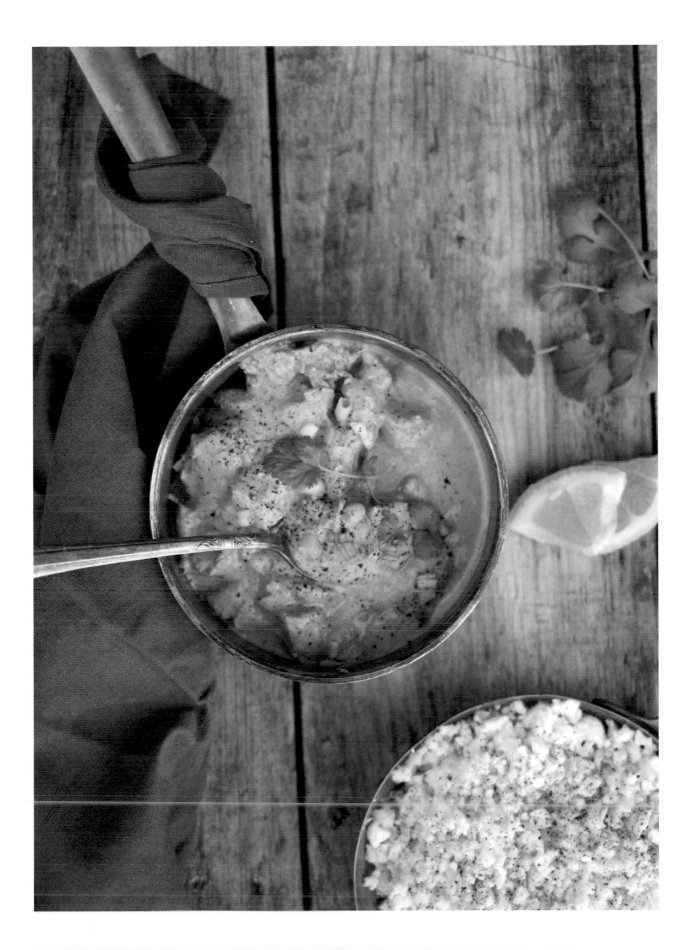

Herb Roasted Chicken

L M H
KETO ✗ ✗ ✗

1 (3- to 4-pound) chicken

Fine sea salt and ground black pepper

3 tablespoons lard or coconut oil (or unsalted butter if not dairy-sensitive), softened

1 tablespoon chopped fresh thyme

2 teaspoons chopped fresh rosemary

1 lemon, sliced

1 onion, quartered

3 cloves garlic, whacked with the side of a knife

This chicken works great in Turkey Tetrazzini (page 158) or Buffalo Chicken Casserole (page 190). If you prefer extra-crispy and tasty skin, after seasoning the chicken well with salt and pepper, place it in the refrigerator overnight, uncovered, to allow the skin to dry. I also suggest trussing the legs with kitchen twine.

prep time: 5 minutes   *cook time:* 1 hour 15 minutes   *yield:* 12 servings

1. Preheat the oven to 425°F.

2. Season the inside and outside of the chicken with a generous amount of salt and pepper. Place the lard in a medium-sized bowl and add the herbs. Mix until combined. Slather the herby lard under the layer of skin so it can penetrate the chicken. Stuff the lemon slices, onion quarters, and garlic into the cavity.

3. Place the chicken in a large roasting pan and roast for 1 hour 15 minutes or until a meat thermometer inserted into the thickest part of the chicken reads 170°F.

4. Allow the chicken to rest for 10 minutes before slicing and serving. Discard the lemon, onion, and garlic.

5. Store extras in an airtight container in the refrigerator for up to 3 days. Reheat on a baking sheet in a preheated 350°F oven for 5 minutes or until warmed through.

nutritional info (per serving)				
calories	fat	protein	carbs	fiber
320	23g	25g	2g	0.4g

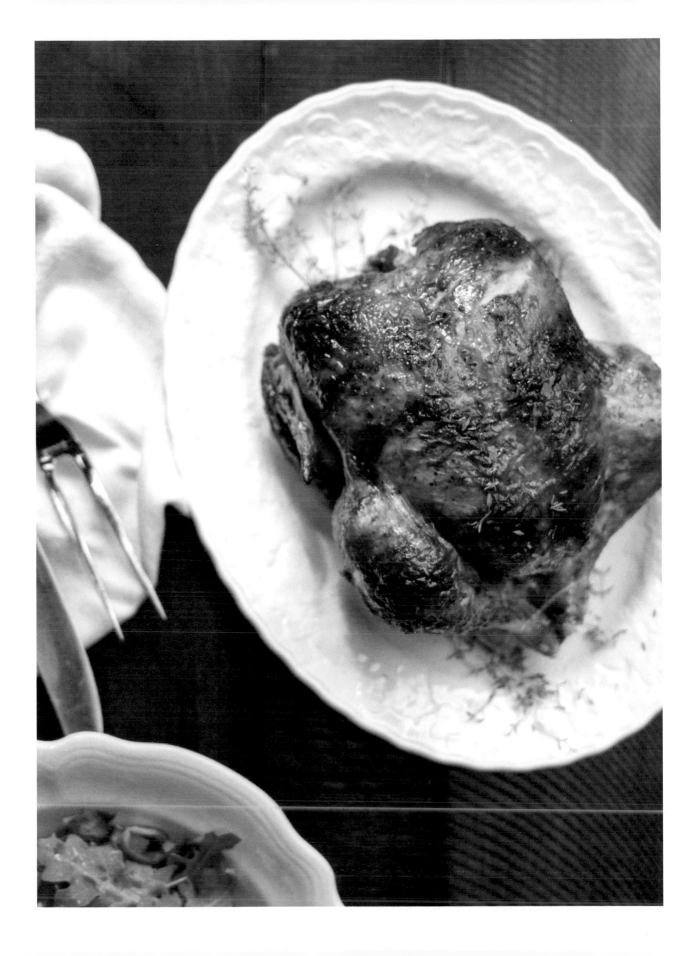

Chicken Cordon Bleu

L→H M KETO ✕ ✕

I love this recipe. I'm not a huge poultry fan, but even I will say that this dish is divine.

prep time: 10 minutes   *cook time:* 15 minutes   *yield:* 8 servings

browned butter cheese sauce

½ cup (1 stick) unsalted butter

½ cup beef or chicken bone broth, homemade (page 356) or store-bought

1 ounce cream cheese (2 tablespoons)

10 ounces Swiss cheese, shredded

Fine sea salt

8 boneless, skinless chicken thighs

½ teaspoon ground black pepper

8 slices Swiss cheese

8 slices cooked deli ham

1 cup powdered Parmesan cheese (see page 13)

2 teaspoons Italian seasoning

1 tablespoon ghee or coconut oil, for the skillet

Chopped fresh parsley, for garnish

1. To make the sauce, heat the butter in a large saucepan over high heat for about 5 minutes, whisking. The butter will start to sizzle and foam up. Watch for brown (but not black!) flecks; when you start to see them, remove the pan from the heat and whisk vigorously.

2. While whisking, slowly add the broth, cream cheese, and shredded cheese. Heat lightly, just until the cheese is melted. Add salt to taste. Remove from the heat, place in a blender, and blend until very smooth. Allow the sauce to cool a bit before serving.

3. Preheat the oven to 350°F. Grease a 13 by 9-inch baking dish.

4. Place the chicken thighs between 2 pieces of parchment paper and pound them to ¼-inch thickness.

5. Sprinkle each piece of chicken on both sides with the pepper (salt isn't needed because the ham and Parmesan cheese are salty enough). Place 1 slice of Swiss cheese and 1 slice of ham on top of each thigh. Roll up each thigh and secure with a toothpick. Place in a bowl, sprinkle the Parmesan cheese and Italian seasoning over the top, and turn to coat all sides of the chicken well.

6. Heat the ghee in a large skillet over medium-high heat. Place the chicken rolls in the hot skillet and cook until browned on one side, about 4 minutes. Turn the chicken and cook for 2 more minutes, until golden brown.

7. Transfer the chicken rolls to the greased baking dish. Bake until the cheese is melted and the chicken is cooked through, about 5 minutes. Remove the toothpicks and allow to rest for 5 minutes. Slice crosswise and serve hot, with warm cheese sauce drizzled over each piece. Sprinkle with chopped parsley, if desired.

8. Store extras in an airtight container in the refrigerator for up to 3 days. Reheat the chicken rolls on a rimmed baking sheet in a preheated 350°F oven for 5 minutes or until warmed through. Rewarm the sauce on the stovetop over medium-low heat.

tip: The cheese sauce can be made up to 3 days ahead and stored in the refrigerator, then rewarmed on the stovetop over medium-low heat.

note: If you prefer to skip the frying, you can skip Step 6, place the chicken rolls in the greased baking dish, and bake them for 20 minutes or until the chicken is no longer pink inside.

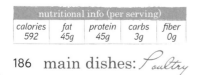

nutritional info (per serving)				
calories	fat	protein	carbs	fiber
592	45g	45g	3g	0g

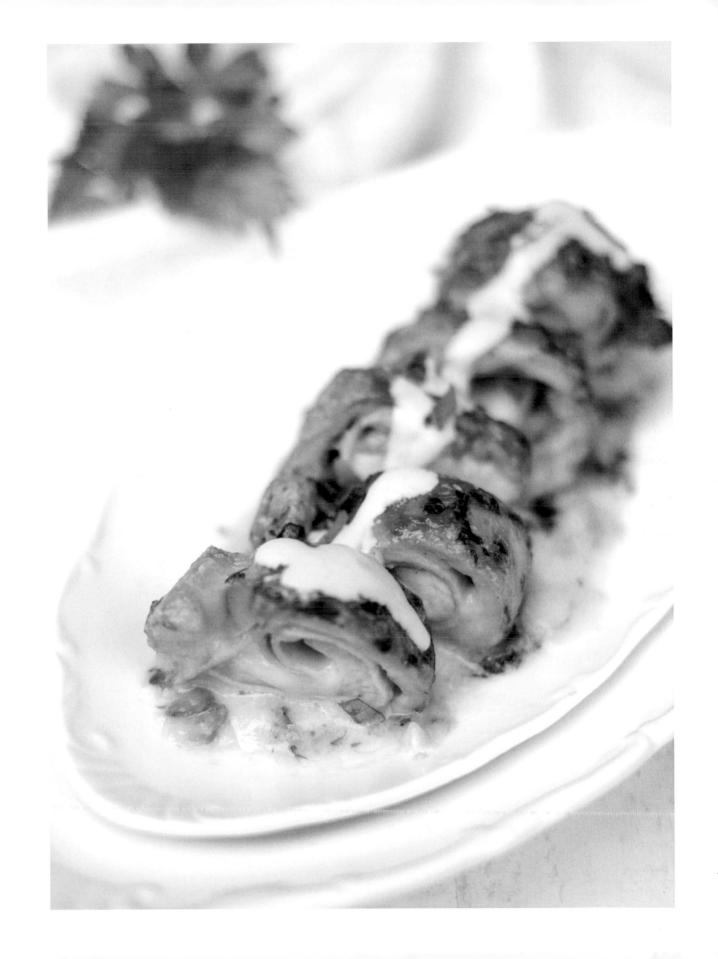

Slow Cooker Creamy Picante Chicken

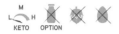

KETO   OPTION

3 cups salsa

1 (8-ounce) package cream cheese (Kite Hill brand cream cheese style spread if dairy-free)

2 teaspoons fine sea salt

6 boneless, skinless chicken thighs

Double batch Cauliflower Rice (page 362), for serving

This recipe is a family classic! If you are always stressed out about making dinner, this is an awesome, simple go-to dish. I suggest doing some prep work the night before. I make cauliflower rice and store it in an airtight container in the refrigerator for easy additions to meals such as this one. I also recommend putting all the ingredients in the slow cooker insert the night before. In the morning, all you have to do is remember to take it out of the fridge and turn on the slow cooker. Dinner will be ready when you get home!

prep time: 5 minutes   *cook time:* 6 to 8 hours   *yield:* 6 servings

1. Place the salsa and cream cheese in a 4-quart slow cooker. Add the salt and stir to combine. Top with the chicken thighs. Cover and cook on low for 6 to 8 hours, until the chicken can easily be shredded with 2 forks. Shred the meat and combine it with the creamy sauce in the slow cooker. Serve over cauliflower rice.

2. Store extras in an airtight container in the refrigerator for up to 3 days. Reheat in a saucepan over medium heat for 5 minutes or until warmed through.

nutritional info (per serving)				
calories	fat	protein	carbs	fiber
348	21g	27g	9g	2g

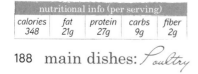

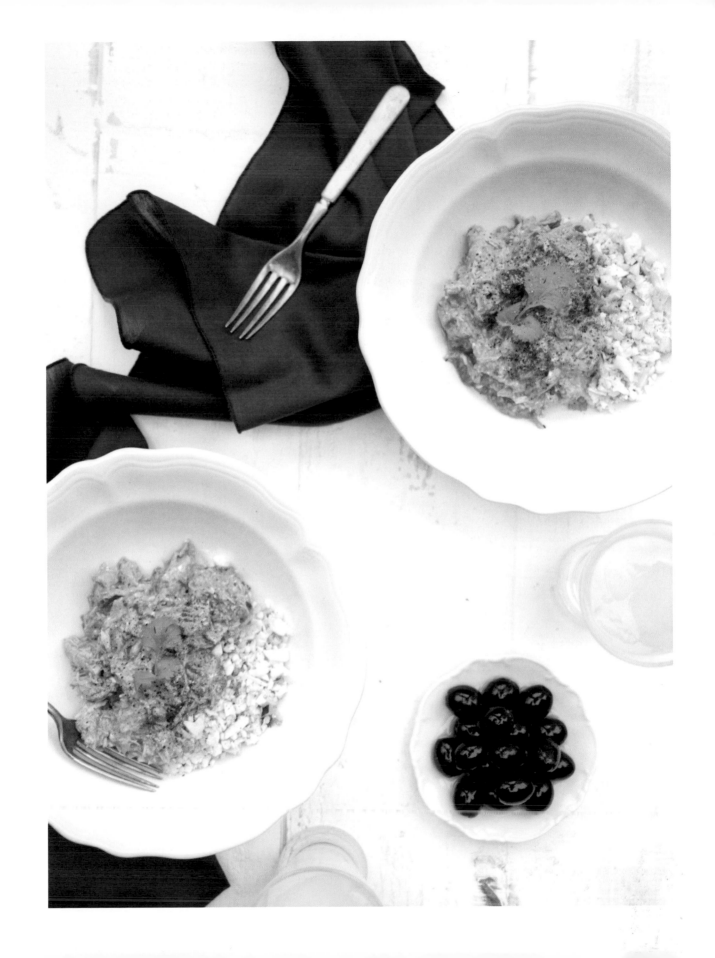

Buffalo Chicken Casserole

L M H   KETO   OPTION

prep time: 10 minutes   *cook time:* 30 minutes   *yield:* 4 servings

2 tablespoons unsalted butter or ghee (or coconut oil if dairy-free)

1 cup diced celery

½ cup diced onions

3 cloves garlic, smashed to a paste

4 boneless, skinless chicken thighs, cut into ¾-inch cubes

1 teaspoon fine sea salt

¼ teaspoon ground black pepper

4 cups cauliflower florets, cut into ½-inch pieces

1 tablespoon wing sauce or other medium-hot hot sauce, or more to taste

2 ounces cream cheese (¼ cup) (Kite Hill brand cream cheese style spread if dairy-free), softened

3 tablespoons chicken bone broth, homemade (page 356) or store-bought

½ cup crumbled blue cheese (omit for dairy-free)

Chopped fresh herbs, such as thyme, for garnish

Celery sticks, for serving

1. Preheat the oven to 350°F.

2. Melt the butter in a large cast-iron skillet or Dutch oven over medium-high heat. Add the celery and onions and sauté for 2 minutes, stirring often. Add the garlic and sauté for another minute.

3. Season the chicken on all sides with the salt and pepper. Add the chicken to the skillet and sauté for 7 minutes or until the chicken is cooked through. Add the cauliflower to the skillet.

4. Place the wing sauce, cream cheese, and broth in a blender and puree until smooth. Add the mixture to the skillet and stir well to combine. Top the skillet with the blue cheese crumbles. Transfer the skillet to the oven and bake, uncovered, for 20 minutes or until the cauliflower is soft. Remove from the oven and garnish with fresh herbs. Serve with celery sticks.

5. Store extras in an airtight container in the refrigerator for up to 3 days. Reheat in a baking dish in a preheated 350°F oven for 5 minutes or until warmed through.

nutritional info (per serving)				
calories	*fat*	*protein*	*carbs*	*fiber*
430	29g	32g	8g	2g

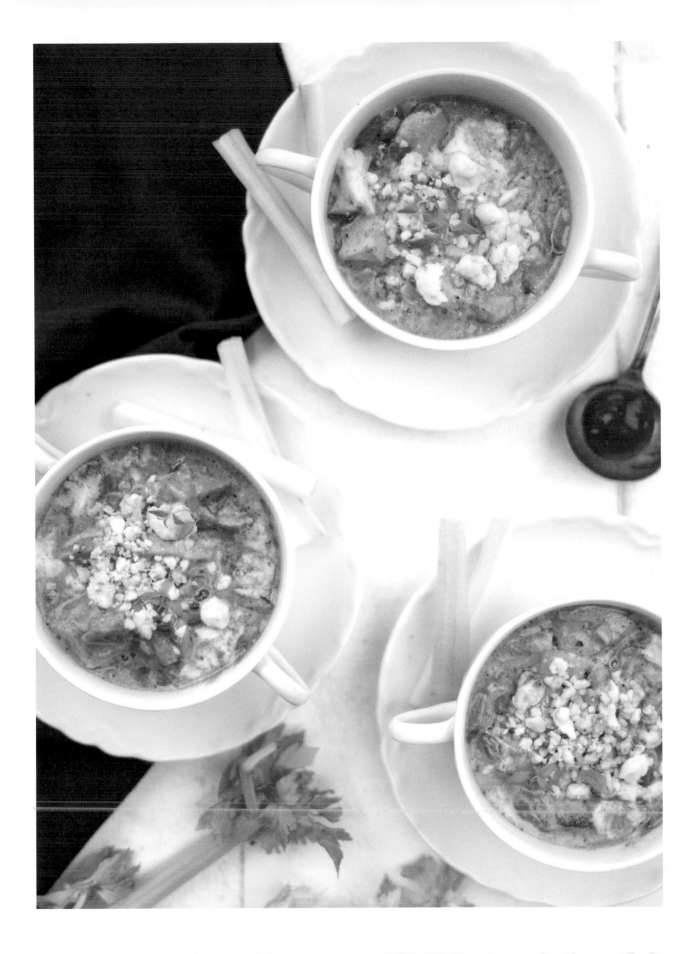

Duck à l'Orange

1 (5-pound) duck

1 tablespoon fine sea salt

1 teaspoon ground black pepper

Rind from 1 orange

4 sprigs fresh thyme

4 sprigs fresh marjoram

Unsalted butter, softened

1 onion, sliced thin

1 stalk celery, chopped

1 cup duck or chicken bone broth, homemade (page 356) or store-bought

sauce

2 cups duck or chicken bone broth, homemade (page 356) or store-bought

½ cup (1 stick) unsalted butter or duck fat

¼ cup Swerve confectioners'-style sweetener or equivalent amount of liquid or powdered sweetener (see page 24), or more to taste

2 tablespoons coconut vinegar or sherry wine vinegar

2 tablespoons minced shallots

Grated zest of 2 oranges, plus extra for garnish (optional)

Juice of 3 lemons

6 drops food-grade orange oil, or more to taste

Fresh thyme leaves, for garnish

Orange slices, for garnish

prep time: 7 minutes *cook time:* 2 hours 15 minutes *yield:* 8 servings

1. Preheat the oven to 475°F.

2. Pat the duck dry and season the inside and outside well with the salt and pepper. Place the orange rind, thyme, and marjoram inside the cavity. Rub the outside of the duck with butter.

3. Place the onion slices and chopped celery in a roasting pan. Set the duck on top. Add the broth and bake for 30 minutes.

4. Meanwhile, make the orange sauce: Combine all the ingredients in a small saucepan. Simmer over medium heat (not high or it will burn) until reduced by half, stirring often, 30 to 45 minutes. Taste and add more sweetener and/or orange oil, if desired. Strain the sauce and discard the orange zest.

5. After the duck has been in the oven for 30 minutes, reduce the oven temperature to 350°F. Pour the sauce into the roasting pan and cook the duck for 80 more minutes or until the internal temperature reaches 170°F.

6. Turn the oven to broil and broil the duck for 4 minutes or until the skin is crisp. Remove the duck from the roasting pan and drain the juices from the cavity. Place on a serving platter and allow the duck to rest for 10 minutes before carving. Serve topped with the orange sauce and garnished with thyme leaves, orange slices, and extra orange zest, if desired.

7. Store extras in an airtight container in the refrigerator for up to 3 days. Reheat on a rimmed baking sheet in a preheated 350°F oven for 5 minutes or until warmed through.

nutritional info (per serving)				
calories	*fat*	*protein*	*carbs*	*fiber*
478	41g	20g	7g	2g

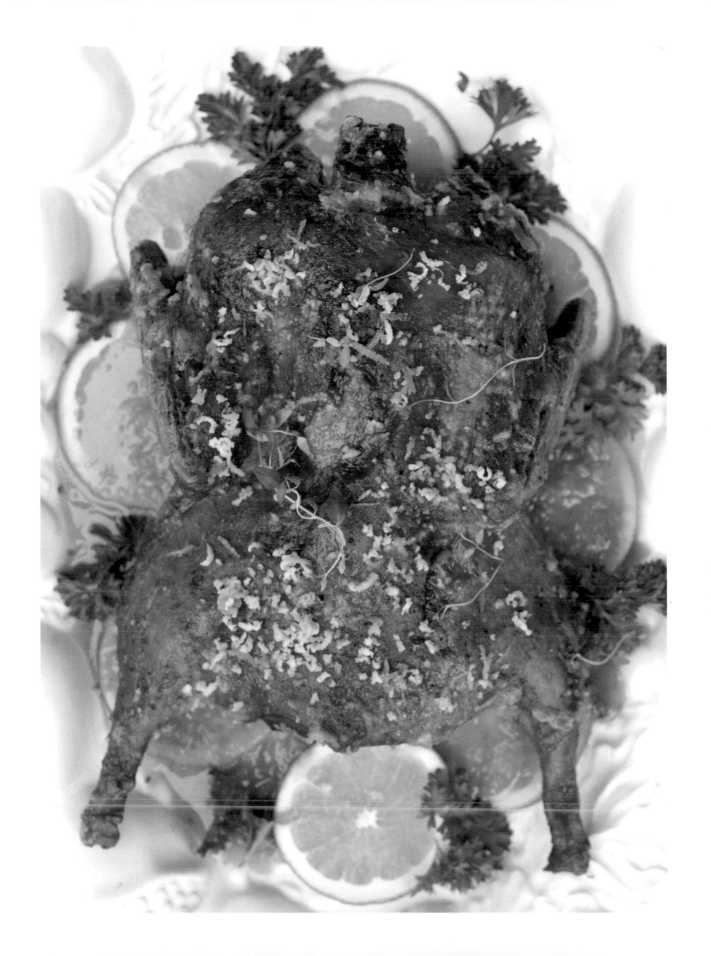

Braised Duck Legs
with Bacon and Mushrooms

This dish is amazingly flavorful on its own, but if you'd like to make it even more decadent, I suggest serving it over Mashed Fauxtatoes (page 129).

L M H
KETO ✖ ✖

2 tablespoons ghee or unsalted butter

4 duck leg quarters (legs and thighs)

Fine sea salt and ground black pepper

½ cup diced onions

1 leek, cleaned and diced

2 bay leaves

2 sprigs fresh rosemary

2 sprigs fresh thyme

4 cups duck or chicken bone broth, homemade (page 356) or store-bought

2 strips bacon, diced

8 ounces mushrooms, sliced

prep time: 10 minutes   *cook time:* 1½ hours   *yield:* 4 servings

1. Melt the ghee in a Dutch oven or large stockpot over medium heat. Season the duck legs generously with salt and pepper. Place the duck legs skin side down in the pot and brown for 3 minutes. Flip and brown on the other side for 3 minutes. Remove the duck legs and set aside.

2. Add the onions and leek to the pot and cook for 3 minutes. Meanwhile, tie the bay leaves, rosemary, and thyme together with kitchen twine. Add the bouquet of herbs and the broth to the pot. Return the duck legs to the pot, bring to a simmer, cover, and simmer for 75 minutes or until the duck is very tender. Remove the duck legs and set aside. Continue to cook the sauce until reduced and thickened to your liking, then return the duck to the sauce.

3. Meanwhile, make the bacon and mushrooms: Place the diced bacon in a skillet over medium-high heat and fry until it is starting to brown and get crispy and there is a bit of bacon fat in the pan. Add the mushrooms and brown with the crisped bacon.

4. Remove the bay leaves and herbs from the pot. Serve the duck with the sauce and onion mixture, topped with the bacon and mushrooms.

5. Store extras in an airtight container in the refrigerator for up to 3 days. Reheat the duck on a rimmed baking sheet in a preheated 350°F oven for 5 minutes or until warmed through. Warm the sauce in a small saucepan on the stovetop over medium-low heat.

nutritional info (per serving)				
calories	*fat*	*protein*	*carbs*	*fiber*
393	33g	19g	6g	1g

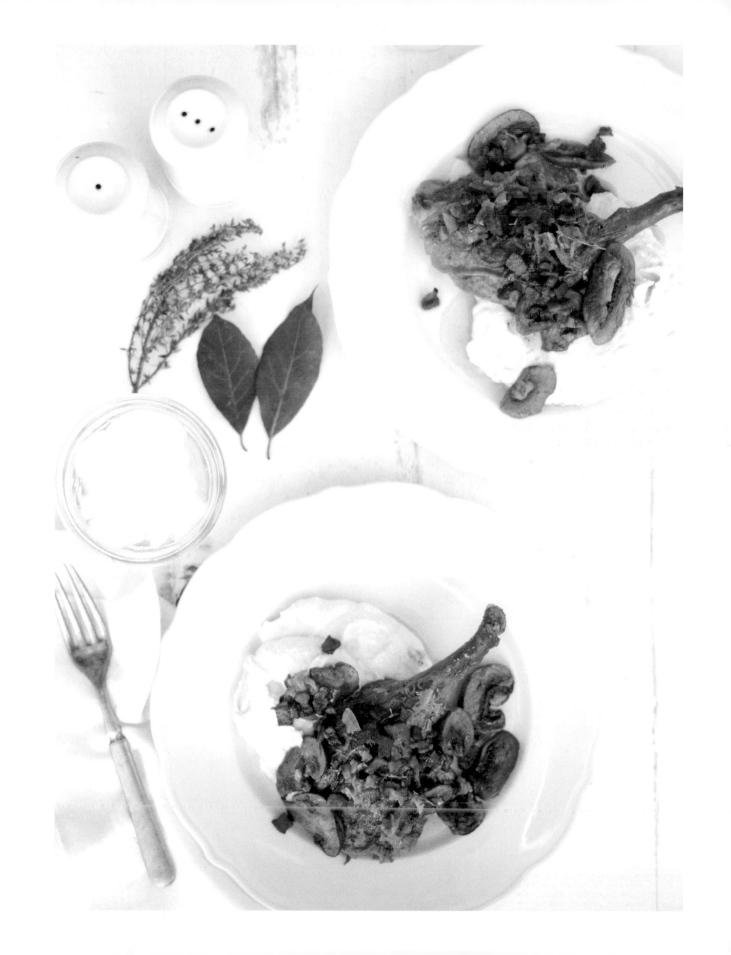

Chicken Pot Pies

L M H
KETO

dough

1¾ cups shredded mozzarella cheese

2 tablespoons unsalted butter

1 large egg, beaten

¾ cup blanched almond flour

⅛ teaspoon fine sea salt

filling

2 tablespoons unsalted butter

¼ cup diced celery

¼ cup diced onions

¼ teaspoon minced fresh oregano

¼ teaspoon minced fresh thyme

¼ teaspoon fine sea salt

3 boneless, skinless chicken thighs, cut into ¼-inch pieces

4 ounces cream cheese (½ cup), softened

½ cup chicken bone broth, homemade (page 356) or store-bought

for garnish

Fresh thyme sprigs

prep time: 10 minutes, plus 1 hour to chill dough, if needed

cook time: 15 minutes   *yield:* 4 servings

1. Preheat the oven to 425°F.

2. To make the dough, place the mozzarella and butter in a microwave-safe bowl and microwave for 1 to 2 minutes, until the cheese is entirely melted. Stir well. Add the egg and combine well using a hand mixer. Add the almond flour and salt and combine well with the mixer. Use your hands and work it like a traditional dough, kneading for about 3 minutes. (*Note:* If the dough is too sticky, chill it in the refrigerator for an hour or overnight.)

3. While the dough is chilling, make the filling: Melt the butter in a sauté pan over medium heat. Add the celery, onions, herbs, and salt and cook until the veggies are soft, about 4 minutes. Add the chicken and sauté until cooked through, about 4 more minutes. Add the cream cheese and stir until well combined. While stirring, slowly pour in the broth. Divide among four 14-ounce oven-safe bowls or ramekins.

4. Grease a piece of parchment paper. Place one-quarter of the dough on the greased parchment and pat it out with your hands to form a small circle, slightly larger than the diameter of the bowls or ramekins you're using. Repeat with the remaining dough. Place a circle of dough on top of each filled bowl or ramekin. Seal each pie closed by crimping the dough around the edge with your fingers.

5. Place the bowls on a rimmed baking sheet and place in the oven. Bake for 15 to 20 minutes, until the pies are golden brown and the dough is fully cooked. Serve the pies garnished with fresh thyme.

6. Store extras in an airtight container in the refrigerator for up to 3 days. Reheat on a rimmed baking sheet in a preheated 350°F oven for 5 minutes or until warmed through.

nutritional info (per pie)				
calories	fat	protein	carbs	fiber
631	50g	38g	9g	3g

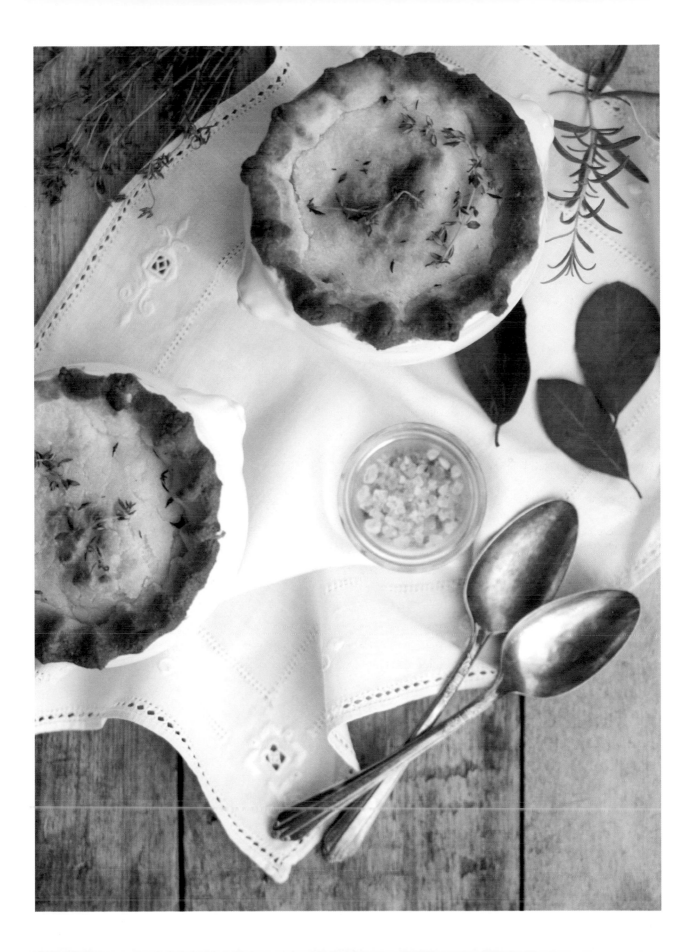

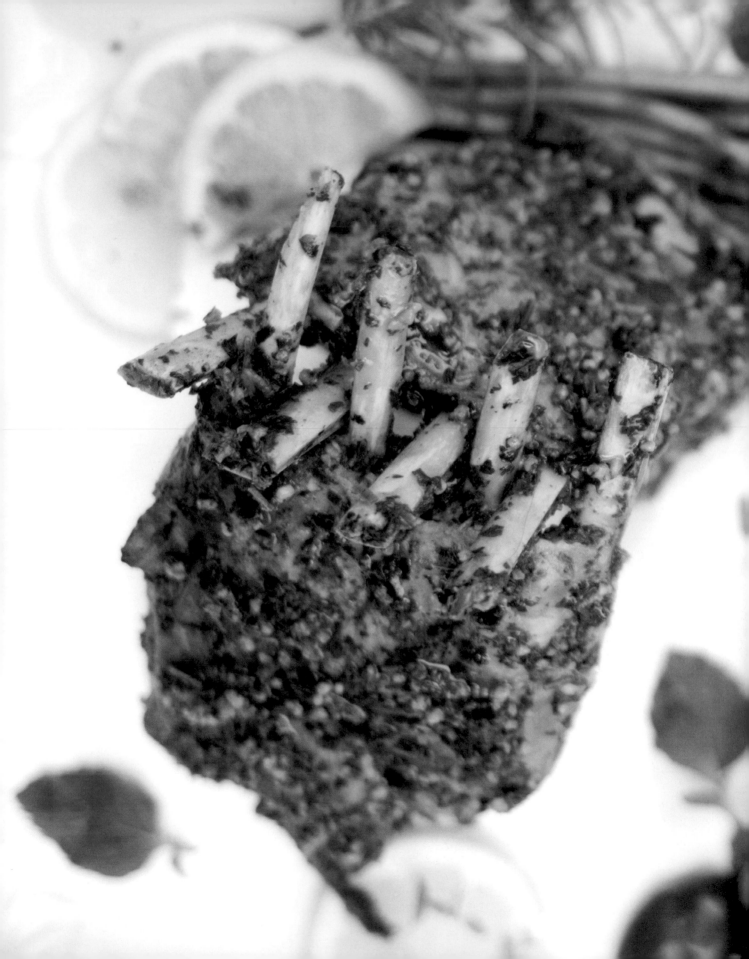

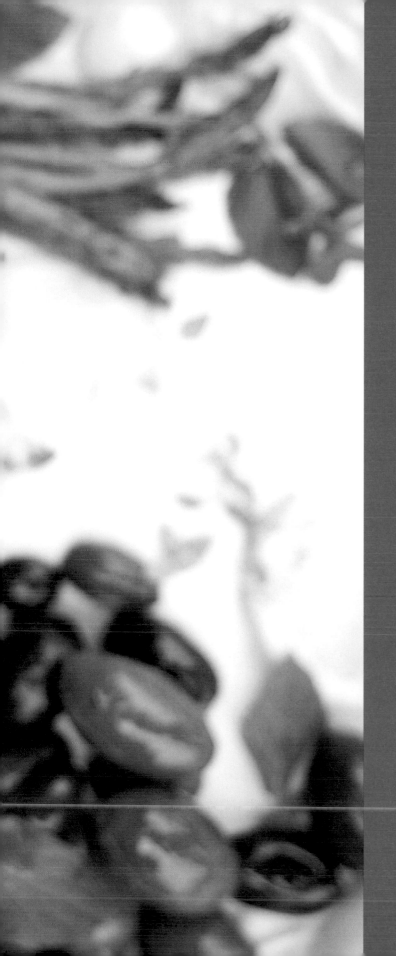

main dishes
Beef and Lamb

Sunday Supper Pot Roast
Over Mashed Fauxtatoes

L M H
KETO OPTION (icons)

prep time: 15 minutes (not including time to make fauxtatoes)
cook time: 6 hours   *yield:* 8 servings

1 (5-pound) bone-in beef chuck roast

Fine sea salt and ground black pepper

3 tablespoons ghee (or coconut oil if dairy-free), divided

2 stalks celery, cut into ½-inch pieces

2 sprigs fresh thyme

1 sprig fresh rosemary

8 ounces sliced mushrooms

1 cup chopped onions

2 cloves garlic, minced

2 tablespoons tomato paste

2½ cups beef bone broth, homemade (page 356) or store-bought

1 batch Mashed Fauxtatoes (page 129) (or Cauliflower Rice, page 362, if dairy-free), for serving

1. Season both sides of the roast liberally with salt and pepper.

2. Heat 2 tablespoons of the ghee in a large skillet over medium-high heat. When hot, sear the roast for 5 minutes on each side, or until browned.

3. Place the celery in a 4-quart slow cooker. Set the roast on top of the celery and pour in any juices from the skillet. Add the thyme and rosemary sprigs.

4. Reduce the heat under the skillet to medium, add the mushrooms and the remaining tablespoon of ghee, and sauté the mushrooms for 3 to 4 minutes. Add the onions and sauté for 5 minutes, until the onions are translucent and beginning to brown. Add the garlic and sauté for another minute. Add the tomato paste and cook for 1 more minute. Add the beef broth, stir to combine, and bring to a simmer; then remove from the heat.

5. Pour the onion and mushroom mixture over the top of the roast in the slow cooker. Cover the slow cooker, turn the heat to high, and cook the roast for 5 to 6 hours, until the meat is fork-tender.

6. Pull the meat off the bones and discard the bones. Taste and add more salt and pepper, if needed. Serve over mashed fauxtatoes.

7. Store extras in an airtight container in the refrigerator for up to 3 days. Reheat in a skillet over medium heat for 3 minutes or until warmed through.

nutritional info (per serving)				
calories	fat	protein	carbs	fiber
597	40g	51g	4g	1g

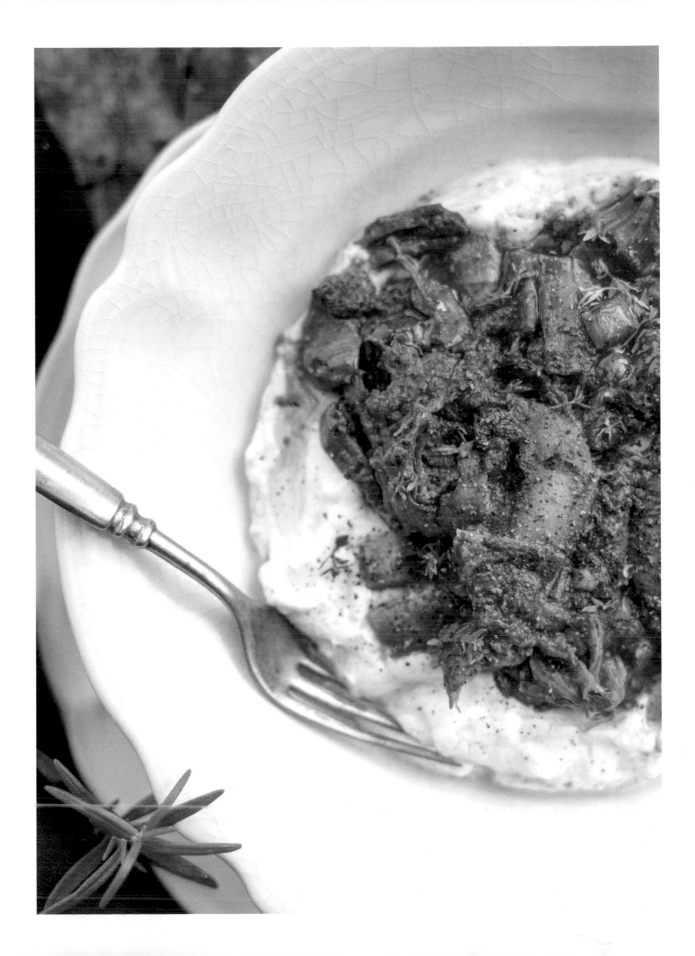

Skillet Moussaka

Moussaka is a Greek lasagna layered with eggplant. If you love feta and other Greek flavors, you must try it!

I assembled this dish one Sunday afternoon, covered it, and stored it in the freezer, unbaked. The other day, I knew I was going to be too busy to prepare a meal when I got home, so I took the moussaka out of the freezer in the morning and pop it in the fridge to thaw for an easy dinner that night.

prep time: 10 minutes   *cook time:* 50 minutes   *yield:* 8 servings

eggplant layer

1 small eggplant (about 12 ounces)

1 teaspoon fine sea salt

1 teaspoon ground black pepper

meat layer

1 tablespoon ghee or coconut oil

½ cup chopped onions

2 cloves garlic, smashed to a paste or minced

1 lemon, thinly sliced

1 cup fresh oregano leaves, chopped

1 cup fresh flat-leaf parsley leaves, chopped

1½ pounds ground lamb or beef

2 cups finely diced mushrooms

1 teaspoon fine sea salt

½ teaspoon ground black pepper

¼ teaspoon ground nutmeg

1 cinnamon stick

1 cup tomato sauce

cheese sauce

¼ cup ghee or unsalted butter

½ cup beef bone broth, homemade (page 356) or store-bought

2 large eggs, separated

8 ounces feta cheese, crumbled

Pinch of ground nutmeg

Fresh oregano leaves, for garnish

Melted ghee, avocado oil, or extra-virgin olive oil, for drizzling

1. Preheat the oven to 350°F.

2. To prepare the eggplant layer, cut the stem off the eggplant and remove the skin with a vegetable peeler. Slice the eggplant lengthwise into ⅛-inch-thick planks. Season both sides of the slices with the salt and pepper. Place the eggplant on a greased rimmed baking sheet and bake for 15 minutes or until soft. Remove the eggplant from the oven, but leave the oven on if you are baking the lasagna right away.

3. Meanwhile, make the meat layer: Heat 1 tablespoon of ghee in an 8-inch cast-iron skillet over medium heat. Add the onions, garlic, lemon slices, oregano, and parsley. Cook, stirring often, until the onions are soft, about 3 minutes. Add the ground lamb and mushrooms. Stir to crumble the meat. Add the salt, pepper, nutmeg, and cinnamon stick, then stir in the tomato sauce. Simmer, uncovered, for 10 minutes, then remove from the heat.

4. Remove half of the meat mixture from the skillet and place a layer of eggplant slices over the remaining meat mixture in the skillet. Top the eggplant layer with the rest of the meat mixture, then add another layer of eggplant. Set the skillet aside.

5. Make the cheese sauce: In a saucepan over low heat, combine the ¼ cup of ghee and the broth. When the ghee is melted, whisk in the egg yolks, feta cheese, and nutmeg and stir just until combined. Beat the egg whites until stiff, then fold them into the sauce. Pour the cheese sauce over the eggplant in the skillet.

6. Place the skillet in the oven and bake the moussaka for 30 to 40 minutes, until the top is golden. Let cool for 10 minutes before serving. Garnish with oregano leaves and a drizzle of melted ghee.

7. Store extras in an airtight container in the refrigerator for up to 4 days. Reheat in a baking dish in a preheated 350°F oven for 5 minutes or until warmed through.

nutritional info (per serving)				
calories 428	*fat* 33g	*protein* 23g	*carbs* 9g	*fiber* 3g

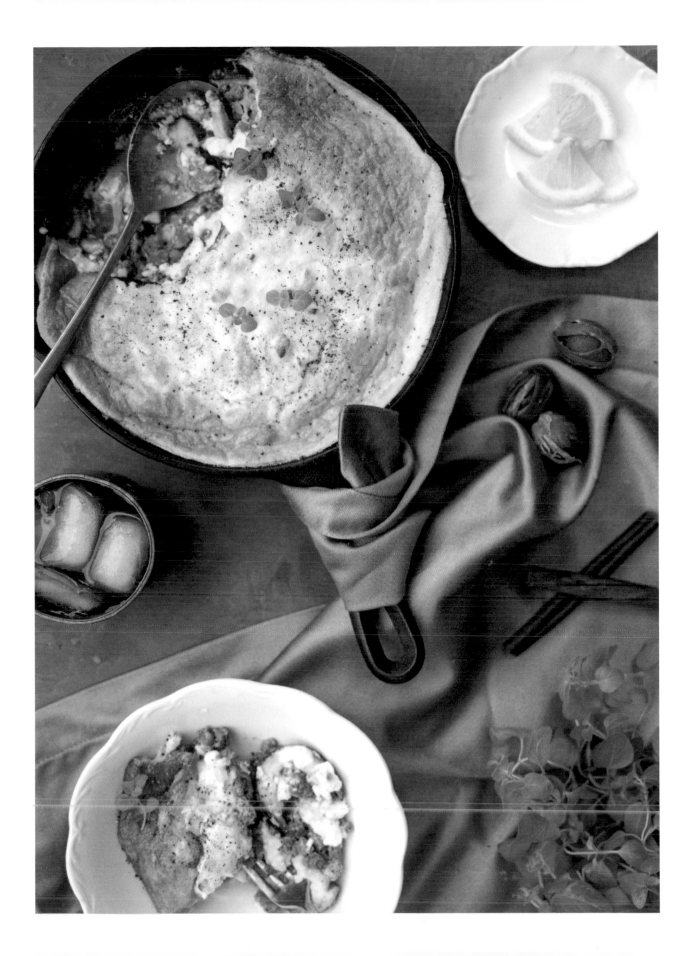

Philly Cheesesteak Cupcakes

prep time: 10 minutes   cook time: 16 minutes
yield: 6 jumbo or 12 regular-size cupcakes (1 jumbo or 2 regular-size per serving)

2 tablespoons coconut oil or unsalted butter

1½ cups diced green bell peppers

¾ cup chopped onions

1 clove garlic, smashed to a paste

1½ pounds ground beef or lamb

1 large egg, beaten

½ cup powdered Parmesan cheese (see page 13)

½ teaspoon fine sea salt

½ teaspoon ground black pepper

½ teaspoon dried basil

½ teaspoon chili powder

½ teaspoon dried ground marjoram

½ teaspoon paprika

½ teaspoon dried thyme leaves

1½ cups cubed provolone or fontina cheese

1. Preheat oven to 350°F. Line a jumbo 6-well muffin pan or a standard-size 12-well muffin pan with paper liners.

2. Heat the oil in a skillet over medium-high heat. Add the bell peppers and onions and sauté until soft, about 3 minutes. Add the garlic and sauté for another minute. Remove from the heat and transfer the vegetable mixture to a large bowl. Add the ground beef, beaten egg, and Parmesan cheese. Season with the salt and spices. Add the cubes of cheese and mix well to combine.

3. Form the mixture into six 2½-inch balls or twelve 1½-inch balls. Place a ball in each lined muffin cup. Bake until the cupcakes' internal temperature reaches 160°F, about 12 minutes for jumbo cupcakes or 9 minutes for regular-sized ones. Remove from the oven and serve warm.

4. Store extras in an airtight container in the refrigerator for up to 3 days. Reheat in a baking dish in a preheated 350°F oven for 5 minutes or until warmed through.

nutritional info (per serving)				
calories	fat	protein	carbs	fiber
504	39g	33g	5g	1g

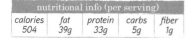

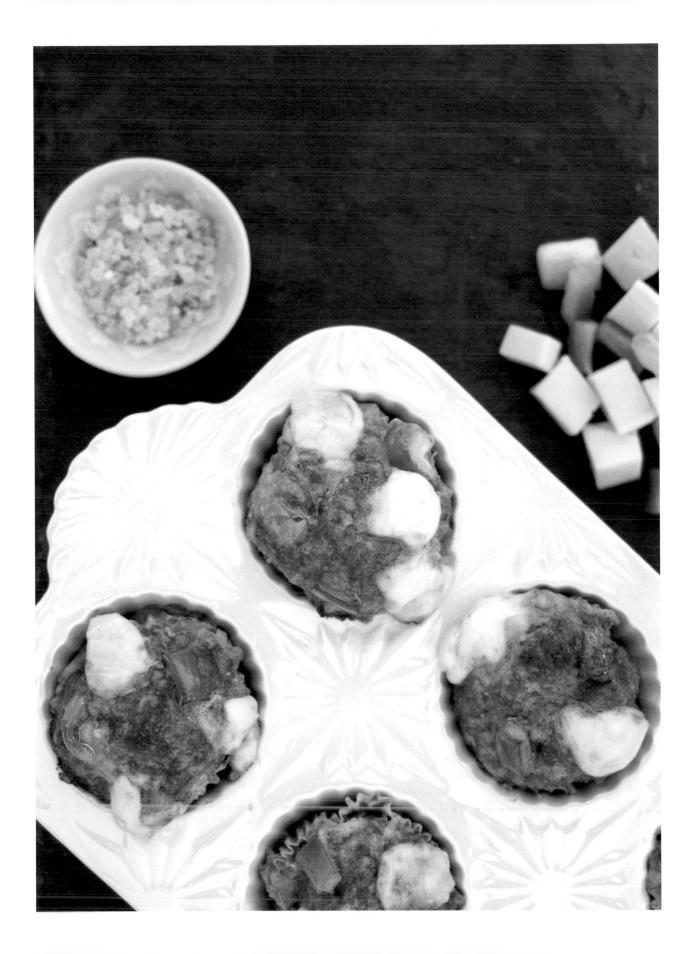

Gyro Loaf
with Tzatziki Sauce

When I was little, I dreaded meatloaf night. I probably would have liked it if I had given it a chance, but seriously, I think the name turned me off. I love meatloaf now. It's like a gigantic hamburger. Who wouldn't want that? I am officially renaming meatloaf "Gigantic Hamburger Loaf"!

Instead of using breadcrumbs or cracker crumbs, I use an egg for the binder, along with finely chopped mushrooms (you won't taste them, but mushrooms make the meatloaf very moist!) and grated Parmesan cheese. Mushrooms and aged cheeses have something called "umami," a pleasant savory taste produced by glutamate and ribonucleotides, which are chemicals that occur naturally in many foods. Umami is subtle, but it blends well with other tastes to intensify and enhance flavors, and it plays an important role in making food taste delicious.

prep time: 10 minutes, plus at least 1 hour to chill tzatziki sauce
cook time: 55 minutes   *yield:* 6 servings

tzatziki sauce

1 cup sour cream

1 medium cucumber, peeled, seeded, and finely chopped or shredded and squeezed dry

½ teaspoon garlic powder

½ teaspoon fine sea salt

1 tablespoon finely chopped fresh parsley

1 tablespoon finely chopped fresh dill, or ¼ teaspoon dried dill weed

gyro loaf

1½ pounds ground lamb or beef

¾ cup finely chopped mushrooms

½ cup diced red onions

¼ cup diced black olives

8 ounces feta cheese, cut into ¼-inch dice, plus extra for garnish

½ cup powdered Parmesan cheese (see page 13)

¼ cup tomato sauce

1 large egg

1 teaspoon Greek seasoning

1 teaspoon dried oregano leaves

1 clove garlic, smashed to a paste

Diced red onions, for garnish

Diced tomatoes, for garnish

1. To make the tzatziki sauce, place all the ingredients for the sauce in a small bowl. Stir well. Set the sauce in the refrigerator to chill for 1 to 2 hours. (*Note:* It can be made up to 3 days ahead.)

2. Preheat the oven to 350°F. Have on hand an 8 by 4-inch loaf pan.

3. Place the ingredients for the gyro loaf in a large bowl and, using your hands, mix together until well combined.

4. Press the meat mixture into the loaf pan. Bake for 55 minutes or until the internal temperature of the loaf reaches 160°F. Allow to rest for 10 minutes before slicing. Serve with the tzatziki sauce, garnished with red onions, tomatoes, and extra feta cheese.

5. Store extras in an airtight container in the refrigerator for up to 3 days. Reheat the gyro loaf in a baking dish in a preheated 350°F oven for 5 minutes or until warmed through.

nutritional info (per serving)				
calories	fat	protein	carbs	fiber
539	41g	33g	6g	1g

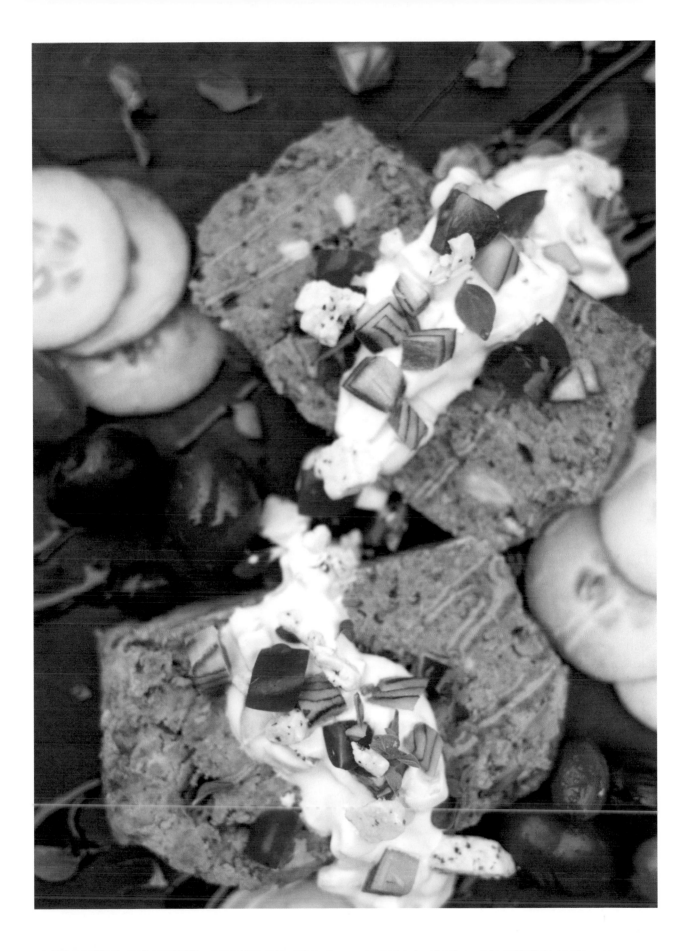

Joe's Special

I once heard Food Network star Tyler Florence describe in detail one of the best dishes he ever ate at a restaurant. He called it Joe's Special. It sounded not only delicious, but also very easy to make, so I decided to try it. He was right! It is delicious *and* easy!

KETO OPTION

prep time: 5 minutes   *cook time:* 25 minutes   *yield:* 2 servings

2 tablespoons MCT oil, avocado oil, or lard

¼ cup diced onions

½ pound ground beef

2 cups fresh spinach

½ teaspoon fine sea salt

¼ teaspoon ground black pepper

2 large eggs

Grated Parmesan cheese, for garnish (omit if dairy-sensitive)

1. Heat the oil in a large cast-iron skillet over medium-low heat. Add the onions and cook for 10 to 20 minutes, until the onions are soft and light brown.

2. Increase the heat to medium and add the ground beef. Brown the meat, crumbling it with a spoon, until cooked through, about 5 minutes. Add the spinach, salt, and pepper and cook for another minute, until the spinach is wilted.

3. Crack the eggs into the center of the skillet and scramble them. Serve warm, garnished with Parmesan cheese, if desired.

4. This dish is best served fresh, but any leftovers can be stored in an airtight container in the refrigerator for up to 3 days. Reheat in a baking dish in a preheated 350°F oven for 5 minutes or until warmed through.

nutritional info (per serving)				
calories	fat	protein	carbs	fiber
495	41g	28g	4g	1g

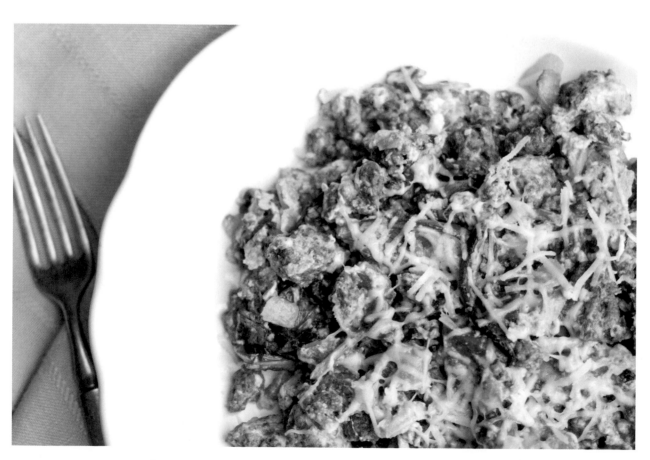

Meatloaf Cordon Bleu

L M H
KETO ✗

prep time: 7 minutes *cook time:* 1 hour 15 minutes *yield:* 8 servings

2 pounds ground beef

2 large eggs, beaten

1 small onion, chopped

½ cup chopped mushrooms

½ cup grated Parmesan cheese

1 clove garlic, smashed to a paste

1 teaspoon fine sea salt

1 teaspoon ground black pepper

4 ounces thinly sliced cooked ham

4 ounces thinly sliced provolone cheese

1. Preheat the oven to 350°F.

2. In a medium-sized bowl, mix together the ground beef, beaten eggs, onion, mushrooms, and Parmesan cheese. Season with the garlic, salt, and pepper and mix to combine.

3. Place a large piece of waxed paper on a work surface and dump the meat mixture out onto it. Pat the mixture into a rectangle about 9 inches wide and ½ inch thick.

4. Lay the slices of ham on top of the flattened meat, then top the ham with the slices of provolone. Pick up the edge of the waxed paper to roll the flattened meat into a log.

5. Remove the waxed paper, press the seam and ends to seal the loaf, and place the loaf in a 9 by 5-inch loaf pan. Bake for 1 hour 15 minutes or until the meatloaf is no longer pink inside.

6. Store extras in an airtight container in the refrigerator for up to 3 days. Reheat in a baking dish in a preheated 350°F oven for 5 minutes or until warmed through.

nutritional info (per serving)				
calories	fat	protein	carbs	fiber
437	32g	31g	3g	1g

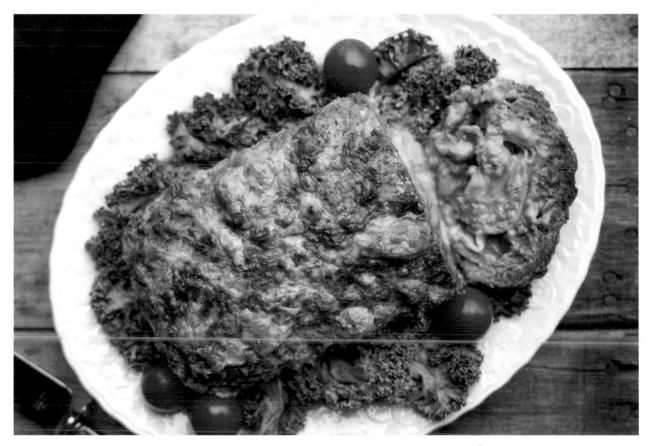

Steak Frites
with Béarnaise Sauce

Don't throw away those cauliflower stems; use them to make keto French fries! You can use the whole head of cauliflower if you prefer, but then they won't look like French fries.

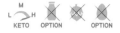

KETO   OPTION   OPTION

prep time: 6 minutes (not including time to make béarnaise)
cook time: 25 minutes   *yield:* 1 serving

fries

1 cauliflower stem

2 teaspoons melted unsalted butter (or melted coconut oil, lard, or avocado oil if dairy-free)

½ teaspoon fine sea salt

¼ teaspoon ground black pepper

steak

1 (4-ounce) boneless rib-eye steak, about ¾ inch thick

1 teaspoon fine sea salt

½ teaspoon ground black pepper

2 tablespoons unsalted butter (or coconut oil, lard, or avocado oil if dairy-free)

for serving

3 tablespoons Béarnaise Sauce (page 357), or 2 tablespoons beef bone broth, homemade (page 356) or store-bought, for a dairy-free, egg-free pan sauce

Fresh thyme leaves (optional)

1. To make the fries, preheat the oven to 425°F. Grease a rimmed baking sheet.

2. Cut the cauliflower stem into French fry shapes and place them on the greased baking sheet. Coat the fries with the melted butter and sprinkle with ½ teaspoon of salt and ¼ teaspoon of pepper. Bake for 25 minutes or until golden brown.

3. Season the steak on both sides with 1 teaspoon of salt and ½ teaspoon of pepper. Place a cast-iron skillet over medium-high heat; when hot, melt the butter in the pan. Add the steak and sear on each side for 1 minute. Reduce the heat to medium and cook for another 6 minutes or until the steak is cooked medium-rare (see chart below). Remove the steak from the pan and allow it to rest before cutting.

4. If you're skipping the béarnaise sauce, use the beef broth to make a quick pan sauce: Pour the broth into the pan and whisk to scrape the bottom of the skillet and combine the drippings and broth.

5. Place the steak on a serving plate, top with the cauliflower fries, and drizzle with the béarnaise sauce or pan sauce. Serve garnished with thyme leaves, if desired.

6. This dish is best served fresh, but any extras can be stored in an airtight container in the refrigerator for up to 3 days. Reheat the steak and fries in a baking dish in a preheated 350°F oven for 5 minutes or until warmed through.

160°F+	Well-done
150°F-155°F	Medium-well
140°F-145°F	Medium
130°F-135°F	Medium-rare
120°F-125°F	Rare

nutritional info (per serving)				
calories	fat	protein	carbs	fiber
655	61g	24g	6g	2g

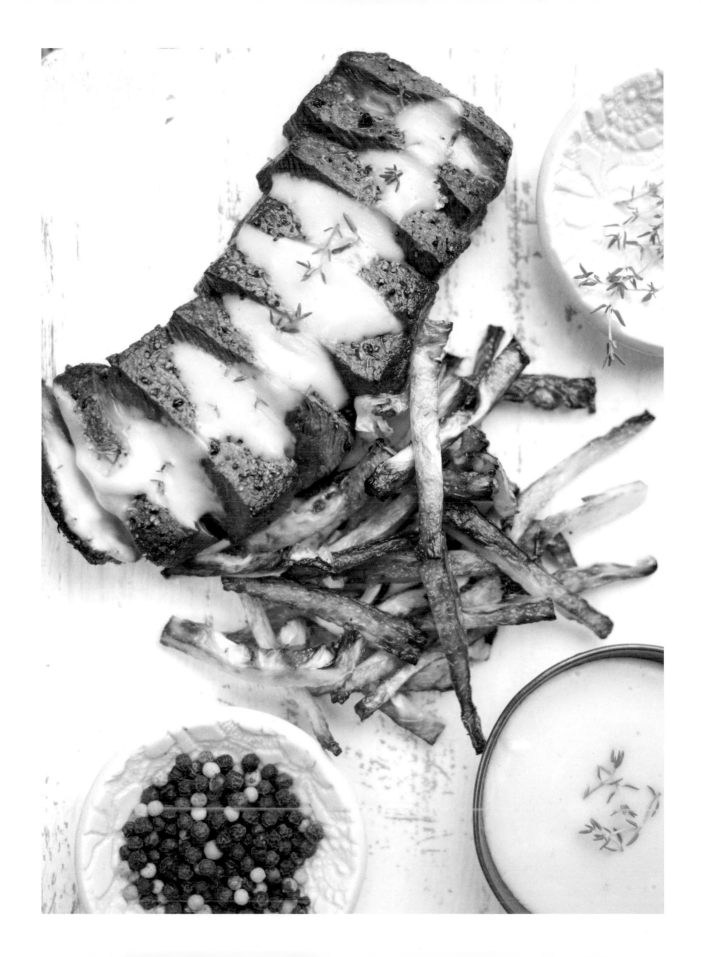

Rib-Eye Steak
with Asparagus Puree and Bacon Custard

prep time: 10 minutes, plus time to chill custard (not including time to cook bacon)
cook time: 35 minutes *yield:* 2 servings

6 strips bacon, cooked and diced

1¼ cups heavy cream, divided

¼ teaspoon ground nutmeg

2 large egg yolks

8 asparagus spears

1 (8-ounce) boneless rib-eye steak

Fine sea salt and ground black pepper

1 tablespoon ghee

for garnish

Baby lettuce leaves

Cherry tomatoes

1. To make the bacon custard, combine the cooked bacon, 1 cup of the cream, and the nutmeg in a saucepan and bring to a gentle simmer. Remove from the heat and allow the flavors to infuse for 15 minutes. Strain and discard the bacon.

2. While the bacon soaks in the cream, place the egg yolks in a heatproof bowl (or insert for a double boiler) and whisk for 5 minutes or until doubled in size and lightened in color. Slowly pour a few tablespoons of the bacon cream into the yolks while whisking so the eggs do not curdle. Set the bowl on top of a pot of simmering water (or the base of the double boiler).

3. Pour the rest of the bacon-infused cream into the bowl over the pot of simmering water. Heat gently, while stirring, until the mixture is thick and coats the back of a spoon, about 7 minutes. Transfer the custard to a clean bowl and set that bowl over a bowl of ice water to cool the custard. When cool, place the custard in the refrigerator to chill completely. For a fancy presentation, transfer the custard to a piping bag, if desired. Leave the custard in the refrigerator until you're ready to garnish the plates. (*Note:* The custard can be made 2 days ahead and stored in an airtight container in the refrigerator. Do not freeze.)

4. To make the asparagus puree, trim the woody ends off the stalks and chop the asparagus into 1-inch pieces. Place the asparagus in a pot of boiling water and cook until tender, about 5 minutes (up to 7 minutes for thicker asparagus). Drain well and place in a blender. Add the remaining ¼ cup of heavy cream and puree until smooth. Add salt to taste and set the puree aside. (*Note:* The puree can be made up to 2 days ahead and stored in an airtight container in the refrigerator.)

5. To make the steak, pat the steak dry with a paper towel, season well on all sides with salt and pepper, and allow to sit at room temperature for 10 to 15 minutes. Heat the ghee in a cast-iron skillet over medium heat. When hot, add the steak and sear for 5 minutes. Flip the steak and cook for another 3 to 5 minutes, depending on how well-done you like it (see chart at left). (A total of 8 minutes' cooking time will give you a medium-rare steak.) Remove the steak from the pan and allow it to rest on a cutting board for 10 minutes, then slice the steak into ½-inch-thick slices.

6. Place a dollop of asparagus puree on each plate and smear it with the back of a spoon. Arrange the sliced rib-eye on the plates. Garnish with baby lettuce and tomatoes and squirt circles of bacon custard around each plate.

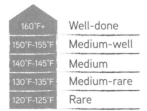

160°F+	Well-done
150°F–155°F	Medium-well
140°F–145°F	Medium
130°F–135°F	Medium-rare
120°F–125°F	Rare

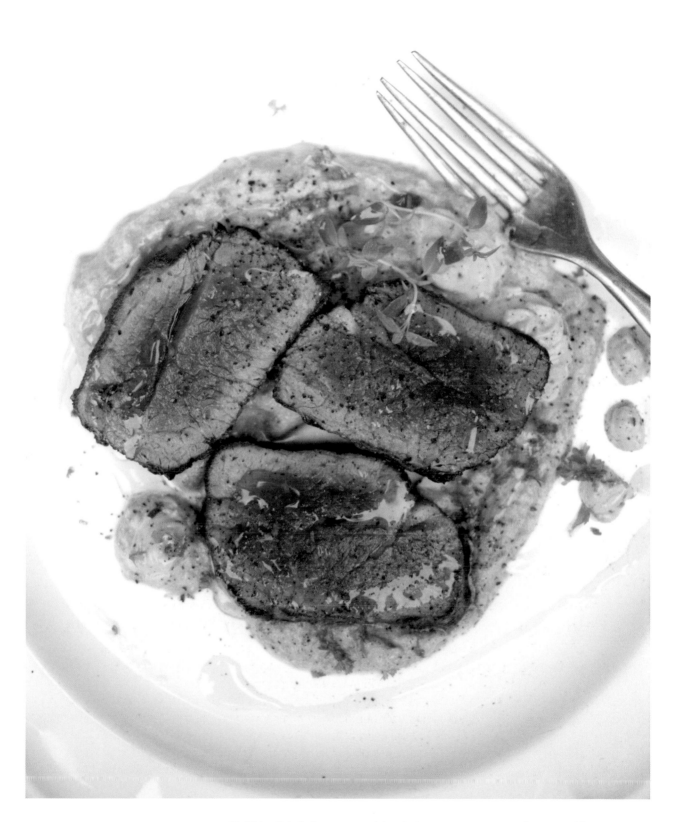

nutritional info (per serving)				
calories	*fat*	*protein*	*carbs*	*fiber*
572	54g	22g	2g	1g

7. This dish is best served fresh, but any extras can be stored in an airtight container in the refrigerator for up to 3 days. Reheat the steak on a rimmed baking sheet in a preheated 350°F oven for 5 minutes or until warmed through.

Filet Mignons Florentine

prep time: 5 minutes (not including time to make hollandaise)

cook time: 10 minutes   *yield:* 2 servings

1 tablespoon keto fat, for frying

2 (3-ounce) filet mignons, about 1¼ inches thick

1½ teaspoons fine sea salt

½ teaspoon ground black pepper

1 large tomato, thinly sliced

2 tablespoons minced shallots

2 cups fresh spinach

¼ cup Easy Basil Hollandaise (page 358)

1. Heat a cast-iron skillet over medium-high heat, then put the fat in the pan. While the skillet is heating, pat the steaks dry with a paper towel and season well with the salt and pepper. Place the steaks in the hot fat and sear on one side for 3 minutes, then flip and sear on the other side for 3 minutes or until done to your liking. (A total of 6 minutes' cooking time will give you medium-rare steaks.) Set the steaks on a cutting board to rest for 10 minutes while you prepare the rest of the meal.

2. Place 3 slices of tomato on each plate. Place the shallots in the skillet in which you cooked the steaks and sauté over medium-high heat for 2 minutes. Add the spinach and sauté for another 2 minutes or until wilted. Season to taste with salt. Top the tomatoes with the wilted greens.

3. Place a rested steak on top of the greens, then drizzle 2 tablespoons of the hollandaise over each steak.

4. This dish is best served fresh, but any extras can be stored in an airtight container in the refrigerator for up to 3 days. Reheat the steak on a baking sheet in a preheated 350°F oven for 5 minutes or until warmed through. To reheat the hollandaise, see page 358.

nutritional info (per serving)				
calories	fat	protein	carbs	fiber
497	43g	20g	6g	2g

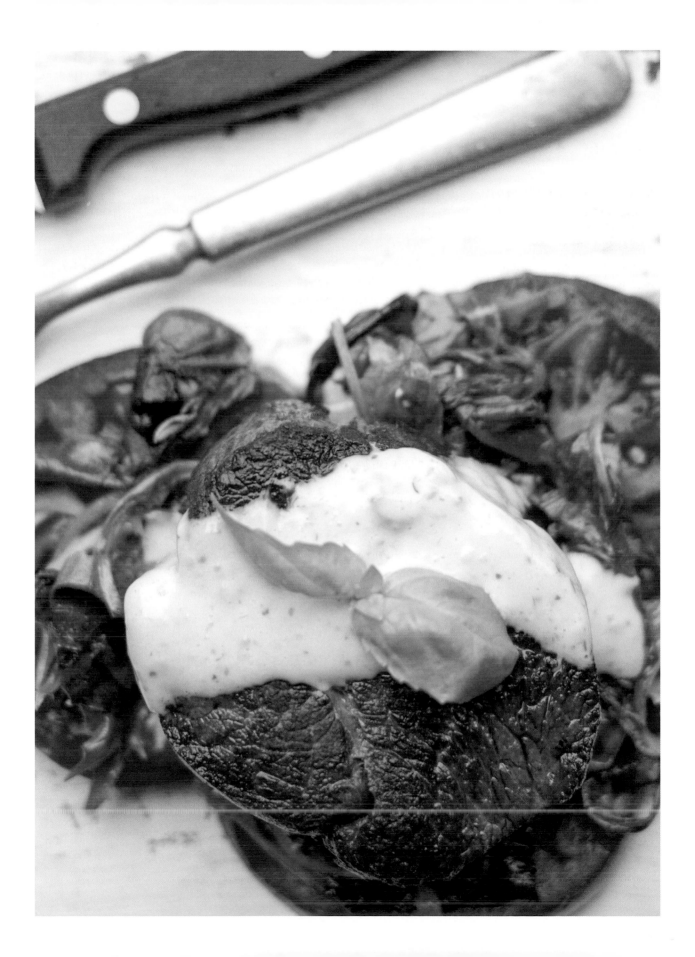

Meatballs
with Brown Gravy

My mom often served meatballs and gravy over white rice when I was a child. This recipe is in her honor! Using homemade beef bone broth creates a nice, thick gravy. If you have only boxed broth or stock, it will work, but you'll need to thicken the gravy with egg yolk (see note below). If you like, replace 1 pound of the ground beef with ground pork to make the recipe even more keto. Serve the meatballs over Zoodles (page 363) or Cauliflower Rice (page 362).

prep time: 5 minutes *cook time:* 35 minutes *yield:* 4 servings

meatballs

1 tablespoon coconut oil (or unsalted butter if not dairy-sensitive)

¼ cup chopped onions

1 teaspoon fine sea salt

2 pounds ground beef

1 cup finely chopped mushrooms

1 cup grated Parmesan cheese (omit for dairy-free)

1 large egg

gravy

2 tablespoons bacon fat or lard (or unsalted butter if not dairy-sensitive)

1 cup beef bone broth, homemade (page 356) or store-bought

1 teaspoon coconut aminos or wheat-free tamari

¼ teaspoon fine sea salt

¼ teaspoon ground black pepper

1 teaspoon fish sauce (optional, for umami flavor)

1. Preheat the oven to 350°F.

2. Heat the coconut oil in a heavy-bottomed skillet. Add the onions, sprinkle with the salt, and cook gently for about 5 minutes, until the onions are translucent. Remove the onions to a bowl to cool.

3. Put the ground beef, mushrooms, Parmesan cheese, and egg in a bowl. When the onion mixture is no longer hot to the touch, add it to the meat mixture and work everything together with your hands.

4. Shape the meat mixture into 2-inch balls and place the balls on a rimmed baking sheet. Bake for 30 minutes or until the meatballs are cooked through.

5. To make the gravy, place all the ingredients for the gravy in a saucepan. Boil, stirring often, for 10 minutes or until the gravy is thick and bubbly. Serve the meatballs with the gravy.

6. Store extras in an airtight container in the refrigerator for up to 3 days. Reheat in a baking dish in a preheated 350°F oven for 5 minutes or until warmed through.

---

note: *If using store-bought broth, pour ½ cup of the broth (unheated) into a small bowl. Add 1 egg yolk and whisk to combine. After the gravy mixture has boiled for 10 minutes, reduce the heat to low and slowly whisk the egg yolk mixture into the hot gravy. Continue to heat while whisking until the sauce has thickened; this is somewhat like how hollandaise is thickened, but in reverse.*

nutritional info (per serving)				
calories	fat	protein	carbs	fiber
550	44g	36g	1g	0.4g

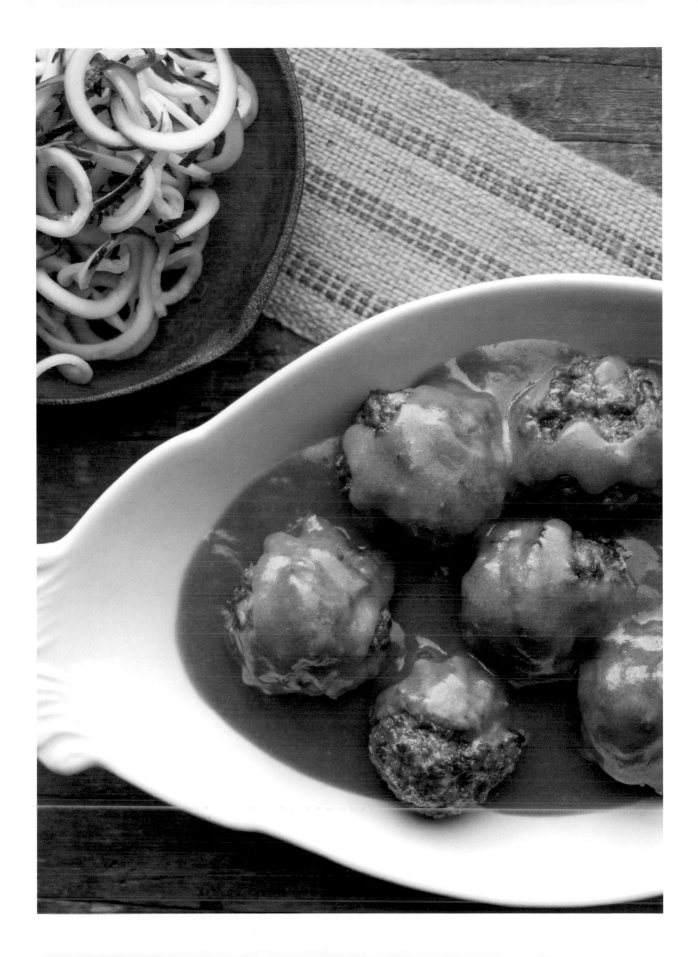

Steak with
Blue Cheese Whip

The blue cheese whip really makes this steak. It tastes great on any cut of steak—or even a piece of chicken! If you are dairy-sensitive, you can serve this steak with dairy-free hollandaise (page 358) instead of the blue cheese whip.

L M H
KETO ✖ ✖

prep time: 5 minutes   *cook time:* about 10 minutes   *yield:* 2 servings

1 (12-ounce) T-bone steak, about ¾ inch thick

1¼ teaspoons fine sea salt

½ teaspoon ground black pepper

1 tablespoon keto fat, for frying

blue cheese whip

¼ cup heavy cream

¼ ounce blue cheese, finely crumbled

⅛ teaspoon fine sea salt

1. Preheat the oven to 400°F.

2. Season the steak generously on all sides with the salt and pepper. Heat a cast-iron skillet over medium-high heat, then melt the fat in the pan. When hot, sear the steak for 3 minutes on each side.

3. Place the skillet in the oven to cook the steak to your desired doneness, using a meat thermometer to determine the internal temperature (see chart below). Remove the skillet from the heat and allow the steak to rest for 10 minutes before slicing and serving.

4. While the steak is resting, make the blue cheese whip: Place the cream in a stand mixer and mix until stiff peaks form. Stir in the blue cheese and salt until well blended. (*Note:* The whip can be made ahead and stored in an airtight container in the refrigerator for up to 3 days.)

5. Serve each portion of steak with 2 tablespoons of the blue cheese whip.

6. This dish is best served fresh, but any extras can be stored in an airtight container in the refrigerator for up to 3 days. Reheat on a rimmed baking sheet in a preheated 350°F oven for 5 minutes or until warmed through.

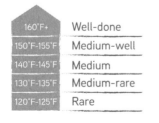

160°F+	Well-done
150°F-155°F	Medium-well
140°F-145°F	Medium
130°F-135°F	Medium-rare
120°F-125°F	Rare

nutritional info (per serving)				
calories	fat	protein	carbs	fiber
566	48g	33g	1g	0.4g

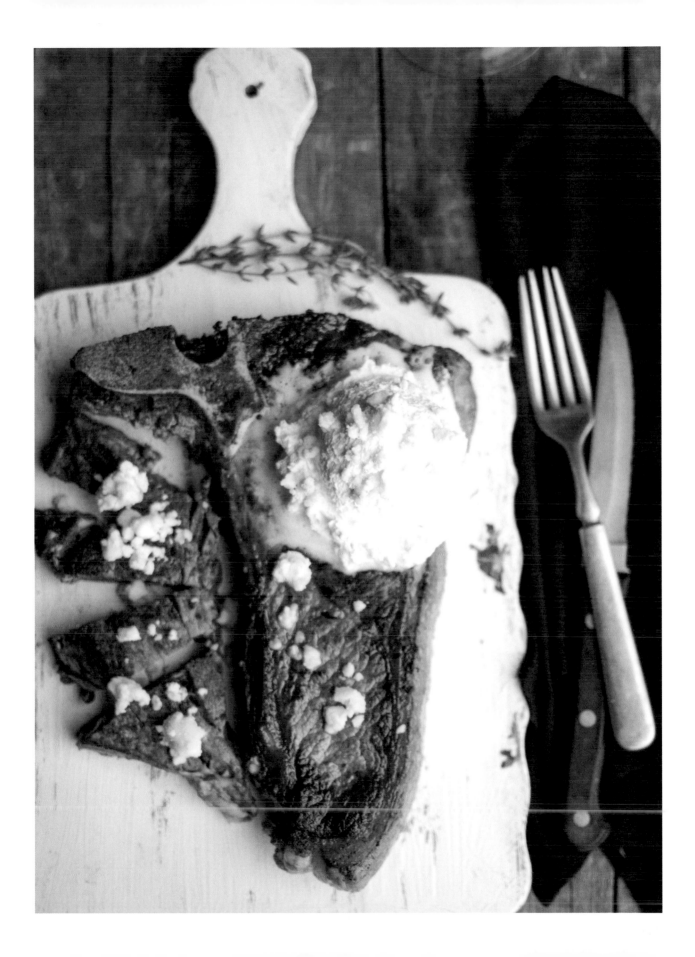

Perfect Reverse-Sear Prime Rib
with Tiger Sauce

Have you ever made prime rib and ended up with a disappointing gray steak? That often happens when you sear the roast first, then slowly cook it through. Never again! The reverse-sear method used in this recipe keeps the prime rib nice and pink, and the sear at the end gets the outside nice and crispy.

For the most tender meat possible, I highly recommend that you roast the prime rib at the ultra-slow-cooking temperature of 150°F. However, because the lowest temperature on some ovens is 200°F, I've included directions for cooking the roast at that higher temperature as well.

prep time: 8 minutes, plus 8 hours to marinate

cook time: 3½ to 5½ hours, depending on lowest available oven temperature

yield: 16 servings

prime rib

1 (8-pound) boneless prime rib roast

2½ tablespoons fine sea salt

1½ tablespoons ground black pepper

½ cup softened ghee or unsalted butter

2 tablespoons chopped fresh rosemary

2 tablespoons chopped fresh thyme

tiger sauce

1 cup sour cream

¼ cup prepared horseradish

2 tablespoons chopped fresh dill or 2 teaspoons dried dill

Fine sea salt (optional)

1. Season the roast liberally with the salt and pepper. Cover the roast with plastic wrap and place it in the refrigerator for at least 8 hours or overnight. Two hours before baking, remove the roast from the fridge and allow it to come to room temperature.

2. Preheat the oven to 150°F (or the lowest available temperature for your oven). Place the roast in a large roasting pan. Rub the softened ghee all over the roast, then sprinkle it with the chopped herbs.

3. Bake the roast for 5½ hours (or 3½ hours in a 200°F oven), or until the internal temperature reaches 115°F for medium-rare or 135°F for medium. The internal temperature will keep rising as the meat rests.

4. While the roast is cooking, make the tiger sauce: Place the sour cream, horseradish, and dill in a small bowl and stir well to combine. Taste and adjust the seasoning, adding more dill or a pinch of salt, if desired. Cover and store in an airtight container in the refrigerator until ready to serve.

5. About 10 minutes before serving, increase the oven temperature to 500°F. Once the temperature is at 500°F, let the roast sear in the oven for 8 minutes or until brown and crispy on the outside. Remove the roast from the oven, allow it to rest for 10 minutes, and then carve it into ¾-inch-thick slices. Serve with the tiger sauce and the pan juices (see note below).

6. Store extra meat and sauce in separate airtight containers for up to 3 days. Reheat the roast on a rimmed baking sheet in a preheated 350°F oven for 5 minutes or until warmed through.

note: You can also use the pan drippings to make Yorkshire Pudding (page 134), a classic accompaniment to prime rib!

nutritional info (per serving)				
calories	*fat*	*protein*	*carbs*	*fiber*
703	49g	60g	2g	1g

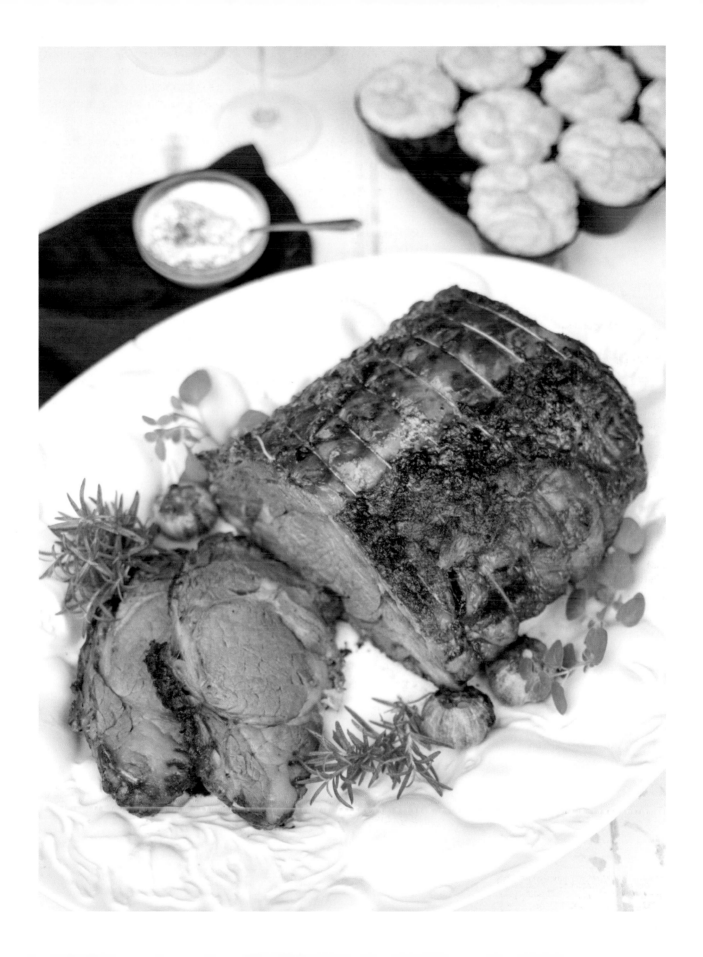

Greek Burgers
with Feta Dressing

L M>H KETO ✖ ✖

1 tablespoon ghee, lard, or coconut oil, for frying

1 pound ground lamb or hamburger

1½ teaspoons fine sea salt

1 teaspoon ground black pepper

for serving

6 leaves lettuce

½ cup thinly sliced red onions

¼ cup thickly sliced cucumbers

6 cherry tomatoes, sliced

½ cup Greek dressing, homemade (page 361) or store-bought

prep time: 15 minutes (not including time to make dressing)

cook time: 6 minutes   *yield:* 3 servings

1. Heat the ghee in a cast-iron skillet over medium-high heat.

2. Using your hands, form the ground meat into 3 patties. Season the outsides of the patties with the salt and pepper. Fry the burgers in the skillet until done to your liking (see chart below).

3. Serve each burger on 2 lettuce leaves, topped with sliced onions, cucumbers, tomatoes, and about 2½ heaping tablespoons of the dressing.

4. This dish is best served fresh, but any extra burgers and dressing can be stored in separate airtight containers in the refrigerator for up to 3 days. Reheat the burgers on a baking sheet in a preheated 350°F oven for 5 minutes or until warmed through.

---

burger tip:

Salt only the outsides of the burgers to keep them moist. Salt removes water from and dissolves some of the meat proteins, which causes the insoluble proteins to bind together. Lots of salt is great for making sausages, but not great for tender, juicy burgers.

160°F+	Well-done
150°F-155°F	Medium-well
140°F-145°F	Medium

nutritional info (per serving)				
calories	fat	protein	carbs	fiber
556	46g	28g	6g	2g

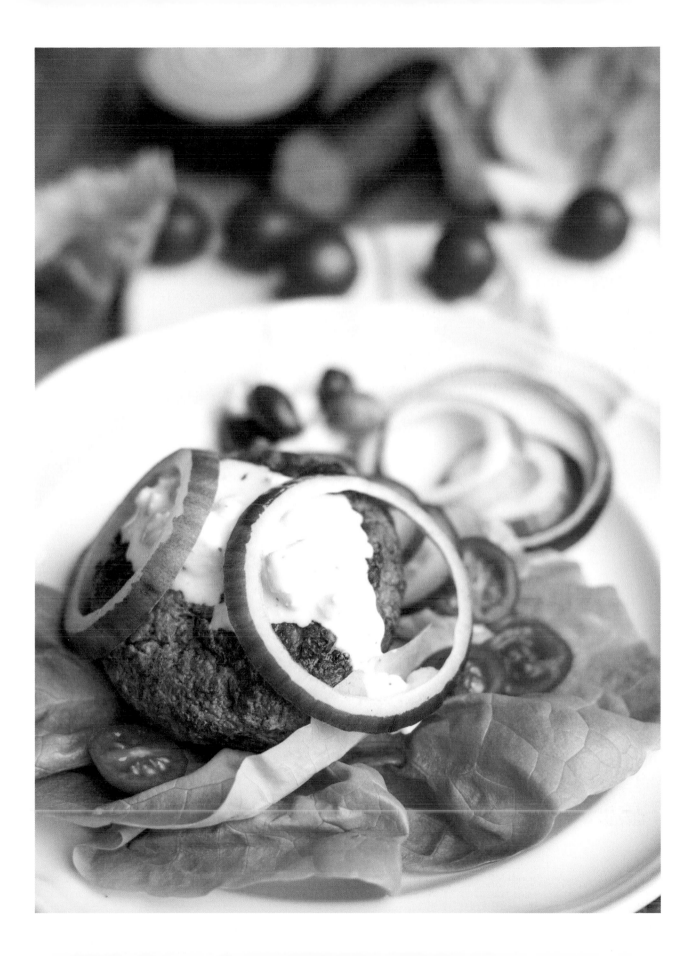

Country-Fried Steak and Gravy

L M H
KETO OPTION

prep time: 10 minutes (not including time to make fauxtatoes or rice)
cook time: 10 minutes   yield: 4 servings

4 (4-ounce) bottom round steaks

2 teaspoons fine sea salt

1 teaspoon ground black pepper

1 large egg

1 cup powdered Parmesan cheese (see page 13) (or pork dust if dairy-free)

½ teaspoon paprika

¼ teaspoon cayenne pepper

¼ cup ghee (or coconut oil if dairy-free), for frying

gravy

1 tablespoon ghee (or coconut oil if dairy-free)

2 tablespoons minced onions

1 clove garlic, minced

4 ounces cream cheese (½ cup) (Kite Hill brand cream cheese style spread if dairy-free), softened

½ cup beef or chicken bone broth, homemade (page 356) or store-bought

Fine sea salt and ground black pepper

1 batch Mashed Fauxtatoes (page 129) (or Cauliflower Rice, page 362, if dairy-free), for serving (optional)

Chopped fresh parsley, for garnish

Melted ghee (or avocado oil if dairy-free), for drizzling

1. To tenderize the steaks, pound them until they are ¼ inch thick. Sprinkle both sides of the steaks with the salt and pepper.

2. Beat the egg in a shallow bowl. Place the Parmesan cheese, paprika, and cayenne pepper in another shallow bowl and stir well to combine. Divide the Parmesan mixture between 2 separate bowls so you can do a dry, wet, dry dipping of the steaks.

3. Dip a steak into the first bowl of Parmesan mixture, then into the egg, then into the second bowl of Parmesan mixture, using your hands to coat all sides of the meat well. Place the coated steak on a clean plate and repeat with the remaining steaks.

4. Place the ¼ cup of ghee in a large cast-iron skillet over medium heat. When hot, add the coated steaks, working in batches if necessary. Cook for 2 minutes or until golden brown, then flip and cook for 2 minutes on the other side. Repeat until all the steaks are cooked. Place the cooked steaks on a warm serving platter and tent with foil to keep warm.

5. To make the gravy, wipe the skillet clean. Melt 1 tablespoon of ghee in the skillet. Add the onions and garlic and sauté over medium heat for 3 minutes or until the onions are translucent. Use a whisk to stir in the cream cheese, whisking until no clumps remain. Slowly add the broth while whisking. Cook, stirring constantly, until the mixture comes to a gentle simmer and is smooth. Reduce the heat to medium-low and continue to simmer, stirring constantly, for 2 minutes or until thickened. Season to taste with salt and pepper.

6. Remove the foil from the serving platter and cover the steaks in the gravy. Serve over mashed fauxtatoes, if desired, and garnish with chopped parsley and a drizzle of melted ghee.

7. Store extras in an airtight container in the refrigerator for up to 3 days. Reheat on a rimmed baking sheet in a preheated 350°F oven for 5 minutes or until warmed through.

busy family tip:

Ask your butcher to tenderize and pound the steaks thin so all you have to do is dip them in the breading and fry them for a tasty dinner!

nutritional info (per serving)				
calories	fat	protein	carbs	fiber
775	58g	50g	12g	5g

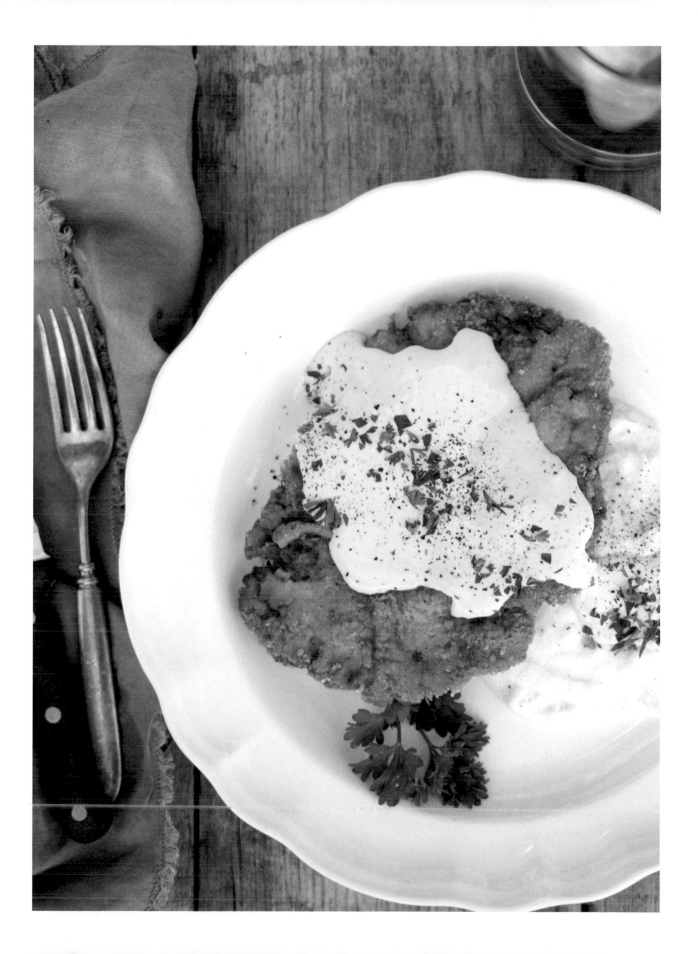

Taco Pizza

There is an amazing pizza place in my hometown of Medford, Wisconsin, called Happy Joe's. One of their specialties is taco pizza. It is topped with a tasty taco sauce instead of pizza sauce and covered with taco fixings such as olives, shredded lettuce, and cilantro. This is my take on it.

L M H
KETO

crust

1¾ cups shredded mozzarella cheese

2 tablespoons unsalted butter

1 large egg, beaten

¾ cup blanched almond flour

⅛ teaspoon fine sea salt

spicy tomato sauce

1 cup tomato sauce

2 tablespoons Swerve confectioners'-style sweetener or equivalent amount of liquid or powdered sweetener (see page 24)

1½ teaspoons chili powder

1 teaspoon ground cumin

1 teaspoon fine sea salt

½ teaspoon paprika

¼ teaspoon garlic powder

¼ teaspoon onion powder

¼ teaspoon dried oregano

toppings

¼ pound ground beef

½ cup shredded sharp cheddar cheese

½ cup shredded mozzarella cheese

¼ cup chopped onions

for garnish

¼ cup sliced black olives

¼ cup shredded lettuce

¼ cup sliced cherry tomatoes

Drizzle of crème fraîche or sour cream thinned slightly with water

Fresh cilantro (optional)

prep time: 10 minutes, plus 1 hour to chill dough, if needed
cook time: 15 minutes   *yield:* 4 servings

1. Place a pizza stone in the cold oven, then turn the oven on to 425°F. (You can use a baking sheet, but a pizza stone will bake the bottom better.)

2. To make the crust, put the mozzarella and butter in a microwave-safe bowl and microwave for 1 to 2 minutes, until the cheese is entirely melted. Stir well. Add the beaten egg and, using a hand mixer, combine well. Add the almond flour and salt and combine well with the mixer. Use your hands and work it like a traditional dough, kneading for about 3 minutes. (*Note:* If the dough is too sticky, chill it in the refrigerator for an hour or overnight.)

3. Place the dough on a greased piece of parchment paper and pat it out with your hands to form a large circle, about 10 inches in diameter. For easy transferring to the oven, slide the sheet of parchment with the dough circle onto an unrimmed baking sheet or pizza peel. Set aside.

4. To make the spicy tomato sauce, place the tomato sauce, sweetener, and seasonings in a bowl and stir well to combine.

5. To make the meat topping, heat a cast-iron skillet over medium heat. Add the beef and 3 tablespoons of the spicy tomato sauce and cook, stirring to break up the clumps, until the meat is browned and crumbly, about 5 minutes. Set aside.

6. Spread the rest of the spicy tomato sauce over the pizza crust. Sprinkle the cheeses over the tomato sauce and top with the beef and onions.

7. Transfer the pizza to the hot pizza stone in the oven by sliding the parchment and pizza off the baking sheet onto the stone. Bake the pizza until the cheese is melted, about 10 minutes. Remove the pizza from the oven and garnish with the black olives, lettuce, tomatoes, crème fraîche, and cilantro, if desired.

8. Store extras in an airtight container in the refrigerator for up to 3 days. Reheat slices on a baking sheet in a preheated 350°F oven for 5 minutes or until warmed through.

nutritional info (per serving)				
calories	fat	protein	carbs	fiber
518	42g	29g	12g	4g

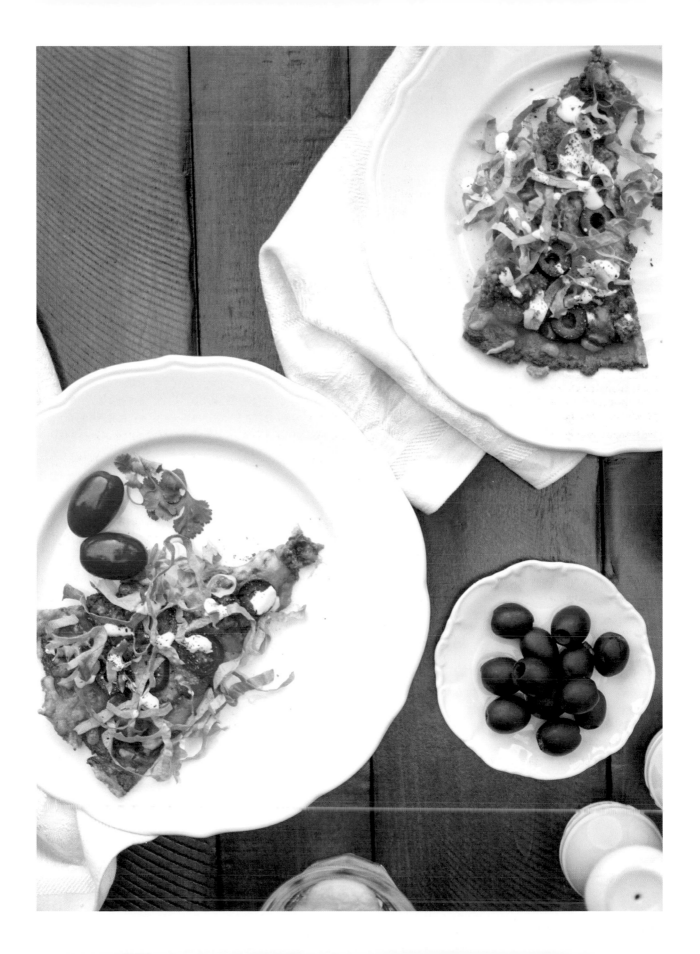

Pizza Supreme

prep time: 10 minutes, plus 1 hour to chill dough, if needed

cook time: 15 minutes   *yield:* 4 servings

crust

1¾ cups shredded mozzarella cheese

2 tablespoons unsalted butter

1 large egg, beaten

¾ cup blanched almond flour

⅛ teaspoon fine sea salt

toppings

¼ pound ground beef

1 teaspoon fine sea salt

1 cup pizza sauce, homemade (page 358) or store-bought

½ cup shredded mozzarella cheese

¼ cup sliced black olives

¼ cup chopped or sliced green bell peppers

¼ cup chopped or sliced red bell peppers

½ cup sliced button mushrooms

¼ cup pepperoni slices

1 (⅛-inch-thick) slice red onion, rings separated

½ teaspoon Italian seasoning (optional)

1. Place a pizza stone in the cold oven, then turn on the oven to 425°F. (You can use a baking sheet, but a pizza stone will bake the bottom better.)

2. To make the crust, put the mozzarella cheese and butter in a microwave-safe bowl and microwave for 1 to 2 minutes, until the cheese is entirely melted. Stir well. Add the egg and, using a hand mixer, combine well. Add the almond flour and salt and combine well with the mixer. Use your hands and work it like a traditional dough, kneading for about 3 minutes. (*Note:* If the dough is too sticky, chill it in the refrigerator for an hour or overnight.)

3. Place the dough on a greased piece of parchment paper and pat it out with your hands to form a large circle, about 10 inches in diameter. For easy transferring to the oven, slide the sheet of parchment with the dough circle onto an unrimmed baking sheet or pizza peel. Set aside.

4. To make the meat topping, heat a cast-iron skillet over medium heat. Add the ground beef, season with the salt, and cook, stirring to break up the clumps, until the meat is browned and crumbly, about 5 minutes. Set aside.

5. Spread the pizza sauce over the crust. Sprinkle the cheese over the sauce and top the pizza with the cooked beef, olives, bell peppers, mushrooms, pepperoni, and red onion. Sprinkle with the Italian seasoning, if desired.

6. Transfer the pizza to the hot pizza stone in the oven by sliding the parchment and pizza off the baking sheet onto the stone. Bake the pizza until the cheese is melted, about 10 minutes.

7. Store extras in an airtight container in the refrigerator for up to 3 days. Reheat slices on a baking sheet in a preheated 350°F oven for 5 minutes or until warmed through.

nutritional info (per serving)				
calories	fat	protein	carbs	fiber
507	42g	28g	10g	4g

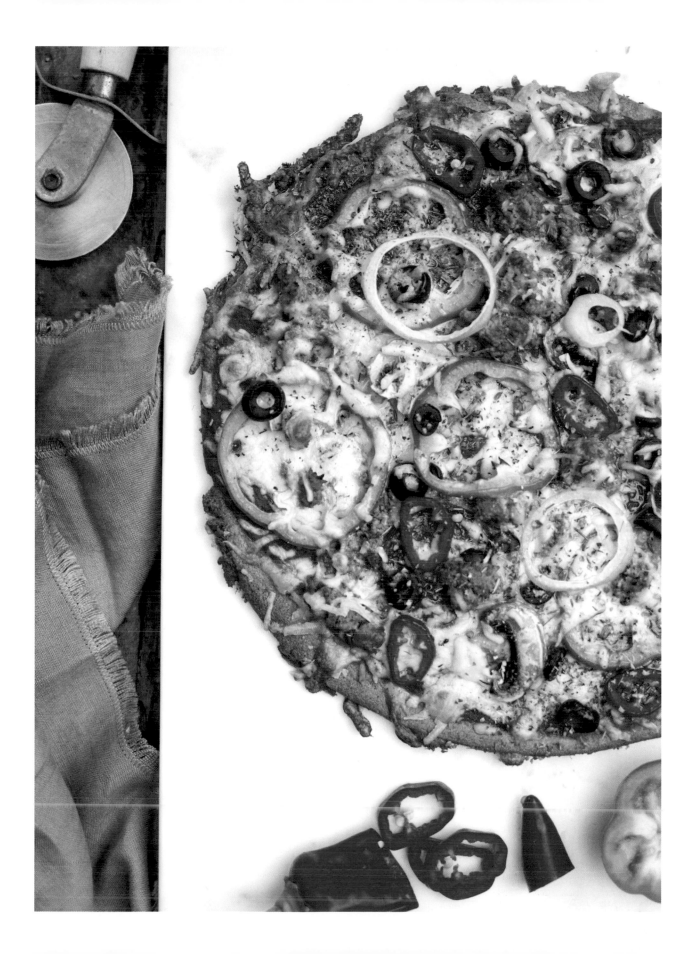

French Dip Sandwiches

One thing I love to do for easy dinners is to make sandwiches using my keto waffles. I make a triple batch of waffles and store them in the freezer for easy additions to meals. To make this recipe even more convenient for a weeknight dinner, I also fill the slow cooker insert the night before and store it in the refrigerator. The meat gets an amazing marinade, and all I have to do when I wake up in the morning is take the insert out of the fridge, put it in the slow cooker, and turn it on. Ta-da! Dinner is ready when I get home!

L M H
KETO

1 (2-pound) boneless beef chuck roast

⅓ cup coconut aminos or wheat free tamari

2 cloves garlic, smashed to a paste, or 1 teaspoon garlic powder

3 whole black peppercorns

1 teaspoon dried rosemary leaves, crushed

½ teaspoon dried thyme leaves

1 bay leaf

4 cups beef bone broth, homemade (page 356) or store-bought

1 batch waffles from the Croque Madame Waffles recipe (page 78)

Softened ghee or unsalted butter

16 slices provolone cheese (omit for dairy-free)

prep time: 10 minutes (not including time to make waffles)
cook time: 6 to 8 hours *yield:* 8 servings

1. Place the roast in a 4-quart slow cooker. In a medium-sized bowl, combine the coconut aminos, garlic, peppercorns, rosemary, thyme, and bay leaf. Pour this mixture over the roast in the slow cooker, then add the beef broth.

2. Cover and cook on low for 6 to 8 hours, until the meat is very tender. Remove the meat from the broth, reserving the broth. Slice or shred the meat.

3. When ready to serve the sandwiches, preheat the oven to 350°F. Place the waffles on a baking sheet. Spread with ghee and bake for 2 to 3 minutes, until barely toasted.

4. To assemble the sandwiches, place the meat on the waffles and top each with 2 slices of provolone cheese, if using. Put the sandwiches in the oven for another 2 to 3 minutes, until the cheese is melted. Serve with the reserved broth in ramekins for dipping the sandwiches.

5. Store extras in an airtight container in the refrigerator for up to 3 days. Reheat the sandwiches on a rimmed baking sheet in a preheated 350°F oven for 5 minutes or until warmed through.

nutritional info (per sandwich)				
calories	fat	protein	carbs	fiber
623	47g	39g	4g	3g

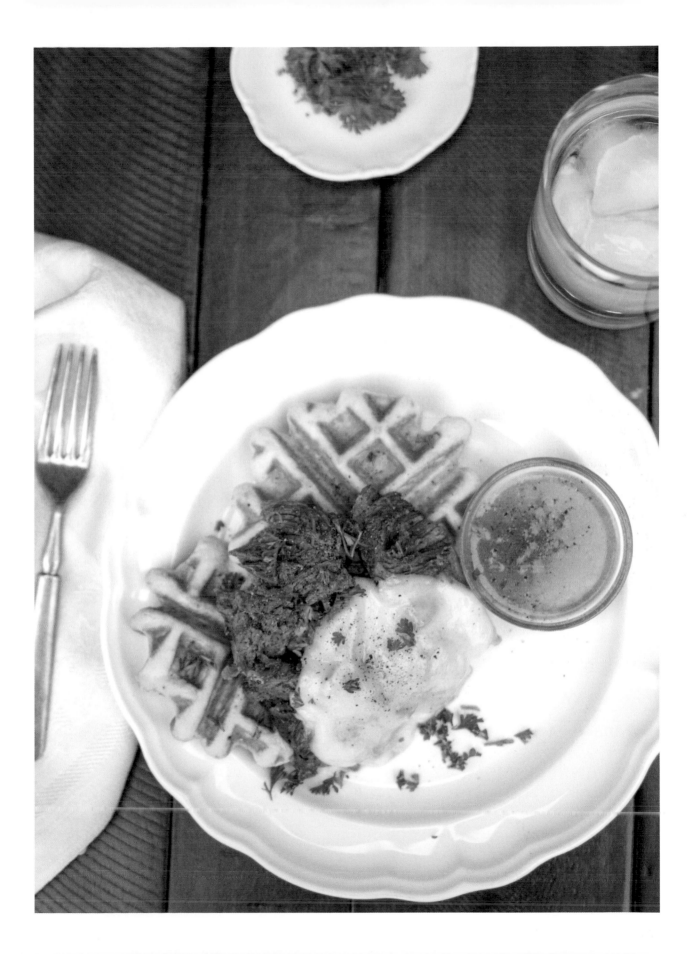

Garlic and Rosemary Rack of Lamb

KETO   OPTION

2 (4-rib) racks of lamb, trimmed and frenched at the tips

1 teaspoon fine sea salt

½ teaspoon ground black pepper

2 teaspoons ghee (or coconut oil if dairy-free)

2 cloves garlic, minced

1 tablespoon finely chopped fresh rosemary

2 teaspoons finely chopped fresh thyme

2 tablespoons avocado oil

Melted ghee or avocado oil, for drizzling

Greek olives, for garnish

Lemon slices, for garnish

Fresh herbs of choice, for garnish

prep time: 10 minutes *cook time:* 30 minutes
yield: 4 servings (2 ribs per serving)

1. Preheat the oven to 350°F.

2. Pat the racks of lamb dry with a paper towel and season them with the salt and pepper. Place the ghee in a cast-iron skillet over medium-high heat. When hot, add the racks of lamb and sear on all sides, about 2 minutes per side. Transfer the seared lamb to a roasting pan.

3. In a small bowl, combine the garlic, rosemary, thyme, and avocado oil. Use your hands to coat the lamb with this mixture.

4. Roast the lamb for 18 minutes or until the internal temperature reaches 125°F. Allow the meat to rest for 10 minutes.

5. Stand the racks of lamb on a serving platter with the frenched tips intertwined at the top. Drizzle with melted ghee and garnish the platter with Greek olives, lemon slices, and the herbs of your choice. To serve, slice the lamb into chops.

6. This dish is best served fresh, but any extras can be stored in an airtight container in the refrigerator for up to 3 days. To reheat, sauté the chops in a greased cast-iron skillet for 2 minutes per side.

nutritional info (per serving)				
calories	fat	protein	carbs	fiber
344	27g	17g	4g	1g

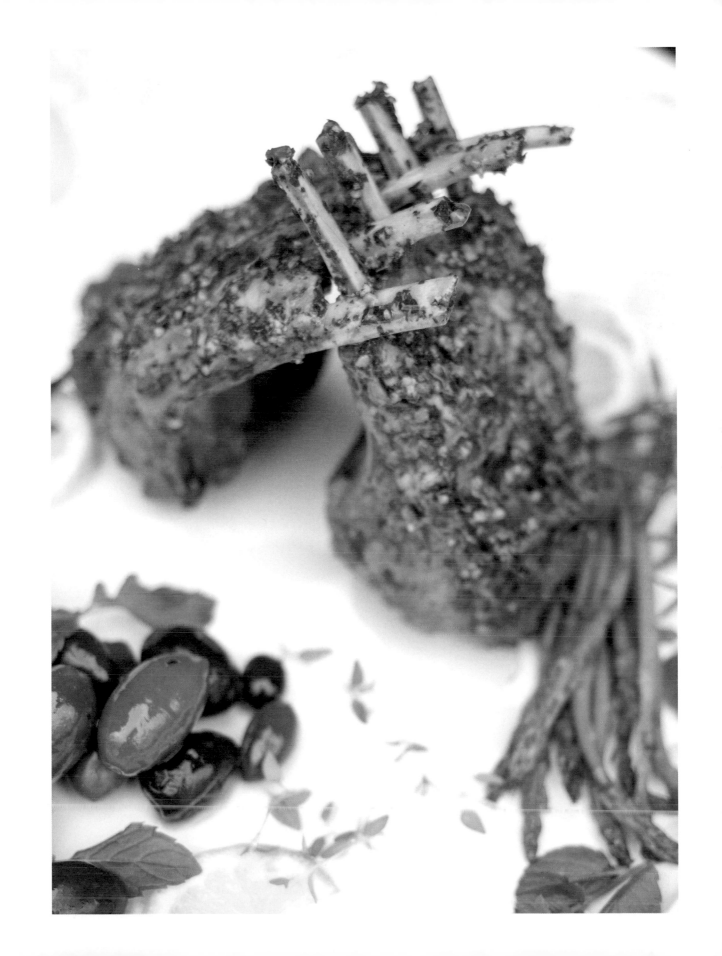

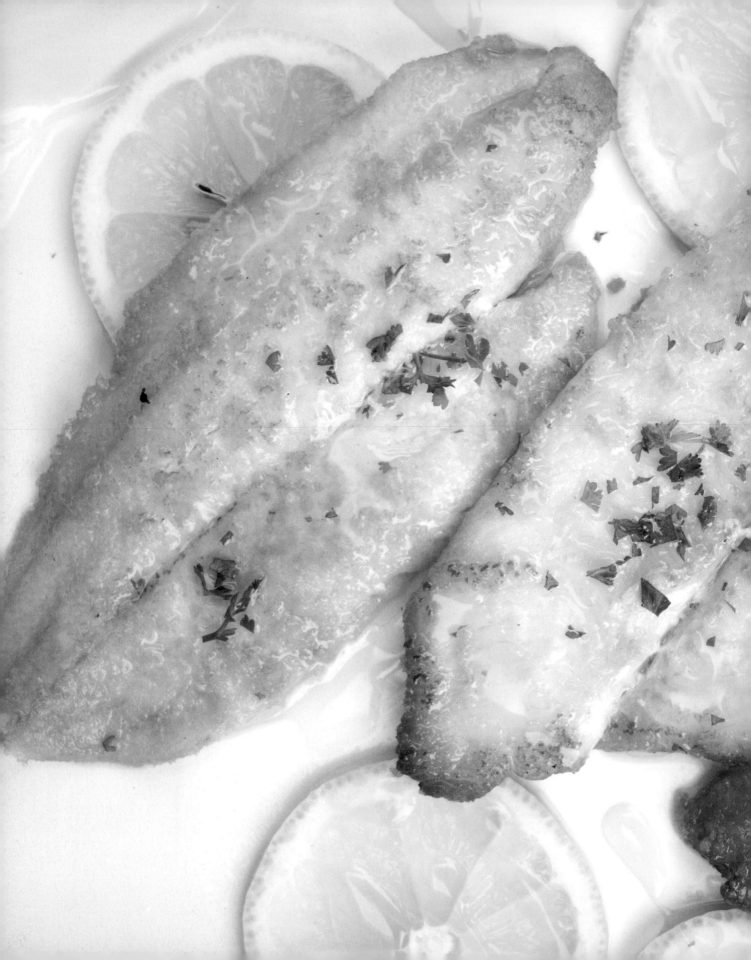

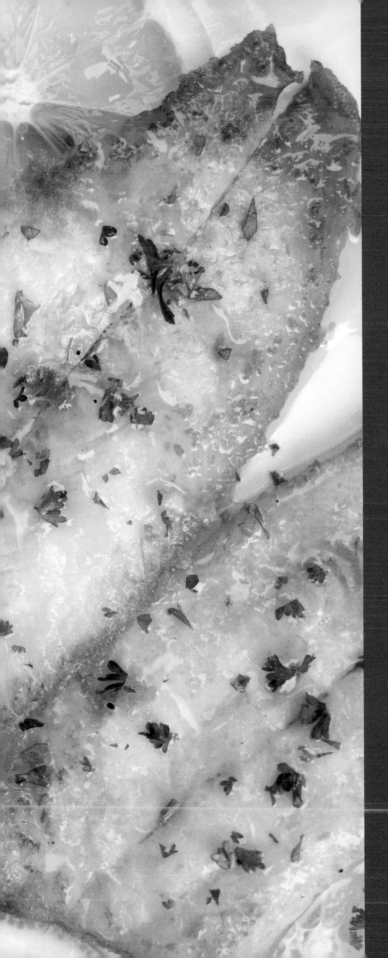

main dishes
Fish and Seafood

Shrimp Thermidor

½ cup ghee or unsalted butter (plus an additional ¼ cup melted ghee or unsalted butter added at the end if using pork rinds)

2 cups sliced button mushrooms

¼ cup diced onions

1 pound large shrimp (about 30), peeled and deveined

1 cup chicken bone broth, homemade (page 356) or store-bought

1 (8-ounce) package cream cheese, softened

¾ cup shredded cheddar cheese

1½ cups crushed pork rinds, divided (optional)

½ cup grated Parmesan cheese

1. Preheat the broiler to high.

2. Melt ½ cup of ghee in a cast-iron skillet over medium-high heat. Add the mushrooms and onions and sauté, stirring occasionally, until the mushrooms are golden brown, about 5 minutes. Add the shrimp and sauté for 4 minutes, until the shrimp are cooked through and no longer translucent.

3. Meanwhile, puree the broth and cream cheese in a blender or food processor until smooth, then add the mixture to the skillet. Add the cheddar cheese and stir in 1 cup of the crushed pork rinds, if using. Pour the mixture into a 9-inch square casserole dish.

4. Cover the top of the casserole with the remaining ½ cup of crushed pork rinds, if using, and the Parmesan cheese. If using pork rinds, drizzle ¼ cup of melted ghee over the top. Place under the broiler for 2 to 4 minutes, until the cheese is melted and turning golden brown.

5. Store extras in an airtight container in the refrigerator for up to 4 days. Reheat in a baking dish in a preheated 375°F oven for 4 minutes or until warmed through.

nutritional info (per serving)				
calories	fat	protein	carbs	fiber
785	57g	56g	5g	1g

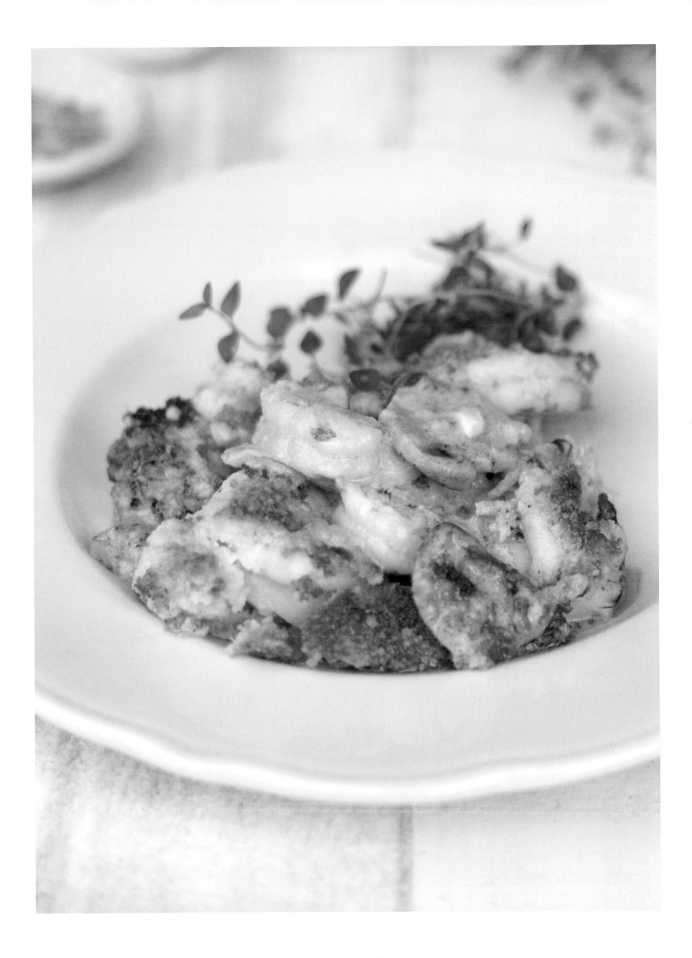

Walleye Simmered in Basil Cream

KETO   OPTION

prep time: 5 minutes   cook time: 10 minutes   yield: 4 servings

¼ cup heavy cream (or full-fat coconut milk if dairy-free)

¼ cup fresh basil leaves, plus extra for garnish

2 tablespoons ghee or unsalted butter (or coconut oil if dairy-free), divided

½ cup chopped onions

1 clove garlic, smashed to a paste

1 pound walleye fillets, skinned and cut crosswise into 1-inch-wide pieces

1 teaspoon fine sea salt

¼ teaspoon ground black pepper

¼ cup fish or chicken bone broth, homemade (page 356) or store-bought

Cherry tomatoes, cut in half, for garnish

1. Place the cream and basil in a food processor or blender and puree until the basil is completely broken down.

2. Heat a cast-iron skillet over medium heat. Melt the ghee in the hot skillet, then add the onions and garlic and sauté for 2 minutes, until the onions are translucent.

3. Season the fish pieces with the salt and pepper. Place the fish in the skillet and add the broth and basil cream. Cook, uncovered, for 7 minutes or until the fish is cooked through and starting to flake.

4. If you prefer a thicker sauce, remove the fish from the pan and continue to boil the sauce for 10 minutes or until thickened to your liking.

5. Place the fish on a serving platter, cover with the sauce, and garnish with additional basil and halved cherry tomatoes.

6. Store extras in an airtight container in the refrigerator for up to 3 days. Reheat in a lightly greased skillet over medium heat until warmed through.

nutritional info (per serving)				
calories	fat	protein	carbs	fiber
210	11g	23g	3g	0.4g

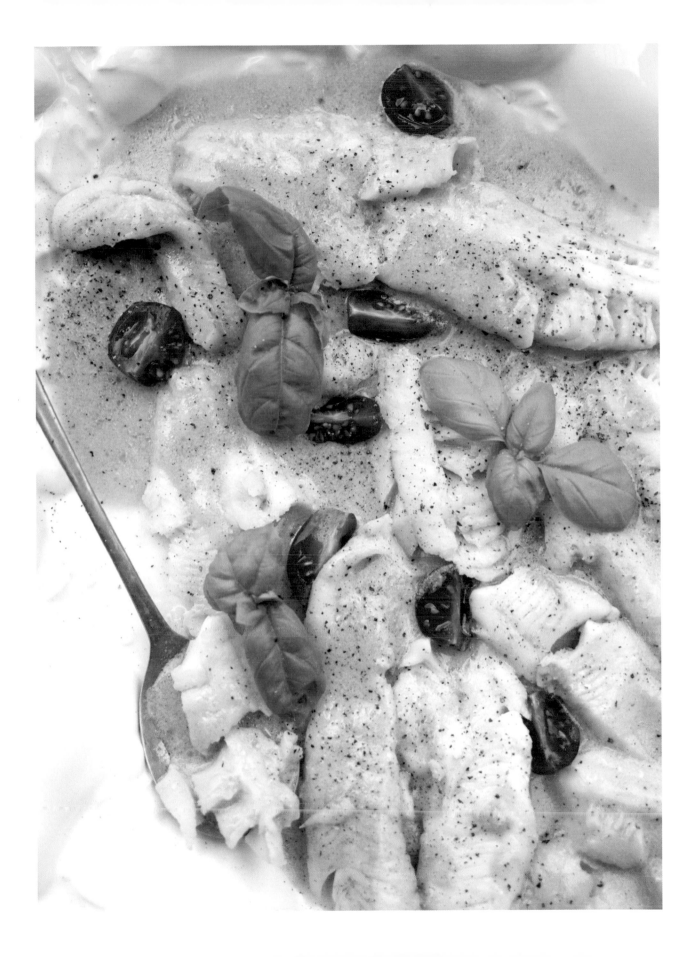

Cheesy Tuna Casserole

L M H KETO · OPTION

If you are a visual learner like me, check out the video about how to smash garlic to a paste on my site, MariaMindBodyHealth.com (type the word *video* in the search field).

prep time: 10 minutes *cook time:* 20 minutes *yield:* 6 servings

1 tablespoon ghee or unsalted butter (or coconut oil or lard if dairy free), plus extra for greasing the dish

1 tablespoon diced celery

1 tablespoon diced onions

1 clove garlic, smashed to a paste

3 (6-ounce) cans tuna, drained

2 cups cauliflower florets, cut into ½-inch pieces

1 cup chopped dill pickles

⅓ cup cream cheese (Kite Hill brand cream cheese style spread if dairy-free), softened

2 tablespoons mayonnaise, homemade (page 359) or store-bought

½ teaspoon fine sea salt

¼ teaspoon ground black pepper

1 cup shredded sharp cheddar cheese (omit for dairy-free)

Sliced green onions, for garnish

Chopped fresh parsley, for garnish

Cherry tomatoes, halved or quartered, depending on size, for garnish

1. Preheat the oven to 375°F. Grease an 11 by 7-inch casserole dish with ghee.

2. Melt 1 tablespoon of ghee in a small skillet over medium-high heat. Add the celery and onions and sauté for 2 to 3 minutes, until the onions are translucent. Add the garlic and sauté for another minute. Move the vegetables to a medium-sized mixing bowl. Add the tuna, cauliflower, pickles, cream cheese, mayonnaise, salt, and pepper to the vegetables and mix to combine.

3. Spoon the tuna mixture into the greased casserole dish. Sprinkle with the cheddar cheese, if using. Bake for 20 minutes or until the cauliflower is tender and the casserole is lightly browned on top. Remove from the oven and allow to stand for 5 minutes. Serve garnished with green onions, parsley, and cherry tomatoes.

4. This dish is best served fresh, but any leftovers can be stored in an airtight container in the refrigerator for up to 3 days. Reheat in a baking dish in a preheated 350°F oven for 3 minutes or until warmed through.

nutritional info (per serving)				
calories	fat	protein	carbs	fiber
344	22g	31g	3g	1g

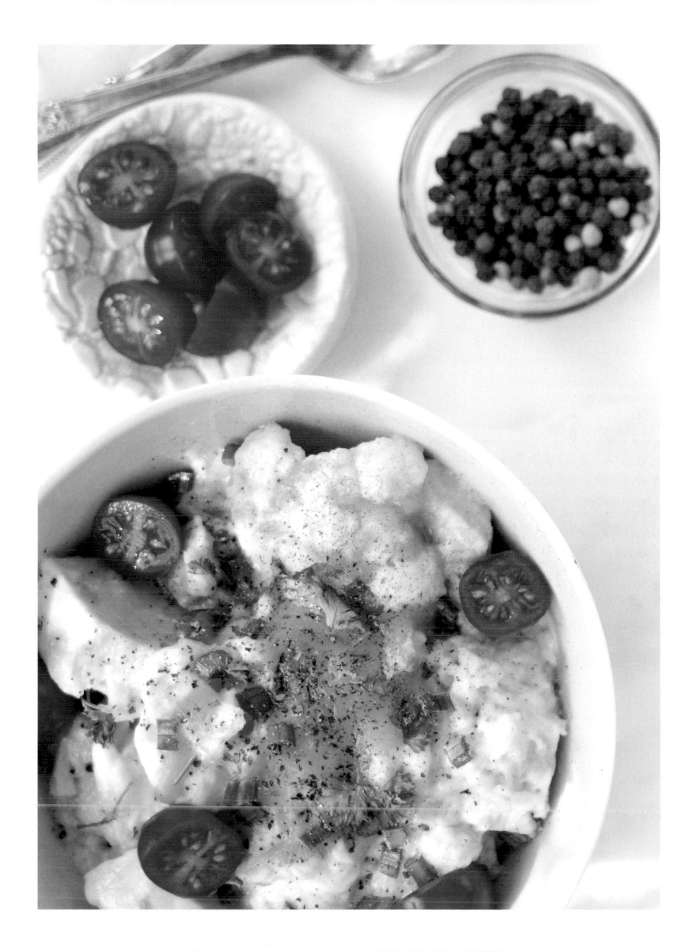

Charleston Shrimp 'n' Gravy Over Grits

L M H
KETO ✖ ✖

prep time: 5 minutes (not including time to make grits)
cook time: 15 minutes   yield: 4 servings

3 strips bacon

2 tablespoons ghee or unsalted butter

1 green bell pepper, chopped

½ cup diced onions

1 clove garlic, smashed to a paste or minced

1 pound large shrimp (about 30), peeled and deveined

2 teaspoons fine sea salt

½ teaspoon ground black pepper

½ cup chicken bone broth, homemade (page 356) or store-bought

Double batch Keto Grits (page 361), for serving

1. Fry the bacon in a cast-iron skillet over medium-high heat until crisp, about 4 minutes. Remove from the skillet and set aside. Leave the drippings in the pan.

2. Add the ghee to the skillet with the bacon drippings and reduce the heat to medium. Add the bell pepper and onions and sauté for 5 minutes or until the onions are soft. Add the garlic and cook for another minute.

3. Season the shrimp with the salt and pepper. Add the shrimp to the skillet, increase the heat to medium-high, and sauté, stirring constantly, for about 4 minutes, until the shrimp are no longer translucent. Using a slotted spoon, remove the shrimp to a warm plate and set aside.

4. Add the broth to the skillet, still over medium-high heat, and whisk the bottom of the skillet to deglaze. Boil the broth until it is thickened to your liking, then remove the skillet from the heat, add the shrimp to the sauce, and stir to coat. Serve the shrimp over keto grits, with the bacon crumbled on top.

5. Store extras in an airtight container in the refrigerator for up to 3 days. Reheat in a lightly greased skillet over medium heat until warmed through.

nutritional info (per serving)				
calories	fat	protein	carbs	fiber
500	34g	41g	5g	1g

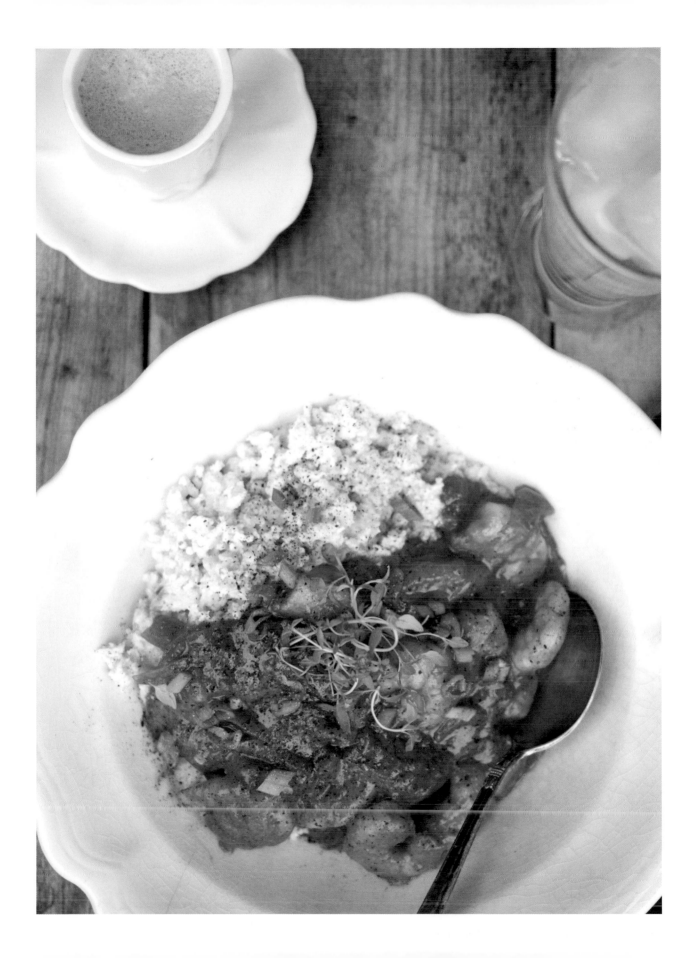

Seafood Risotto

L M H KETO ✖ ✖

1 medium head cauliflower, cored and separated into florets

2 tablespoons ghee, unsalted butter, or coconut oil

2 tablespoons diced onions

1 clove garlic, finely chopped

4 ounces mascarpone or cream cheese (½ cup)

Fine sea salt and ground black pepper

½ cup chicken bone broth, homemade (page 356) or store-bought

¼ cup grated Parmesan cheese

2 cups cooked whole shrimp or cooked crab or langostino pieces

prep time: 10 minutes (not including time to cook shrimp)
cook time: 7 minutes   *yield:* 4 servings

1. To make the "rice," place the cauliflower florets in a food processor and pulse until the cauliflower is rice-sized; set aside.

2. Heat the ghee in a cast-iron skillet over medium heat. When hot, add the onions and garlic and sauté for 2 minutes, stirring often. Add the cauliflower rice and mascarpone and season with a couple of pinches each of salt and pepper. Whisk and cook the mixture until the mascarpone is soft, about 1 minute.

3. Add the broth slowly, while whisking. Cook for 4 minutes or until the "rice" is soft.

4. Add the Parmesan cheese and cooked shrimp and stir to combine; cook for a minute or two to heat through, then season to taste with salt and pepper, if needed, and serve.

5. Store extras in an airtight container in the refrigerator for up to 3 days. Reheat in a lightly greased skillet over medium heat until warmed through.

nutritional info (per serving)				
calories	fat	protein	carbs	fiber
368	24g	29g	9g	4g

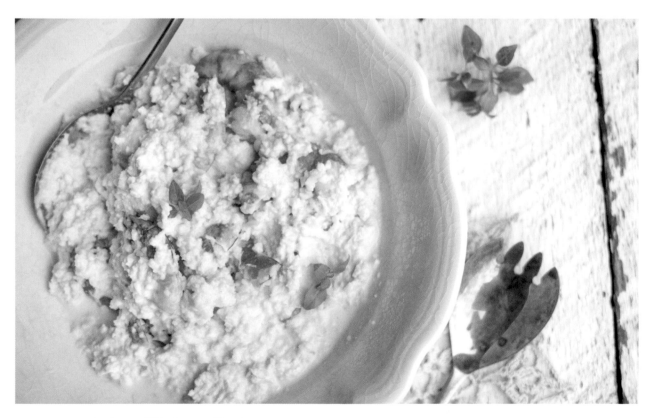

Surf and Turf for Two

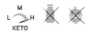

2 (3-ounce) filet mignons

Fine sea salt and ground black pepper

2 jumbo prawns or jumbo shrimp, shell-on, butterflied and deveined

2 tablespoons keto fat of choice, for frying

¼ cup Easy Basil Hollandaise (page 358), for serving

160°F+	Well-done
150°F-155°F	Medium-well
140°F-145°F	Medium
130°F-135°F	Medium-rare
120°F-125°F	Rare

nutritional info (per serving)				
calories	fat	protein	carbs	fiber
526	49g	19g	0.4g	0g

1. Season the filets well on all sides with salt and pepper. Let sit at room temperature for 15 minutes.

2. Heat a cast-iron skillet over medium-high heat. Season the prawns well with salt and pepper.

3. Melt the fat in the hot pan, then add the filets and sear on both sides until cooked to your desired doneness (see chart below).

4. Remove the filets from the skillet and allow them to rest for 10 minutes. While the filets are resting, fry the prawns in the same skillet until the shells have turned pink and the meat is cooked through and no longer translucent, about 3 minutes per side.

5. Place each steak on a plate. Top with a prawn and drizzle each plate with 2 tablespoons of the hollandaise. This dish is best served fresh.

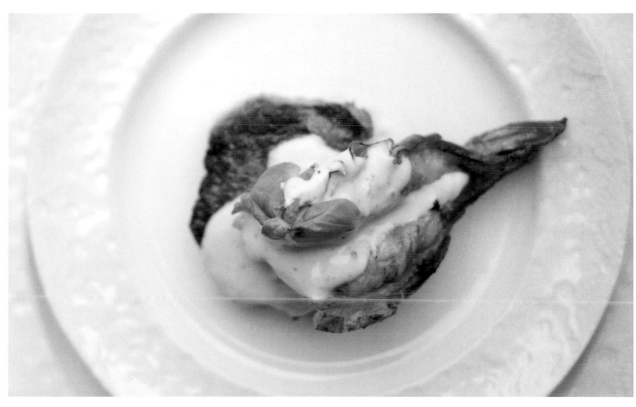

Crawfish Étouffée

The name *étouffée* refers to "smothering" seafood with a heavy sauce. I swapped out the traditional white rice for cauliflower rice to make this very-low-carb yet super-tasty Crawfish Étouffée. You can also omit the rice or serve the étouffée over Keto Grits (page 361).

I purchased frozen crawfish from the freezer section of my local grocery store in the middle of winter in Wisconsin. If you have a hard time finding crawfish, you can ask your market to carry it for you. Usually markets will stock products that you ask for in order to keep your business.

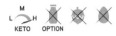

3 tablespoons ghee or unsalted butter (or coconut oil if dairy-free)

3 strips bacon, chopped

½ cup chopped onions

½ green or red bell pepper, chopped

3 cloves garlic, smashed to a paste or minced

¼ cup diced tomatoes

2 bay leaves

1 teaspoon chopped fresh thyme leaves

1 teaspoon paprika

¼ teaspoon cayenne pepper

¼ teaspoon fine sea salt

¼ teaspoon ground black pepper

1 cup chicken bone broth, homemade (page 356) or store-bought

1½ pounds peeled frozen crawfish tails, defrosted

1 to 2 tablespoons sour cream (or Kite Hill brand cream cheese style spread if dairy-free) (helps thicken the sauce)

2 teaspoons hot sauce, or more to taste

Chopped fresh parsley leaves, for garnish

Sliced green onions, for garnish

½ batch Cauliflower Rice (page 362), for serving

Lemon wedges, for serving (optional)

prep time: 10 minutes (not including time to make cauliflower rice)
cook time: 25 minutes *yield:* 4 servings

1. Melt the ghee in a Dutch oven over medium-high heat. When hot, add the bacon and sauté until crisp. Add the onions and bell pepper and sauté for 4 minutes or until soft. Add the garlic and sauté for another minute.

2. Stir in the tomatoes, bay leaves, thyme, paprika, cayenne, salt, and black pepper and cook for 2 minutes. Add the broth and boil until the liquid has reduced a bit, about 10 minutes. Add the crawfish tails to the broth mixture and cook for 10 minutes or until the crawfish are cooked through. Stir in the sour cream and hot sauce and heat through.

3. Transfer the étouffée to a serving dish and garnish with parsley and green onions. Serve over cauliflower rice with lemon wedges, if desired.

4. This dish is best served fresh, but any extras can be stored in an airtight container in the refrigerator for up to 3 days. Reheat in a skillet over medium heat for 3 minutes or until warmed through.

nutritional info (per serving)				
calories	fat	protein	carbs	fiber
372	21g	36g	7g	2g

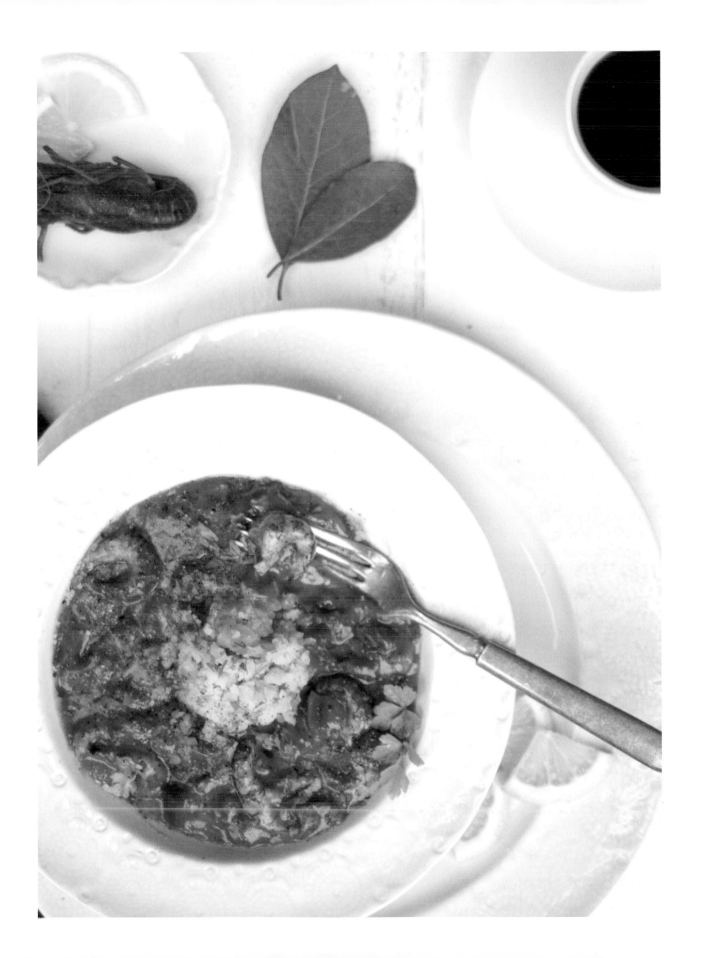

Halibut Smothered
in Creamy Lemon-Dill Sauce

prep time: 5 minutes   *cook time:* 12 minutes   *yield:* 4 servings

4 (4-ounce) halibut fillets

1 teaspoon fine sea salt

¼ teaspoon ground black pepper

2 tablespoons ghee or unsalted butter (or coconut oil if dairy-free), divided

½ cup finely diced red onions

1 clove garlic, smashed to a paste

2 to 3 sprigs fresh dill, plus extra for garnish

¼ cup fish or chicken bone broth, homemade (page 356) or store-bought

¼ cup heavy cream (or full-fat coconut milk if dairy-free)

2 outer leaves of red cabbage, for color (optional)

½ teaspoon lemon juice

Lemon wedges, for garnish

Purple salt, for garnish (optional)

1. Season the fish with the salt and pepper. Melt 1 tablespoon of the ghee in a cast-iron skillet over medium heat. Add the onions and garlic and sauté for 2 minutes. Place the fish in the skillet and top with the dill. Pour the broth and cream into the skillet around the fish. Add the cabbage, if using. Simmer, uncovered, until the fish is no longer translucent in the center and flakes easily, about 10 minutes per inch of thickness. (The exact cook time will depend on how thick the fillets are.) Stir in the lemon juice.

2. Remove the fish to a serving platter; discard the cabbage leaves and sprigs of dill. If you prefer a thicker sauce, boil the sauce for 10 minutes or until thickened to your liking.

3. Cover the fish with the sauce and serve garnished with lemon wedges, more fresh dill, and a sprinkle of purple salt, if desired.

4. Store extras in an airtight container in the refrigerator for up to 3 days. Reheat in a lightly greased skillet over medium heat until warmed through.

nutritional info (per serving)				
calories	*fat*	*protein*	*carbs*	*fiber*
270	17g	24g	4g	1g

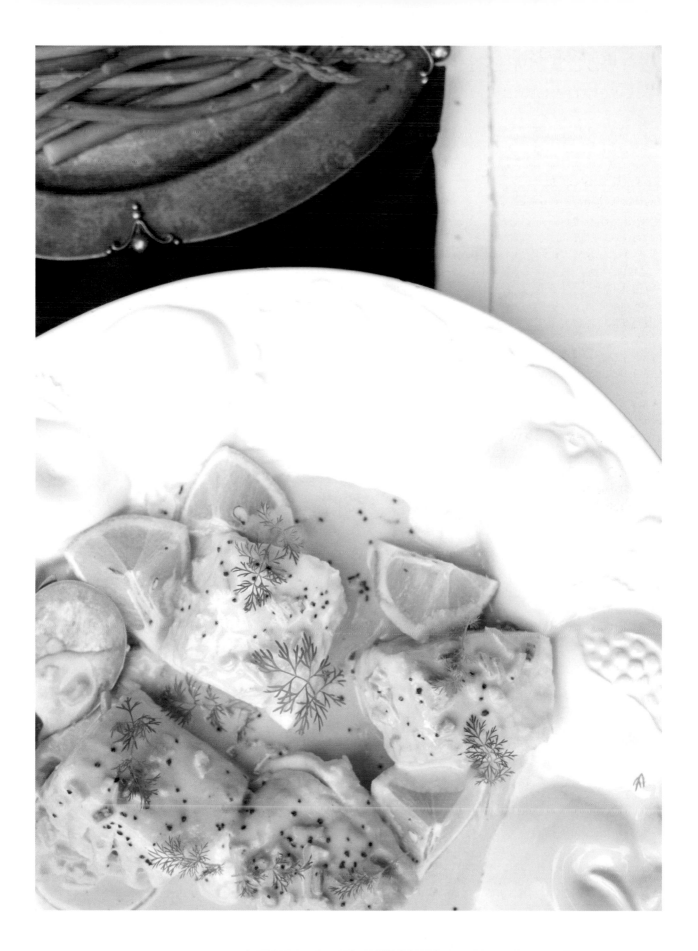

Sole Meunière

One of my favorite scenes in the movie *Julie and Julia* is when Julia Child arrives in France and has her first meal of sole meunière, a dish of pan-fried fish bathed in a beautiful butter sauce. She swoons over how lovely the fish is and how much butter the fish is in. It is enough to make even someone who doesn't like fish a fan!

L M H KETO ✕ ✕

4 (4-ounce) sole fillets

Ground black pepper

½ cup powdered Parmesan cheese (see page 13)

2 tablespoons ghee or avocado oil

¼ cup plus 2 tablespoons unsalted butter, divided

1 tablespoon lemon juice

2 tablespoons chopped fresh parsley leaves

Lemon wedges or slices, for serving

prep time: 5 minutes *cook time:* 6 minutes *yield:* 4 servings

1. Rinse the fish and pat it dry. Lightly sprinkle both sides of the fish with pepper.

2. Place the Parmesan cheese in a pie pan. Dredge each fillet on both sides in the Parmesan and set aside on a plate next to the stove.

3. Heat the ghee in a large skillet over medium-high heat. When it is hot and shimmering, add 2 tablespoons of the butter and quickly swirl the skillet to coat the bottom with butter. Once the butter is hot, add the coated fish. Do not move the fillets for 2 minutes. After 2 minutes, gently flip the fish and cook for another 2 minutes, until the fish is cooked through and no longer translucent in the middle. Place the fish on a serving platter and pour the skillet drippings over the fish.

4. Add the remaining ¼ cup of butter to the skillet, still over medium-high heat. Heat, whisking often, until the butter foams up and brown (but not black!) flecks appear, about 2 minutes. Remove the pan from the heat, add the lemon juice and parsley to the browned butter, and stir well. Pour the sauce over the fish. Serve with lemon wedges or slices.

5. Store extras in an airtight container in the refrigerator for up to 3 days. Reheat the fish in a lightly greased skillet over medium heat until warmed through.

nutritional info (per serving)				
calories	fat	protein	carbs	fiber
383	31g	28g	1g	0.2g

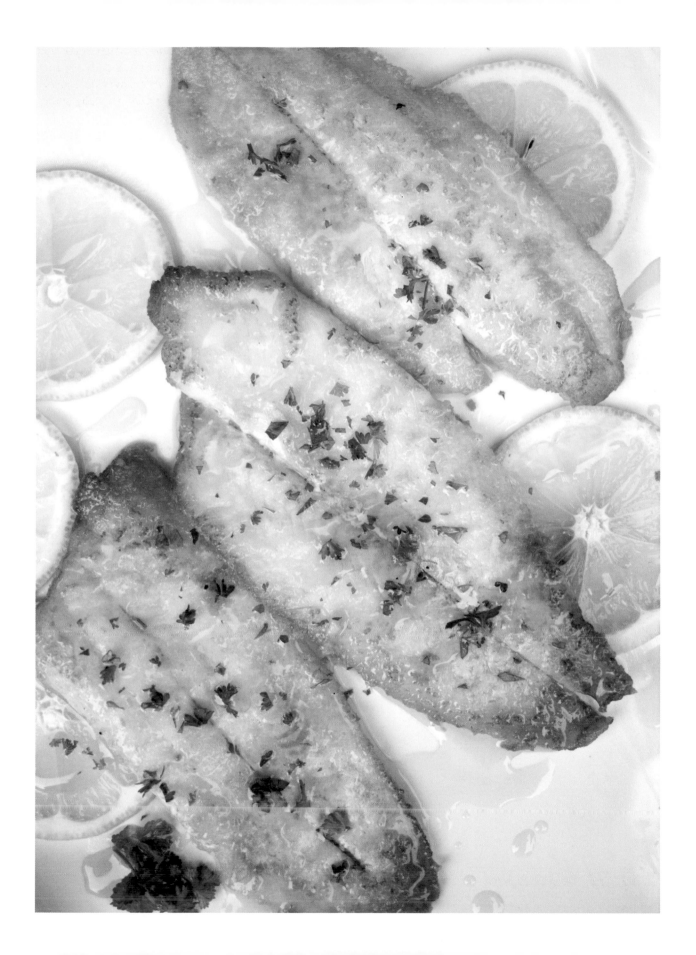

Creole Catfish

KETO   OPTION

prep time: 5 minutes   *cook time:* 15 minutes   *yield:* 4 servings

2 tablespoons ghee (or coconut oil if dairy-free)

¼ cup diced onions

1 clove garlic, smashed to a paste

1 (18.3-ounce) jar crushed tomatoes, with juices

1 teaspoon fine sea salt

½ teaspoon garlic powder

½ teaspoon onion powder

½ teaspoon dried oregano leaves

Pinch of pure stevia powder (optional)

⅛ teaspoon hot sauce, or more to taste

1 pound catfish fillets, cut into 1-inch-wide pieces

Fine sea salt and ground black pepper

1 batch Cauliflower Rice (page 362), or double batch Keto Grits (page 361), for serving (optional)

1. In a medium-sized saucepan, melt the ghee over medium heat. Add the onions and sauté for 2 minutes or until soft. Add the garlic and sauté for another minute. Add the tomatoes (with juices), salt, garlic powder, onion powder, oregano, stevia powder (if using), and hot sauce. Bring to a boil, then stir in the catfish pieces.

2. Cover the pan and cook for 5 to 8 minutes, until the fish flakes and is cooked all the way through. Taste and add more salt and pepper, if desired.

3. Serve the fish mixture over cauliflower rice or grits, if desired. Store extras in an airtight container in the refrigerator for up to 3 days. Reheat the fish in a lightly greased skillet over medium heat until warmed through.

nutritional info (per serving)				
calories	*fat*	*protein*	*carbs*	*fiber*
210	11g	19g	10g	3g

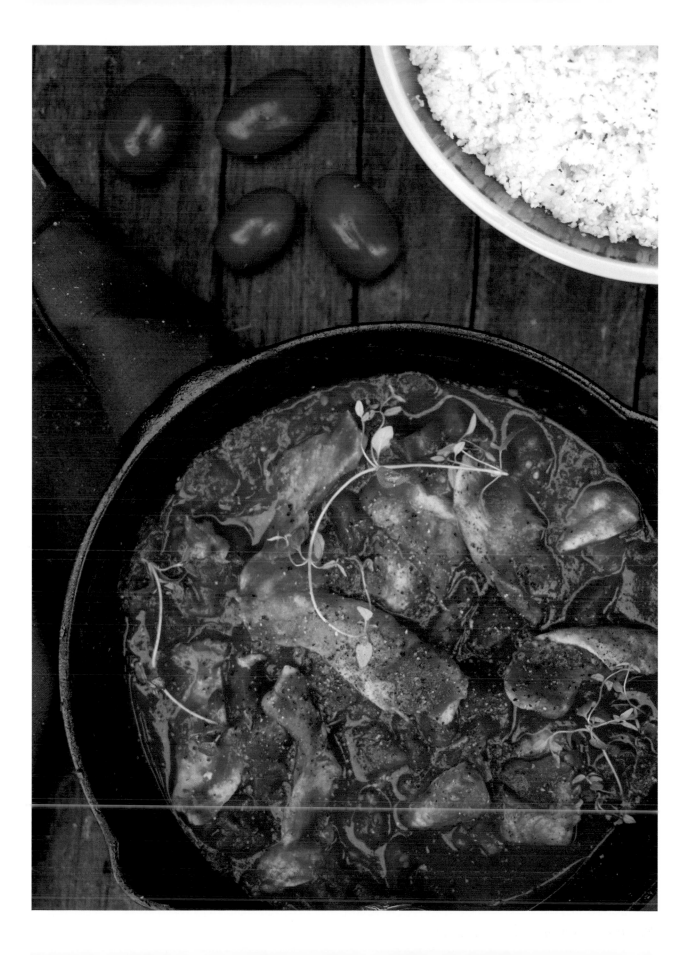

Butter-Poached Lobster Tails Over Creamy Keto Risotto

Beurre monte is a thick, creamy, decadent butter sauce that is wonderful for poaching meats, low-carb vegetables, and seafood such as lobster. It is super-easy to make, but it's very delicate. If you heat it above 160°F, it will break and the butter will separate. Don't be nervous about trying your hand at this sauce, though; just take it slow. You will not be disappointed!

You can make the beurre monte up to an hour ahead and keep it warm on the stove until you're ready to use it. You can also make the keto risotto after you poach the lobster tails, using the leftover beurre monte in place of the ghee or butter in the risotto for extra lobster-infused flavor.

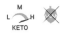

2 lobster tails

creamy keto risotto

4 large eggs

¼ cup beef bone broth, homemade (page 356) or store-bought

½ teaspoon fine sea salt

¼ cup ghee or unsalted butter

¼ cup grated Parmesan cheese

beurre monte

¾ cup to 1½ cups (1½ to 3 sticks) unsalted butter

prep time: 5 minutes *cook time:* 10 minutes *yield:* 2 servings

1. Remove the lobster tails from the refrigerator and allow them to come to room temperature. Using a pair of kitchen shears, cut down the middle of the shell on the underside (concave side) of the tail. Pull the shell open along the sides to expose the meat, avoiding the spines (they can be sharp). Gently wriggle the meat from the shell.

2. To make the risotto, whisk together the eggs, broth, and salt in a small bowl. In a medium-sized saucepan, melt the ghee over medium heat. Add the egg mixture to the pan and cook until the mixture thickens and small curds form, scraping the bottom of the pan and stirring to keep large curds from forming. (A whisk works well for this task.)

3. Add the Parmesan cheese to the risotto and stir until well combined. Remove from the heat and transfer the risotto to a serving bowl.

4. To find out how much butter you will need for poaching, place the peeled lobster tails in a pot just large enough to fit them snugly. Add water to just cover the tails. Remove the tails and set aside. Measure the water in the pan—that is the amount of butter you will need for poaching (see notes). Cut that amount of butter into ½-inch cubes.

5. To make the beurre monte, place 1 tablespoon of water in the pot and bring it to a boil over high heat. Reduce the heat to low and add a few chunks of the butter while whisking to emulsify; keep whisking or the butter will break. Once the emulsion has started, you can add the butter faster without it breaking. Using a thermometer to monitor the temperature, hold the temperature of the beurre monte at 160°F for poaching. If it gets too hot, the butter will break (but the sauce will still taste good). The sauce should have a thick, creamy consistency.

6. Place the lobster tails in the pot (making sure they aren't too cold) and poach for 5 to 7 minutes, depending on how large the tails are. They are cooked when the meat has turned white and has a soft consistency; if you overcook them, the meat will be rubbery. Serve the lobster over the risotto with 2 tablespoons of the beurre monte per serving.

7. This dish is best served fresh, but any extras can be stored in an airtight container in the refrigerator for up to 3 days. To reheat, gently warm the beurre monte in a saucepan over medium-low heat, then add the lobster and heat until warmed through.

nutritional info (per serving)				
calories	fat	protein	carbs	fiber
775	69g	38g	1g	0g

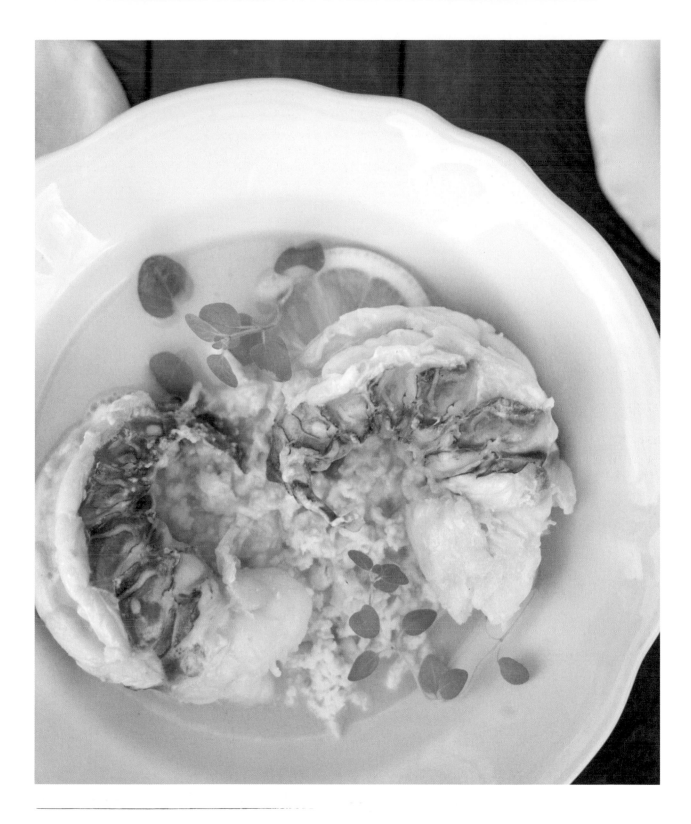

notes: Do not forget to remove the shells from the lobster tails. In my first attempt at poaching lobster, I didn't remove the shells and the lobster didn't poach like it should have . . . an expensive mistake!

This recipe uses a lot of butter, but the leftover poaching sauce is great over cauliflower rice, vegetable noodles, or fish.

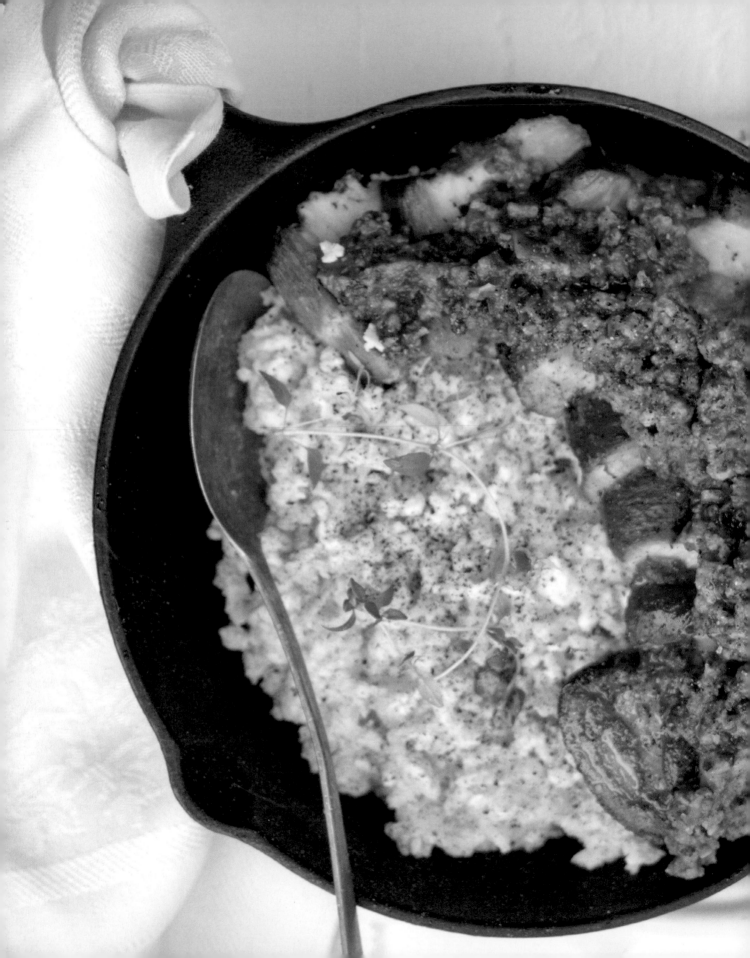

main dishes
Pork

BBQ Pulled Pork Sandwiches with
Wilted Bacon Slaw

This recipe yields a lot of meat, but the leftover pulled pork makes great BBQ Pulled Pork Hash with Eggs (page 74).

prep time: 15 minutes (not including time to make buns) *cook time:* 8 hours *yield:* 12 servings

BBQ pulled pork

1 (6-pound) boneless pork shoulder roast

2 cups tomato sauce

¼ cup diced onions

8 cloves garlic, minced

¼ cup Swerve confectioners'-style sweetener or equivalent amount of liquid or powdered sweetener (see page 24) (optional)

2 tablespoons coconut vinegar or apple cider vinegar

2 teaspoons liquid smoke

2 teaspoons fine sea salt

1 teaspoon ground black pepper

wilted bacon coleslaw

2 cups shredded green and/or red cabbage

2 strips bacon, cut into small dice

2 tablespoons avocado oil (or melted ghee if not dairy-sensitive)

1½ tablespoons coconut vinegar or apple cider vinegar

2 teaspoons Swerve confectioners'-style sweetener or equivalent amount of liquid or powdered sweetener (see page 24)

Fine sea salt and ground black pepper

Double batch round Keto Buns (page 362)

1. To make the pulled pork, place the pork roast in a slow cooker. In a bowl, combine the rest of the ingredients for the pork. Pour the mixture over the roast in the slow cooker. Cover and cook on low for 8 hours or until the meat shreds easily with 2 forks.

2. When the meat is nearly done, make the coleslaw: Place the cabbage in a large bowl and set aside. In a large sauté pan, cook the bacon slowly over medium heat until it is browned and crispy, 8 to 10 minutes. Add the oil, vinegar, and sweetener, if using, to the pan and bring to a boil, then remove the pan from the heat. Pour the hot dressing over the cabbage, tossing to wilt the cabbage and coat it with the dressing. Season the coleslaw with salt and pepper to taste.

3. Assemble the sandwiches and serve hot. Store leftover pulled pork and coleslaw in separate airtight containers in the refrigerator for up to 3 days. Leftover pork can be frozen for up to a month. Reheat the pork on a rimmed baking sheet in a preheated 350°F oven for 5 minutes or until warmed through.

nutritional info (per serving)				
calories	fat	protein	carbs	fiber
645	47g	45g	5g	1g

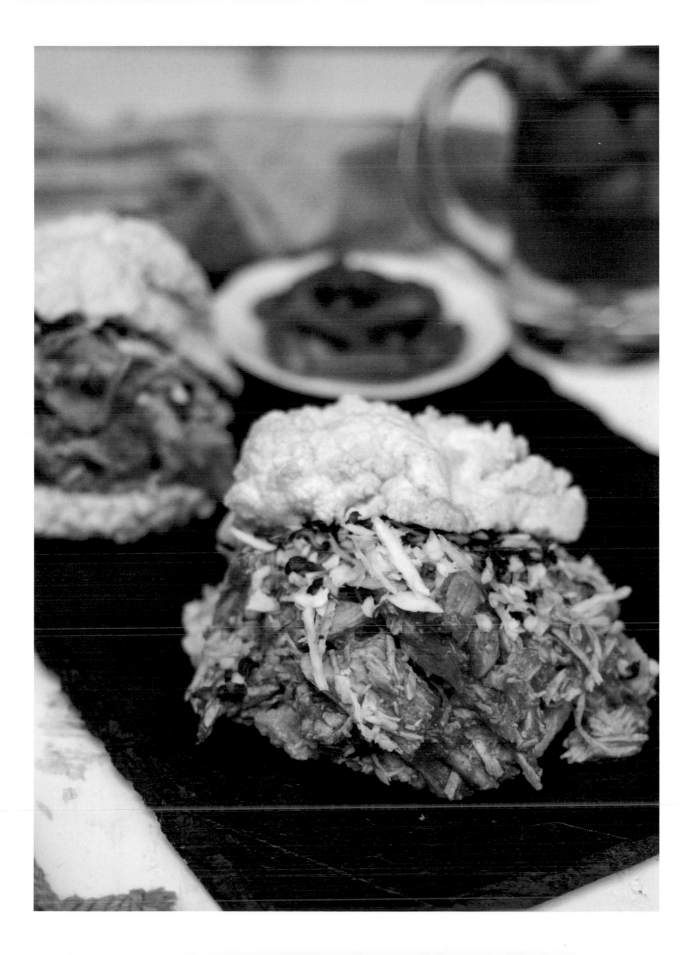

Saucy Stuffed Cabbage Rolls

KETO · OPTION

When I was growing up, my mom often made stuffed cabbage rolls with rice. Instead of rice, I add a few eggs. When scrambled into small pieces as they cook, eggs resemble rice. I think cabbage rolls taste even better this way!

1 large head green cabbage

2 tablespoons ghee (or coconut oil if dairy-free)

1 cup finely chopped onions

1 clove garlic, minced

1 pound ground pork

2 large eggs, beaten

2 tablespoons paprika

1 teaspoon fine sea salt

½ teaspoon ground black pepper

¼ teaspoon dried ground marjoram

2 cups sauerkraut

2 cups tomato sauce

1 cup sour cream (omit for dairy-free)

prep time: 10 minutes   *cook time:* 30 minutes   *yield:* 8 servings

1. Preheat the oven to 375°F.

2. In a stockpot, bring to a boil enough salted water to cover the head of cabbage. Add the cabbage, reduce the heat to low, and simmer for 8 minutes or until the leaves are soft and easily bendable. Remove the cabbage from the pot and let it drain and cool. When it is cool enough to handle, pull off 16 large leaves and lay them on paper towels to dry.

3. Melt the ghee in a large skillet over medium heat, then add the onions and garlic and sauté until the onions are lightly colored. Add the ground pork, beaten eggs, paprika, salt, pepper, and marjoram and sauté until cooked through, stirring to crumble the pork and break up the eggs into small pieces. Remove the skillet from the heat.

4. Place 2 tablespoons of the pork mixture in the center of a soft cabbage leaf and, beginning with the thick end of the leaf, fold over the sides, then roll the whole leaf tightly, as you would a small burrito. Repeat until all the stuffing has been used.

5. Spread the sauerkraut in a 5-quart casserole dish and arrange the cabbage rolls on top of it.

6. Mix together the tomato sauce and sour cream, if using, and use it to cover the cabbage rolls. Bake the rolls for 20 minutes or until hot and bubbly.

7. Store extras in an airtight container in the refrigerator for up to 3 days. Reheat on a rimmed baking sheet in a preheated 350°F oven for 5 minutes or until warmed through.

nutritional info (per serving)				
calories	fat	protein	carbs	fiber
317	23g	14g	14g	5g

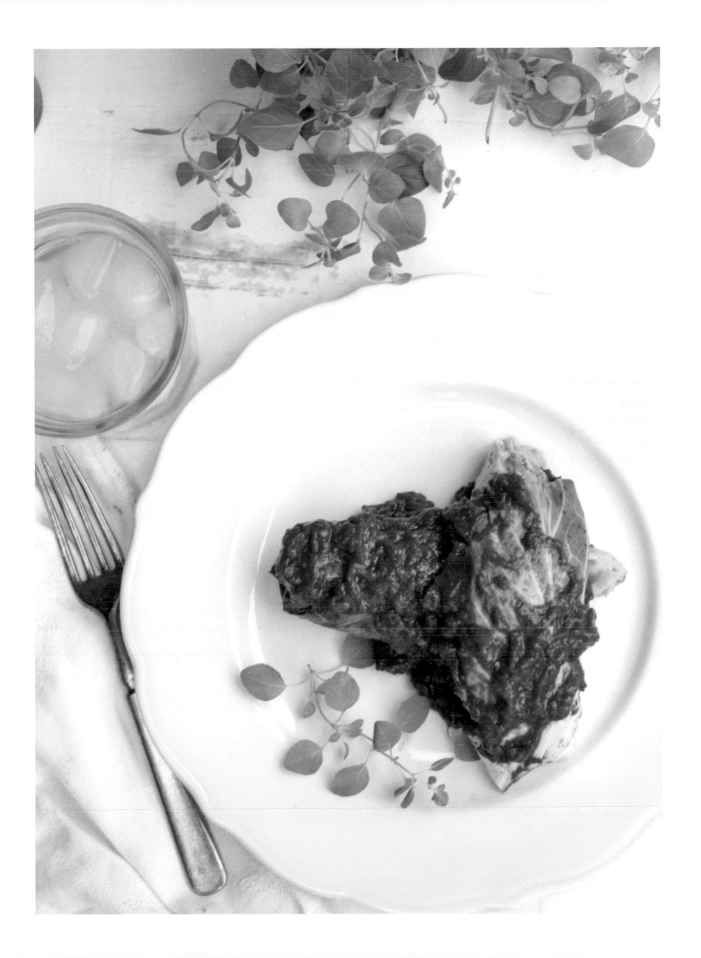

Schnitzel

I am a true German girl, and I was lucky enough to travel to Germany with Craig when he and I were first married. I dined on schnitzel almost every day! There's nothing like sitting among the people of Fussen on long picnic tables overlooking a beautiful lake, with mountains in the background.

When schnitzel is made with pork cutlets, it's called Schweine Schnitzel; when made with veal cutlets, it's called Wiener Schnitzel. This recipe works with either type of meat.

4 boneless pork chops or veal cutlets

Fine sea salt and ground black pepper

2 large eggs

¾ cup powdered Parmesan cheese (see page 13) (or pork dust if dairy-free)

¼ cup coconut oil or avocado oil, for frying, plus more if needed

for serving

1 lemon, sliced into wedges

Chopped fresh parsley

prep time: 7 minutes   *cook time:* 12 minutes   *yield:* 4 servings

1. Place the pork chops between 2 sheets of plastic wrap and pound them with the flat side of a meat tenderizer until they're ¼ inch thick. Lightly season both sides of the chops with salt and pepper.

2. Lightly beat the eggs in a shallow bowl. Divide the Parmesan cheese between 2 bowls so you can do a dry, wet, dry dipping of the chops.

3. Place a chop in the first bowl of Parmesan, then dip the chop in the eggs, and then in the second bowl of Parmesan, coating both sides and all edges. Repeat with the remaining chops.

4. Heat the oil to about 330°F in a large cast-iron skillet. When hot, add the schnitzel two at a time and fry for 2 to 3 minutes on each side, until deep golden brown. Transfer the schnitzel briefly to a plate lined with paper towels. Before making the second batch, add more oil if needed to maintain about ⅛ inch of oil in the skillet. Serve the schnitzel immediately with lemon wedges and sprinkled with parsley.

5. Store extras in an airtight container in the refrigerator for up to 3 days. Reheat on a rimmed baking sheet in a preheated 350°F oven for 5 minutes or until warmed through.

busy family tip:
Ask your butcher to tenderize and pound the chops thin so all you have to do is dip them in the breading and fry them for a tasty dinner!

nutritional info (per serving)				
calories	fat	protein	carbs	fiber
464	36g	37g	2g	0.5g

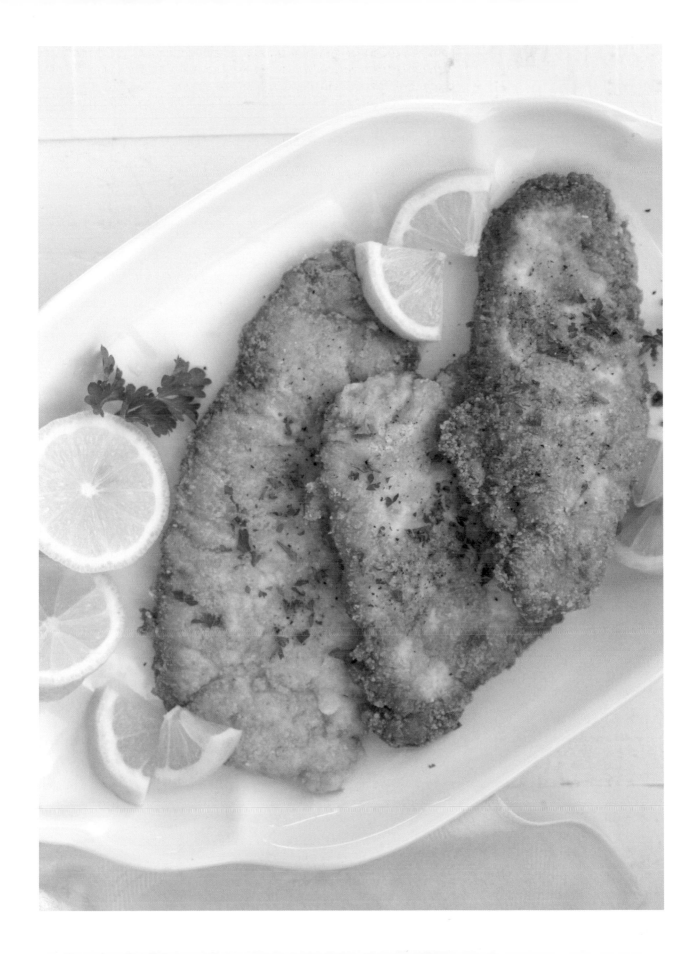

Smothered Pork Chops
in Mushroom and Onion Gravy

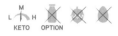

prep time: 10 minutes   *cook time:* 30 minutes   *yield:* 4 servings

4 tablespoons ghee, divided (or lard or coconut oil if dairy-free)

2 cups thinly sliced onions

2 cups chicken or beef bone broth, homemade (page 356) or store-bought

4 (8-ounce) bone-in pork loin chops

½ teaspoon fine sea salt

¼ teaspoon ground black pepper

2 cups sliced button mushrooms

1. To make the gravy, melt 2 tablespoons of the ghee in a large skillet over medium heat. Add the onions and sauté for 5 minutes, stirring occasionally. Add the broth and cook for 20 to 30 minutes, until the broth has reduced by almost half, then slide the skillet off the heat.

2. Meanwhile, sprinkle the pork chops with the salt and pepper. Melt the remaining 2 tablespoons of ghee in a large cast-iron skillet over medium-high heat. Add the mushrooms and sauté for 6 minutes or until brown. Season the mushrooms with salt and pepper to taste. Move the mushrooms to the skillet with the gravy, then place the chops in the hot cast-iron skillet. Sear on one side for 3 minutes, then flip and cook for another 7 to 10 minutes, until the internal temperature of the chops reaches 135°F (the temperature will rise after cooking). Let the chops rest for about 8 minutes before serving.

3. Place the chops on a serving platter and smother with the mushroom and onion gravy. Store extras in an airtight container in the refrigerator for up to 3 days. Reheat on a rimmed baking sheet in a preheated 350°F oven for 5 minutes or until warmed through.

nutritional info (per serving)				
calories	fat	protein	carbs	fiber
691	59g	30g	10g	2g

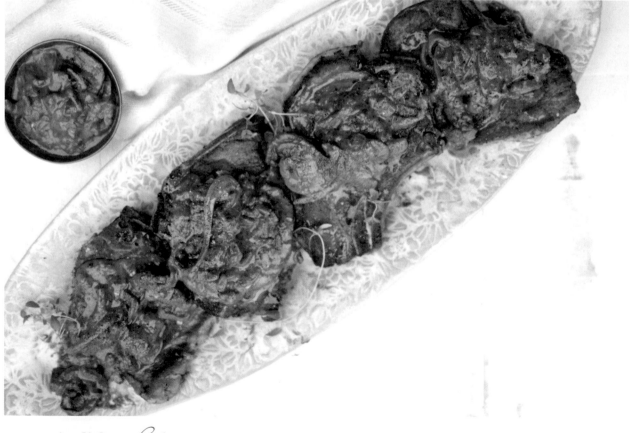

Ham 'n' Grits
with Redeye Gravy

prep time: 8 minutes (not including time to make grits)
cook time: 20 minutes *yield:* 2 servings

2 tablespoons ghee or unsalted butter, plus extra for serving

2 (½-inch-thick) ham steaks (about 1½ pounds total), cut into ½-inch cubes

¼ cup diced onions

½ cup brewed decaf coffee, or 1 shot decaf espresso diluted with ¼ cup water

1 batch Keto Grits (page 361), for serving

Sliced green onions, for garnish

1. Melt the ghee in a large cast-iron skillet over medium-high heat. Place the ham and onions in the pan and cook, stirring often, for 6 minutes or until the cubes of ham are brown and crispy. Remove the ham to a warm serving plate.

2. Pour the coffee into the skillet with the onions and, using a whisk, scrape up any browned bits from the bottom of the skillet. Cook for 10 minutes or until the gravy has reduced a bit and thickened.

3. Place the keto grits on a serving platter. Top them with the ham and gravy and garnish with green onions. Store extras in an airtight container in the refrigerator for up to 3 days. Reheat in a baking dish in a preheated 350°F oven for 5 minutes or until warmed through.

nutritional info (per serving)				
calories	fat	protein	carbs	fiber
454	38g	24g	4g	1g

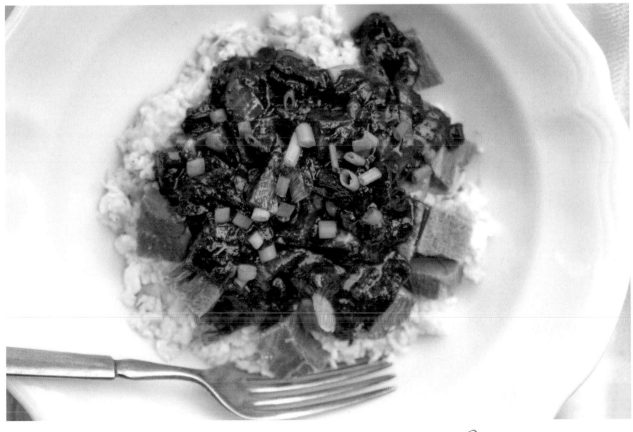

Pork and Cheddar Sausages

L M H
KETO ✗ ✗

2½ pounds pork butt

½ pound pork fat

½ cup coconut vinegar

6 feet medium hog casings

⅓ cup ice-cold beef or chicken bone broth, homemade (page 356) or store-bought

2 cups finely diced sharp cheddar cheese

¼ cup chopped green onions or 2 tablespoons dried chives

Cloves squeezed from 1 head roasted garlic, or 2 cloves raw garlic, smashed to paste

1 tablespoon fine sea salt

1 tablespoon lard or coconut oil, for the pan

Keto dipping sauce(s) of choice, such as stone-ground mustard, for serving (optional)

prep time: 20 minutes, plus 3 to 4 hours to chill meat, soak casings, and rest sausage
cook time: 10 minutes   *yield:* 12 sausages (1 per serving)

1. Line a rimmed baking sheet with parchment paper. Cut the pork butt and fat into 1-inch cubes and spread them out on the lined baking sheet. Freeze for 1 hour.

2. After the meat and fat have been in the freezer for 30 minutes, fill a large bowl with the coconut vinegar and 2 quarts of water. Place the casings in the liquid to soak for 30 minutes.

3. Remove the pork meat and fat from the freezer and grind it using the coarse disk of a meat grinder (I use my KitchenAid food grinder attachment). In a large bowl, place the ground pork butt and fat, broth, cheese, green onions, garlic, and salt; combine well using your hands. Cook up a small dab of the sausage mixture in a skillet over medium heat; taste the cooked sausage and add more salt to the raw sausage mixture, if desired. Place the bowl of sausage in the freezer for 30 minutes to chill and firm up before stuffing the casings.

4. Load a sausage stuffer (I use my KitchenAid sausage stuffer attachment) with the presoaked casings and stuff the casings by pushing the sausage mixture through the attachment. Twist the sausages into links about 5 inches in length. (*Note:* If you do not have a sausage stuffer, you can form the sausage mixture into 12 large patties instead.) Refrigerate the sausages for a few hours to allow the flavors to meld. Cook them within 3 days.

5. To cook the sausages, melt 1 tablespoon of lard or coconut oil in a large skillet over medium heat. Poke a few small holes in each sausage link. Sauté the sausages for 10 minutes or until their internal temperature reaches 160°F. Serve with keto dipping sauce, if desired. Once cooked, the sausages will keep in an airtight container in the refrigerator for up to 5 days. They can also be frozen for up to a month.

busy family tip:
Make a double batch of these sausages and freeze them for easy meals.

nutritional info (per sausage)				
calories	fat	protein	carbs	fiber
413	36g	21g	1g	0g

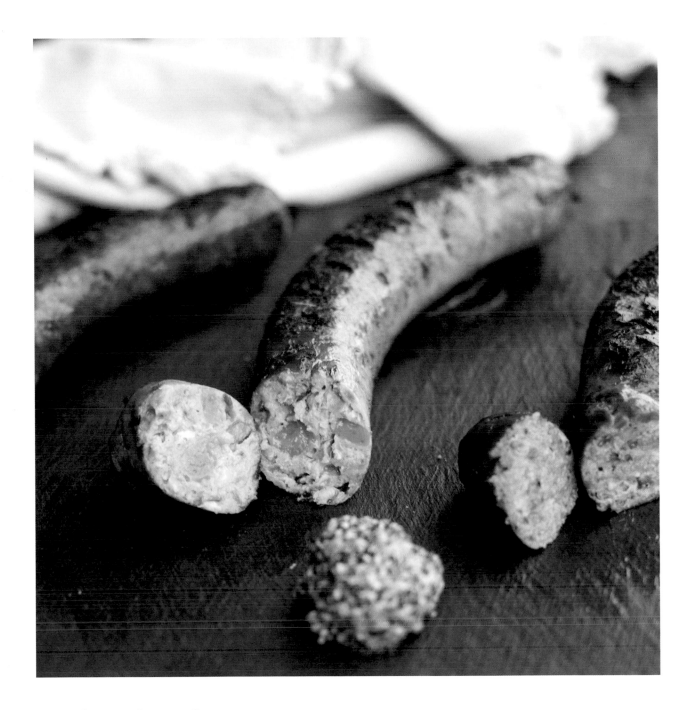

tips for making the best sausages:

Liquid is needed to bind protein to fat; the more liquid you add, the more fat you can add—to a point.

For great flavor and nutrients, I suggest using homemade bone broth as the liquid. However, good-quality store-bought broth will work, too.

Use cold meat and fat when making sausage. Cold meat won't turn mushy. Commercial sausage makers often add dry ice to the meat to keep it cold, but there's no need to go to that extreme. After cubing the meat, either place the cubes in the freezer for an hour, as directed, or place them in the refrigerator for 4 hours or overnight before grinding. After grinding and mixing the meat with the other ingredients, I place the bowl in the freezer for 30 minutes so that the meat mixture stays cold while stuffing.

If the sausage pops out of the casing when you bite into it, you cooked it too fast and at too high a temperature.

Bangers and Mash with Onion Gravy

KETO

4 (4-ounce) banger sausages

onion gravy

2 tablespoons unsalted butter

1 cup sliced onions

2 cups beef bone broth, homemade (page 356) or store-bought

1 teaspoon chopped fresh thyme or other herb of choice

Fine sea salt and ground black pepper

1 batch Mashed Fauxtatoes (page 129), for serving

When making this recipe, be sure to use all-natural sausages with natural casings. If you can't find bangers, this dish is equally good with just about any type of sausage. I love it with my Pork and Cheddar Sausages (page 266) or with bratwurst. If using brats, avoid brands made with corn syrup or other undesirable ingredients.

prep time: 8 minutes (not including time to make fauxtatoes)
cook time: 20 minutes *yield:* 4 servings

1. Preheat a grill or broiler to high heat.

2. Bring a pot of water to a boil. Add the sausages and boil for 8 minutes.

3. Meanwhile, make the onion gravy: Melt the butter in a skillet over medium-high heat. Add the onions and cook until translucent and just starting to brown, about 6 minutes. Add the broth and increase the heat to a boil. Boil for 10 minutes or until the liquid is reduced by half. Add the thyme and season with salt and pepper.

4. Place the boiled sausages on the grill or, if using the oven broiler, on a rimmed baking sheet and grill or broil for 1 to 2 minutes, until the outsides are charred to your liking.

5. To serve, place ½ cup of mashed fauxtatoes on each plate. Top with a sausage and cover with the onion gravy.

6. Store extras in an airtight container in the refrigerator for up to 3 days. Reheat the sausages on a rimmed baking sheet in a preheated 350°F oven for 5 minutes or until warmed through. Reheat the gravy in a small saucepan over medium heat until warmed.

busy family tip:
You can skip the step of browning the sausages on the grill or under the broiler. Once they are boiled, they are fully cooked, but I prefer the charred taste of grilled or broiled sausages.

nutritional info (per serving)				
calories	fat	protein	carbs	fiber
641	50g	33g	13g	5g

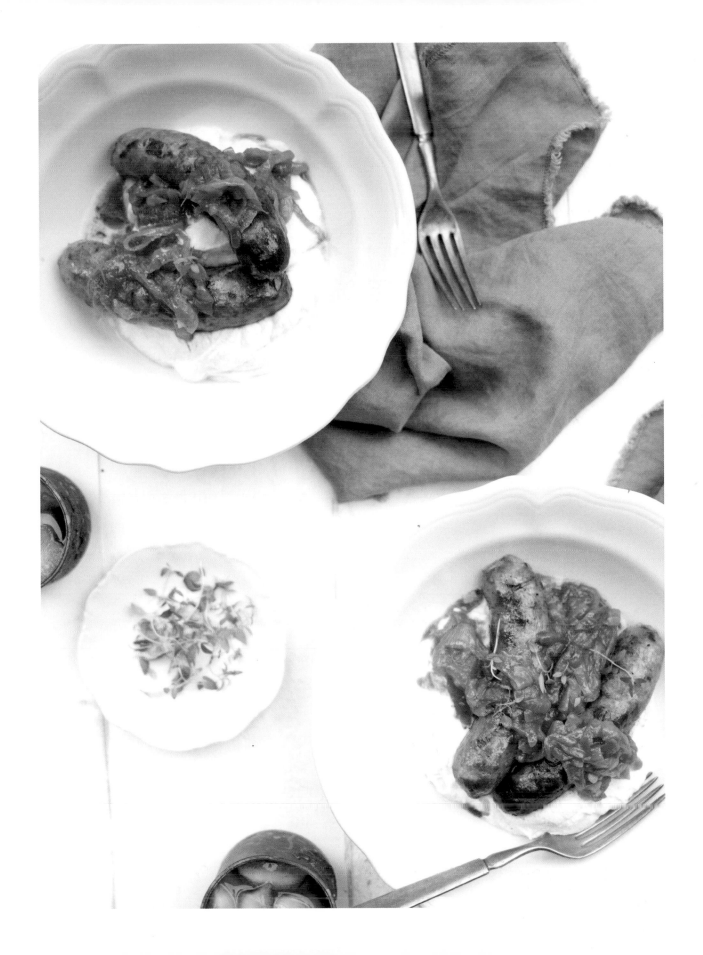

Crispy Pork Belly Over Grits
with Bacon Jam

prep time: 7 minutes (not including time to make grits) cook time: 40 minutes
yield: 4 servings

bacon jam

¼ pound bacon, cut into small dice

¼ cup diced onions

½ cup beef bone broth, homemade (page 356) or store-bought

pork belly

1 tablespoon ghee or coconut oil

1 (12-ounce) package fully cooked pork belly (see note)

1 batch Keto Grits (page 361), for serving

Chopped fresh herbs of choice, for garnish (optional)

1. To make the bacon jam, cook the bacon in a large cast-iron skillet over medium-high heat until crisp-tender, about 10 minutes. Add the onions and cook for about 5 more minutes. Add the broth and bring to a simmer, scraping the bits off the bottom of the pan. Increase the heat to high and boil, while stirring, until the liquid has evaporated and the jam has a spreadable texture, about 10 minutes. (*Note:* Once cool, the jam can be stored in a sealed jar in the refrigerator for up to 6 days.)

2. To make the pork belly, heat the ghee in a cast-iron skillet over medium-high heat. Place the slab of pork belly in the hot pan and sear on all sides for about 2 minutes per side, until crispy. Remove from the heat and cut into ½-inch-thick slices.

3. To serve, divide the grits among 4 plates or bowls and top with the pork belly. Cover the pork with the bacon jam and garnish with fresh herbs, if desired.

4. Store extras in an airtight container in the refrigerator for up to 3 days. Reheat on a rimmed baking sheet in a preheated 350°F oven for 5 minutes or until warmed through.

---

note: *Vacuum-sealed packages of fully cooked pork belly are available at Trader Joe's.*

nutritional info (per serving)				
calories	fat	protein	carbs	fiber
551	48g	27g	1g	0g

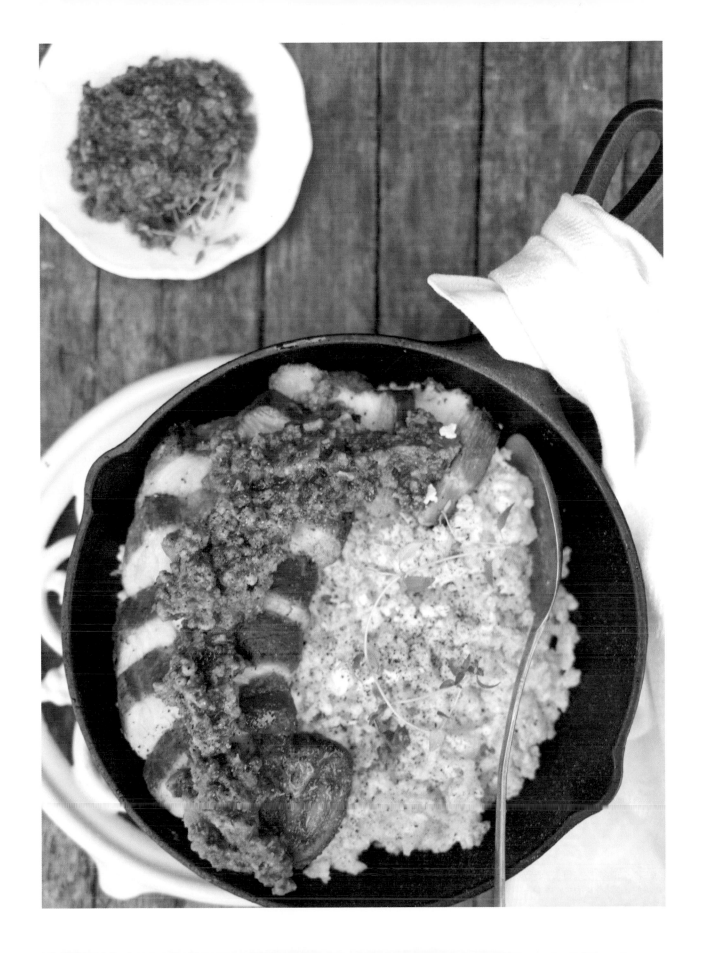

Creamy Cajun Pasta

prep time: 10 minutes (not including time to make zoodles)
cook time: 10 minutes *yield:* 4 servings

cajun seasoning

1 teaspoon smoked paprika

¾ teaspoon fine sea salt

½ teaspoon onion powder

½ teaspoon dried ground oregano

½ teaspoons dried ground thyme

¼ teaspoon ground black pepper

¼ teaspoon cayenne pepper

⅛ teaspoon red pepper flakes

½ pound boneless, skinless chicken thighs

2 tablespoons unsalted butter

1 red bell pepper, cut into ½-inch pieces

¼ cup diced red onions

2 teaspoons minced garlic

½ pound smoked sausage, cut into ½-inch slices

½ cup chicken bone broth, homemade (page 356) or store-bought

1½ cups heavy cream

¼ cup grated Parmesan cheese

½ teaspoon fine sea salt

½ batch Zoodles (page 363), for serving

1. In a small bowl, mix together the ingredients for the Cajun seasoning.

2. Cut the chicken thighs into 1-inch pieces. Coat the chicken pieces with 1 tablespoon of the Cajun seasoning.

3. Heat the butter in a cast-iron skillet over medium heat. Add the bell pepper, onions, and garlic and sauté until the pepper is soft and the onions are translucent, about 4 minutes. Add the seasoned chicken and sear on all sides until cooked through, about 3 minutes per side. Add the sausage and sear on both sides, about 1 minute per side.

4. Add the broth to the pan to deglaze it. Using a whisk, scrape the bits from the bottom of the pan to incorporate them into the sauce. Add the cream and Parmesan cheese and heat until simmering. Season with the salt and remaining Cajun seasoning. Simmer on low until thickened, about 3 minutes. Serve over zoodles.

5. Store extras in an airtight container in the refrigerator for up to 3 days. Reheat in a skillet over medium heat for 5 minutes or until warmed through.

nutritional info (per serving)				
calories	fat	protein	carbs	fiber
669	32g	64g	6g	2g

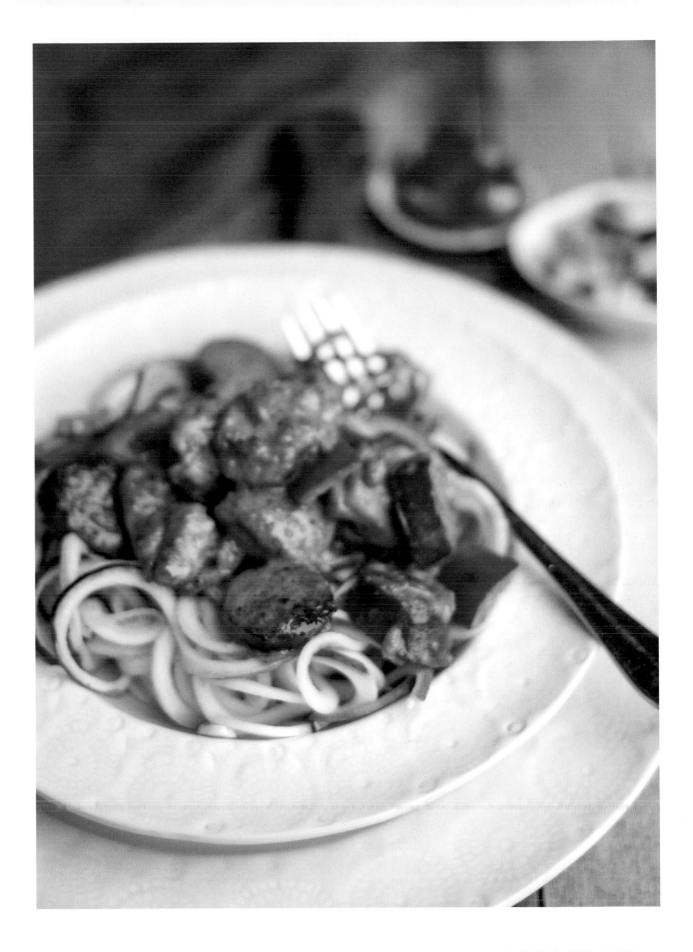

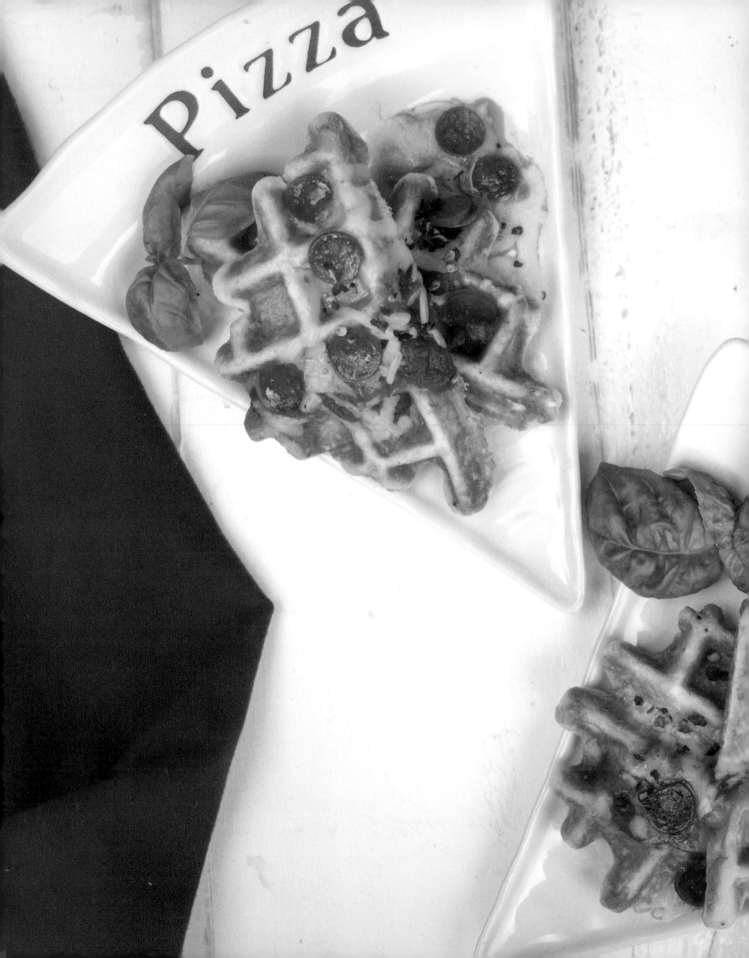

Comfort Food Favorites
for Grown-up Kids

Bomba Burgers

My husband asked me if I'd ever had a pizza burger, and I couldn't really remember. He told me that when he was a kid, pizza burger night was his favorite! He often rode his bike to the local A&W Root Beer stand and ordered a pizza burger with this best friend, Chad. This recipe is in honor of my love, Craig.

prep time: 10 minutes, plus 1 hour to chill dough, if needed
cook time: 16 minutes *yield:* 4 servings

pizza dough

1¾ cups shredded mozzarella cheese

2 tablespoons unsalted butter

1 large egg

¾ cup blanched almond flour

⅛ teaspoon fine sea salt

burgers

1 pound ground beef

Fine sea salt and ground black pepper

4 (½-ounce) slices mozzarella cheese

12 slices pepperoni

4 tablespoons pizza sauce, homemade (page 358) or store-bought, divided, plus extra for serving

1. To make the dough, place the mozzarella and butter in a microwave-safe bowl and microwave for 1 to 2 minutes, until the cheese is entirely melted. Stir well.

2. Add the egg and, using a hand mixer, combine well. Add the almond flour and salt and combine well with the mixer. Use your hands and work it like traditional dough, kneading for about 3 minutes. (*Note:* If the dough is too sticky, chill it in the refrigerator for an hour or overnight.)

3. Place a pizza stone, if using, in the cold oven and preheat the oven to 425°F.

4. Divide the ground beef into four 4-ounce portions, shape into patties, and sprinkle both sides with salt and pepper. In a large greased cast-iron skillet over medium heat, sauté the burgers for 3 to 4 minutes per side, until cooked medium-rare. Remove from the skillet and set aside.

5. Divide the pizza dough into four 4-ounce balls. Place each ball on its own piece of greased parchment paper and top with another piece of greased parchment. Using a rolling pin, roll out each ball into a 5-inch disc. Place 1 slice of cheese in the center, then top with 3 slices of pepperoni, a burger patty, and 1 tablespoon of pizza sauce. (*Note:* If the dough is too sticky to roll out, use your hands to form it around the burger. This dough is very forgiving and can easily be pasted together with your fingers.)

6. Fold the sides of the dough around the burger and seal it, as if you were making a large dumpling. Repeat with the rest of the dough circles and filling ingredients. Place on the hot pizza stone or a large baking sheet and bake for 8 minutes or until the dough is golden brown. Serve with pizza sauce on the side.

7. Store extras in an airtight container in the refrigerator for up to 3 days. Reheat on a rimmed baking sheet in a preheated 350°F oven for 5 minutes or until warmed through.

busy family tip:

I like to make large batches of this pizza dough to store in the refrigerator for up to 4 days or in the freezer for up to a month for easy meals such as these burgers. It also works great for pizza (see pages 226 and 228).

nutritional info (per burger)				
calories	fat	protein	carbs	fiber
689	56g	44g	5g	3g

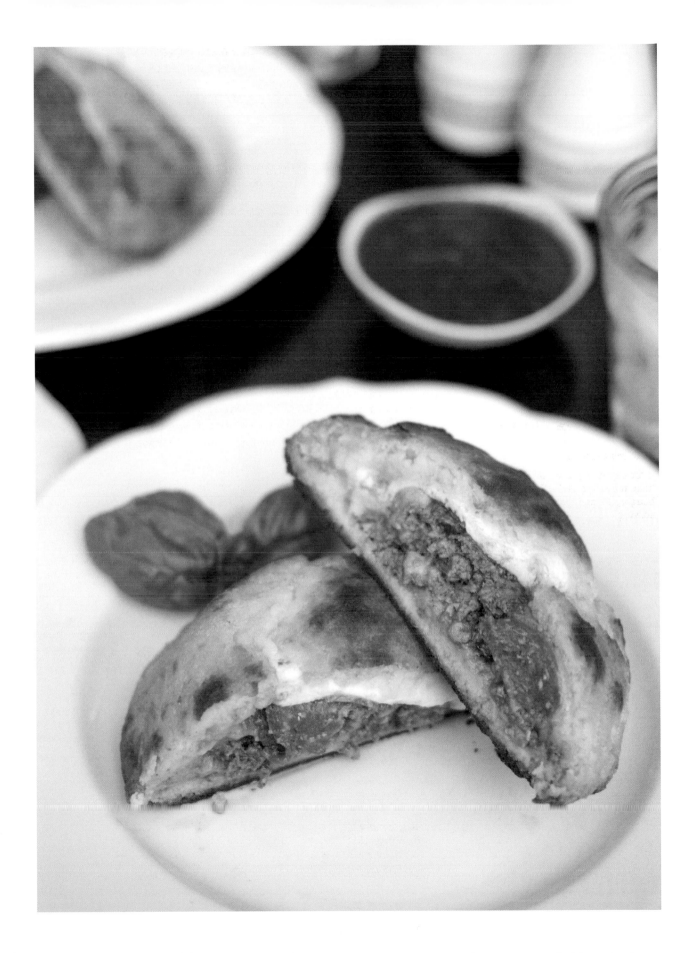

Hot Beef Sundaes

I know that a lot of you have tried mashed cauliflower fauxtatoes and think that the taste is good, but the texture just isn't the same as traditional mashed potatoes. I never really cared for the gritty fake potatoes, either—until we purchased a high-powered blender! We bought it to make pureed baby food, but it has been awesome for so many tasks, including making the smoothest fauxtatoes ever, like the ones used to top these sundaes. If you don't have a high-powered blender, never fear: you can still make the fauxtatoes with a food processor. They may not be as smooth, but they will be just as tasty.

prep time: 10 minutes *cook time:* 3 hours *yield:* 8 servings

hot beef layer

1 tablespoon ghee or coconut oil

1 (4-pound) boneless beef chuck roast

Fine sea salt and ground black pepper

1 cup tomato sauce

½ cup beef bone broth, homemade (page 356) or store-bought, or water

½ cup coconut vinegar or apple cider vinegar

1 tablespoon chili powder

2 cloves garlic, minced

"ice cream" topping (fauxtatoes)

2 cups beef or chicken bone broth, homemade (page 356) or store-bought

1 medium head cauliflower

¼ cup grated Parmesan cheese

1 ounce cream cheese (2 tablespoons), softened, or more if desired

1 clove garlic, smashed to a paste

⅛ teaspoon ground black pepper

for garnish

1 cup shredded cheddar cheese

8 cherry tomatoes

1. To braise the beef, heat the ghee in a Dutch oven over medium-high heat. Season the roast liberally on all sides with salt and pepper. Place the roast in the pot and brown on all sides, about 2 minutes per side.

2. Reduce the heat to medium-low and pour in the tomato sauce, ½ cup of broth, and vinegar. Season with the chili powder, garlic, and more salt and pepper. Cover the pot and simmer for 3 hours or until the meat is fork-tender.

3. Meanwhile, make the "ice cream" topping: Pour the 2 cups of broth into a stockpot and bring to a boil over high heat. Core the cauliflower and cut the florets into bite-sized pieces. Add the florets to the broth, cover, and steam for about 6 minutes, until fork-tender. Drain well; do not let the cauliflower cool. Pat it very dry between several layers of paper towels. In a high-powered blender or food processor, puree the hot cauliflower with the Parmesan, cream cheese, garlic, and pepper until smooth. Set the topping aside.

4. Slice or shred the beef and divide it among 8 sundae cups or bowls. Drizzle some of the accumulated sauce from the Dutch oven onto the meat, then top with the "ice cream," shredded cheddar cheese, and a cherry tomato.

5. Store extras in separate airtight containers in the refrigerator for up to 3 days. Reheat the beef in a skillet over medium heat for 3 minutes or until warmed through. Reheat the cauliflower topping in a saucepan over medium heat for about 3 minutes or until warmed through.

---

busy family tip:

The cauliflower topping can be made up to 3 days ahead and stored in an airtight container in the refrigerator until you're ready to assemble the sundaes.

nutritional info (per sundae)				
calories	*fat*	*protein*	*carbs*	*fiber*
824	65g	50g	8g	3g

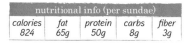

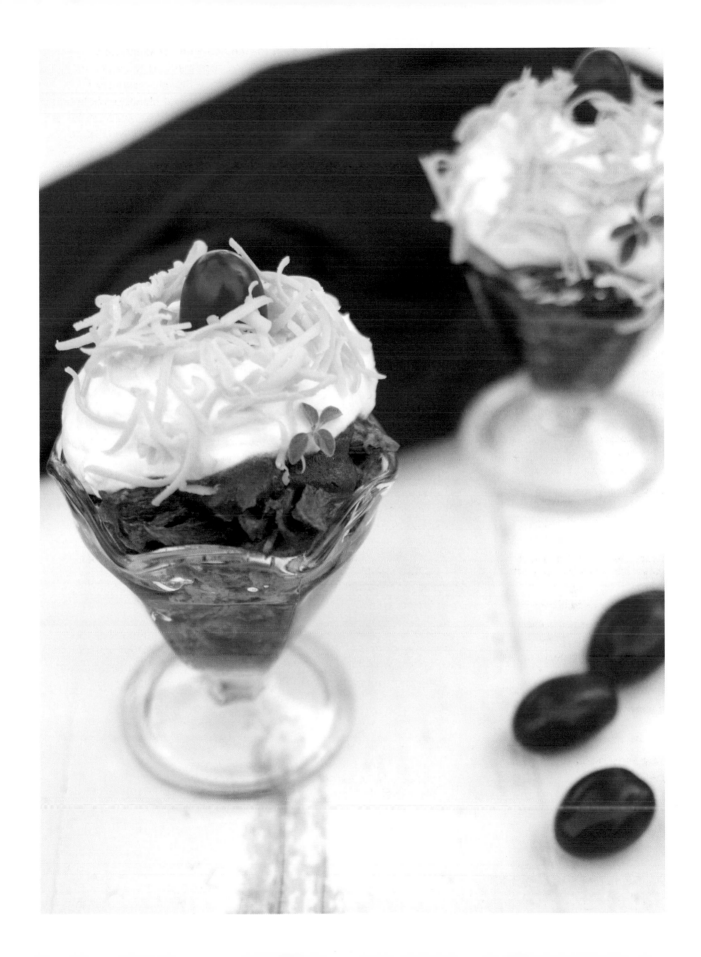

Grilled Cheese Waffles

and Tomato Gorgonzola Bisque

These waffles can be made up to three days ahead and stored in an airtight container in the refrigerator, or frozen for up to a month. I make a triple batch and freeze them for quick and easy sandwiches.

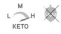

prep time: 15 minutes   *cook time:* 1 hour 5 minutes   *yield:* 8 servings

bisque

1 tablespoon ghee or coconut oil

¼ cup diced onions

2 cloves garlic, minced

¼ cup crumbled Gorgonzola cheese, plus extra for garnish

4 ounces cream cheese (½ cup), softened

1 cup chicken bone broth, homemade (page 356) or store-bought

1 (14½-ounce) can diced tomatoes, with juices

1½ cups tomato sauce

2 teaspoons dried basil

½ teaspoon fine sea salt

¼ teaspoon ground black pepper

Fresh basil leaves, for garnish

Melted ghee or avocado oil, for drizzling

waffles

8 large eggs

4 hard-boiled eggs

¼ cup powdered Parmesan cheese (see page 13)

1 teaspoon onion powder (optional)

1 teaspoon baking powder

½ teaspoon fine sea salt

½ cup ghee or coconut oil, melted but not hot, plus extra for the waffle iron

16 slices cheddar, Gruyère, Swiss, or fontina cheese (or all four!)

1. To make the bisque, heat the ghee in a medium-sized saucepan over medium heat. Add the onions and garlic and cook, stirring, for 4 to 5 minutes, until the onions are soft. Add the Gorgonzola, cream cheese, and broth; heat until the cheeses melt and the mixture is simmering.

2. Stir in the tomatoes (including the juices), tomato sauce, basil, salt, and pepper and bring to a simmer. Continue to simmer for 15 to 20 minutes, stirring constantly; do not allow it to boil. Using an immersion blender or countertop blender, puree the soup until smooth. Slide the pan off the heat and cover with a lid to keep the bisque warm while you make the waffles.

3. To make the waffles, heat a waffle iron to high heat. Place the raw eggs, hard-boiled eggs, Parmesan, onion powder (if using), baking powder, and salt in a blender or food processor and process until smooth and thick. Add the melted ghee and combine well.

4. Grease the hot waffle iron. Place 2½ tablespoons of the waffle batter in the center of the iron and close. (It should be a smaller waffle, about the size of a hamburger bun.) Cook for 3 to 4 minutes, until golden brown and crisp. Repeat with the remaining batter to make 16 small waffles.

5. To assemble the sandwiches, place 2 slices of cheese on a waffle and set another waffle on top. Butter the outsides of the waffle sandwich. Place the sandwich back on the waffle iron and heat until the cheese is melted (the iron won't be able to close completely, but that's okay).

6. To serve, pour the bisque into 8 soup bowls and garnish with crumbled Gorgonzola, fresh basil leaves, and a drizzle of melted ghee. Serve with the grilled cheese waffles.

7. Store extra soup in an airtight container in the refrigerator for up to 3 days. Reheat the soup in a saucepan over medium heat until warmed through, about 3 minutes. Store extra waffles in an airtight container in the refrigerator for up to 3 days or in the freezer for up to 1 month. Reheat the waffles in a preheated 375°F oven or toaster oven for 3 minutes or until warmed through.

nutritional info (per serving)				
calories	fat	protein	carbs	fiber
508	42g	24g	7g	2g

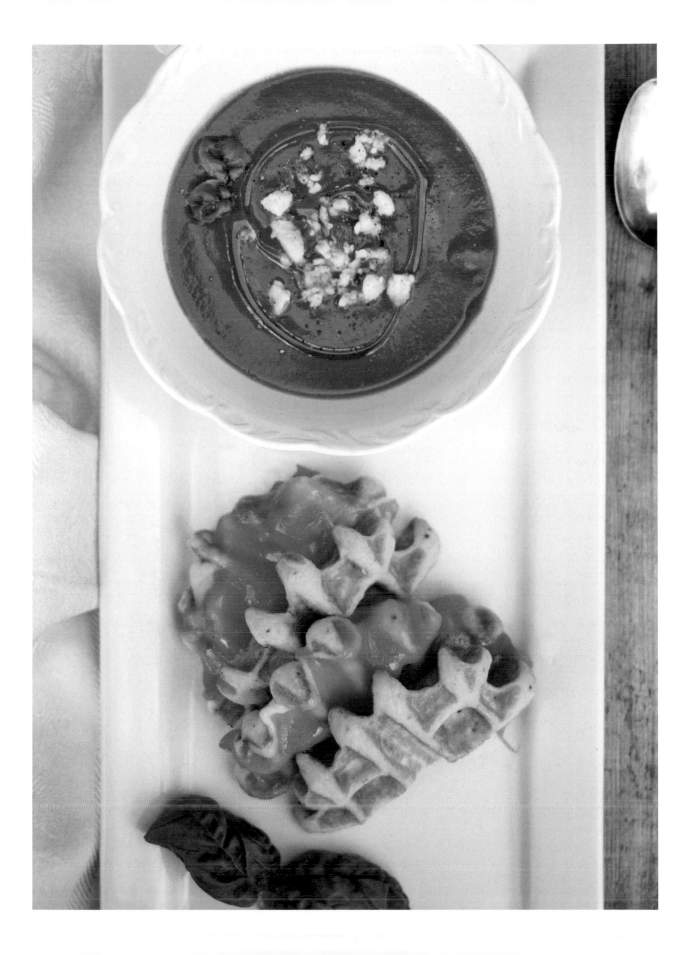

Cheeseburger Soup

What if I told you that when we get a cow from a local farmer, we ask the butcher to make it all into hamburger—even the prize cuts of steak! My family prefers hamburger over steaks. My kids whine when I make steaks, so why push it? I don't want steaks, either. I want hamburgers, sloppy Joes, protein noodle lasagna, keto spaghetti, Paleo chili, easy chipotle taco meat—you name it. Ground beef is how we roll!

4 strips bacon, diced

2 tablespoons unsalted butter, ghee, or lard

½ cup diced onions

1 pound ground beef or venison

1 teaspoon fine sea salt

½ teaspoon ground black pepper

4 ounces cream cheese (½ cup), softened

½ cup shredded sharp cheddar cheese, plus extra for garnish

3 cups beef bone broth, homemade (page 356) or store-bought

for garnish

Diced cherry tomatoes

Sliced green onions

Sliced dill pickles

prep time: 5 minutes   *cook time:* 20 minutes   *yield:* 4 servings

1. Place the bacon in a soup pot over medium heat and sauté until crisp-tender, about 4 minutes. Remove the bacon and reserve for garnish. Leave the drippings in the pot.

2. Add the butter and onions to the pot and sauté for 5 minutes or until translucent. Add the ground beef, salt, and pepper and sauté, while crumbling, until the meat is cooked through and no longer pink, about 5 minutes.

3. Meanwhile, place the cream cheese, shredded cheddar cheese, and broth in a blender and puree until smooth. Add the mixture to the soup pot. Heat for 5 minutes or until warm, but do not allow the soup to boil.

4. Ladle the soup into 4 serving bowls and garnish with diced cherry tomatoes, sliced green onions, shredded cheese, and the reserved bacon. Serve with dill pickle slices on the side.

5. Store extras in an airtight container in the refrigerator for up to 3 days. Reheat in a saucepan over medium heat for a few minutes or until warmed through.

nutritional info (per serving)				
calories	fat	protein	carbs	fiber
586	48g	31g	4g	0.3g

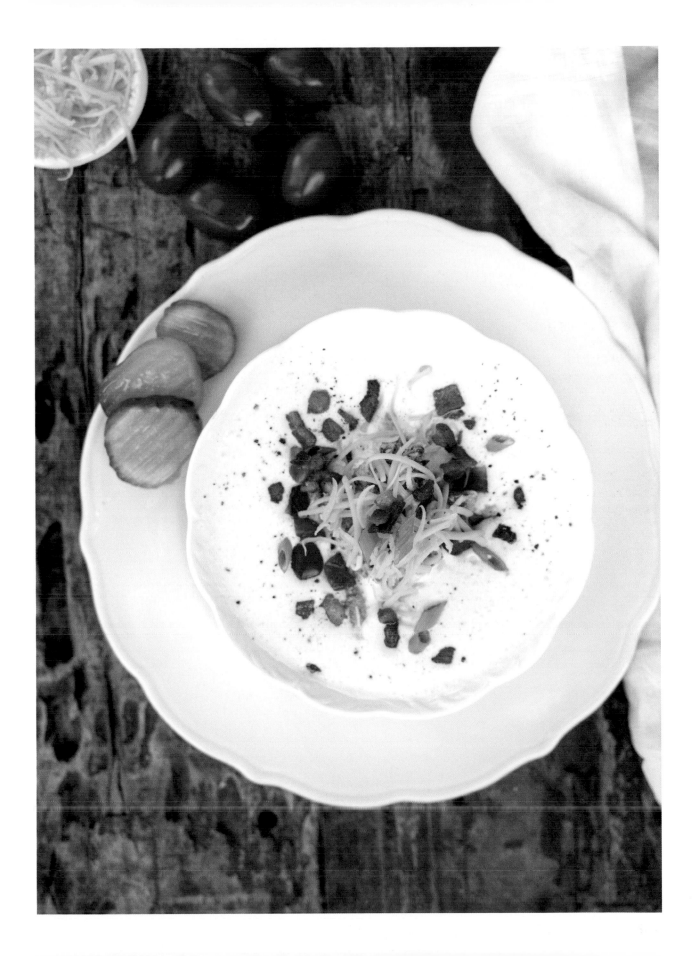

Chili Cheese Dog Casserole

You can find chili cheese dogs on many restaurant menus, including A&W, Burger King, Dairy Queen, and Wendy's. This is my reinvention of those dogs—casserole style. This recipe is so good, there's no need for a hot dog bun. It makes great leftovers, too!

L M H
KETO ✖ ✖

prep time: 10 minutes *cook time:* 40 minutes *yield:* 4 servings

1 pound ground beef

1 large bell pepper (any color), diced

½ cup diced onions

2 cloves garlic, minced

1 cup diced tomatoes (fresh preferred)

1 cup tomato sauce

1 cup beef bone broth, homemade (page 356) or store-bought

1 teaspoon fine sea salt

2 teaspoons chili powder

½ teaspoon ground cumin

¼ teaspoon ground black pepper

2 teaspoons Swerve confectioners'-style sweetener or equivalent amount of liquid or powdered sweetener (see page 24) (optional)

8 uncured hot dogs (see note), sliced lengthwise down the middle and then cut in half

1 cup shredded Monterey Jack or cheddar cheese

1. Preheat the oven to 375°F.

2. Place the ground beef, bell pepper, onions, and garlic in a large cast-iron skillet or other oven-safe skillet over medium heat and cook, while breaking up the beef, until the meat is cooked through, about 5 minutes. Add the tomatoes, tomato sauce, broth, salt, spices, and sweetener, if using. Simmer, uncovered, for 20 minutes.

3. Lay the hot dog slices on top of the casserole mixture in the skillet. Cover the entire mixture with the shredded cheese. Transfer the skillet to the oven and bake for 15 minutes or until the cheese is bubbly and melted.

4. Store extras in an airtight container in the refrigerator for up to 3 days. Reheat in a baking dish in a preheated 350°F oven for a few minutes or until warmed through.

note: I prefer Applegate Farms organic hot dogs.

nutritional info (per serving)				
calories	fat	protein	carbs	fiber
668	48g	43g	10g	2g

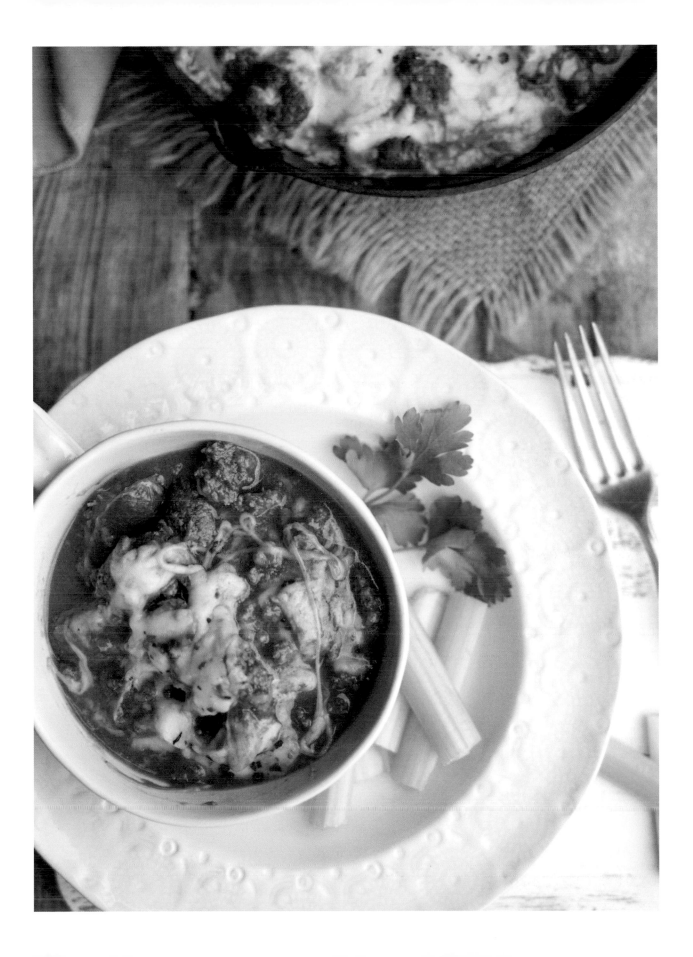

Pizza Waffles

When I was a little girl, my big brother, Cory, taught me how to make pizza toast. It was basically an English muffin topped with pizza sauce and cheese and tossed into the oven for a few minutes. This recipe is in honor of my pizza-lovin' brother, Cory!

L M H
KETO

8 large eggs

4 hard-boiled eggs

¼ cup powdered Parmesan cheese (see page 13)

1 teaspoon Italian seasoning

1 teaspoon baking powder

½ teaspoon fine sea salt

½ cup melted (but not hot) ghee or coconut oil, plus extra for the waffle iron

1 cup pizza sauce, homemade (page 358) or store-bought, plus extra for serving

2 cups shredded mozzarella cheese

½ cup mini pepperoni slices

for garnish (optional)

Fresh basil leaves

Red pepper flakes

prep time: 5 minutes   *cook time:* 35 minutes
yield: 8 pizzas (2 per serving)

1. Heat a waffle iron to high heat. Place the raw eggs, hard-boiled eggs, Parmesan, Italian seasoning, baking powder, and salt in a blender or food processor and combine until smooth and thick. Add the melted ghee and combine well.

2. Grease the hot waffle iron. Place a heaping ¼ cup of the batter in the center of the iron and close. Cook for 3 to 4 minutes, until golden brown and crisp. Repeat with the remaining batter to make 8 waffles.

3. To assemble, preheat the oven to broil. Place the waffles on a baking sheet and top each waffle with 1½ tablespoons of pizza sauce, a few tablespoons of shredded cheese, and a few mini pepperoni. Broil for 1 to 2 minutes, until the cheese is melted. Garnish with fresh basil leaves and/or red pepper flakes, if desired. Serve with additional pizza sauce.

4. Store extras in an airtight container in the refrigerator for up to 3 days. Reheat on a baking sheet in a preheated 350°F oven for a few minutes or until warmed through.

busy family tip:

Make the waffles ahead of time and store them in an airtight container in the refrigerator for up to 3 days or in the freezer for up to 1 month. Reheat the waffles in a preheated 375°F oven or toaster oven for 3 minutes or until warmed through.

nutritional info (per serving)				
calories	fat	protein	carbs	fiber
270	24g	13g	1g	0.3g

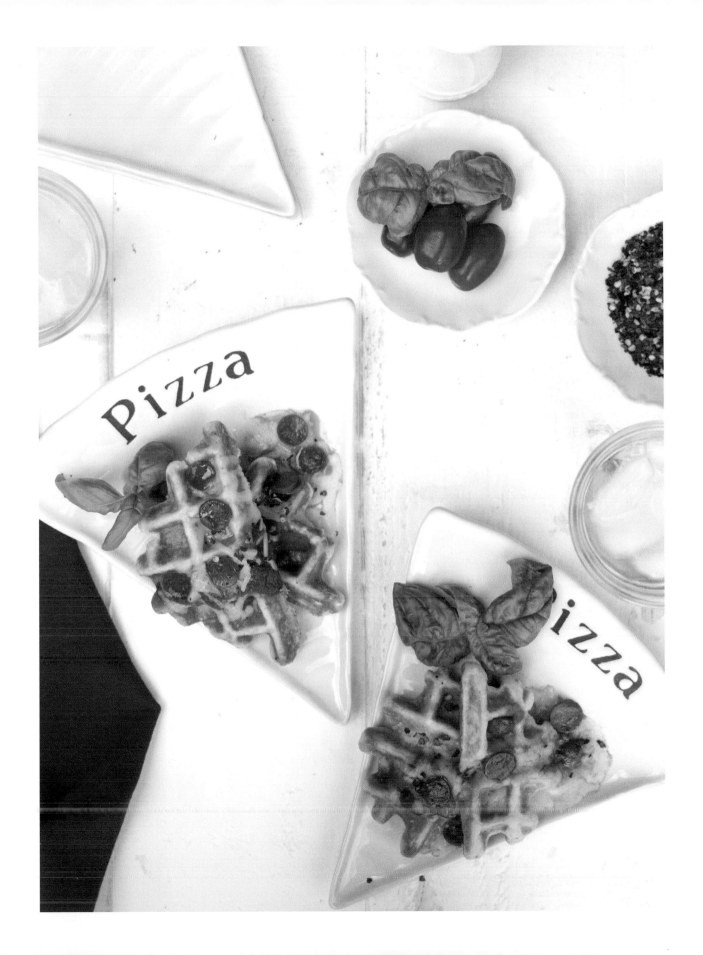

Chicken Parmesan Mini Meatloaves

prep time: 10 minutes   cook time: 22 minutes   yield: 6 servings

1½ pounds ground chicken

¾ cup finely chopped mushrooms

½ cup grated Parmesan cheese (or nutritional yeast if dairy-free)

¼ cup marinara sauce, plus extra for serving

½ cup chopped fresh basil leaves, plus extra whole leaves for garnish

1 teaspoon Italian seasoning

1 teaspoon dried oregano leaves

1 clove garlic, smashed to a paste

1½ cups shredded mozzarella or fontina cheese, plus extra for the top (omit for dairy-free)

1. Preheat the oven to 350°F. Grease six 4 by 2-inch mini loaf pans.

2. In a large bowl, mix together the ground chicken, mushrooms, Parmesan, marinara sauce, and basil. Season with the Italian seasoning, oregano, and garlic, then mix in the shredded cheese.

3. Press the mixture into the greased mini loaf pans. Bake for 20 minutes or until the internal temperature of the meatloaves reaches 160°F. Remove from the oven and sprinkle the tops with shredded cheese, then return to the oven and bake just until the cheese is melted, about 2 minutes. Serve on top of additional marinara sauce, garnished with fresh basil leaves.

4. Store extras in an airtight container in the refrigerator for up to 3 days. Reheat on a rimmed baking sheet in a preheated 350°F oven for 5 minutes or until warmed through.

nutritional info (per mini meatloaf)				
calories	fat	protein	carbs	fiber
254	16g	27g	1g	0.2g

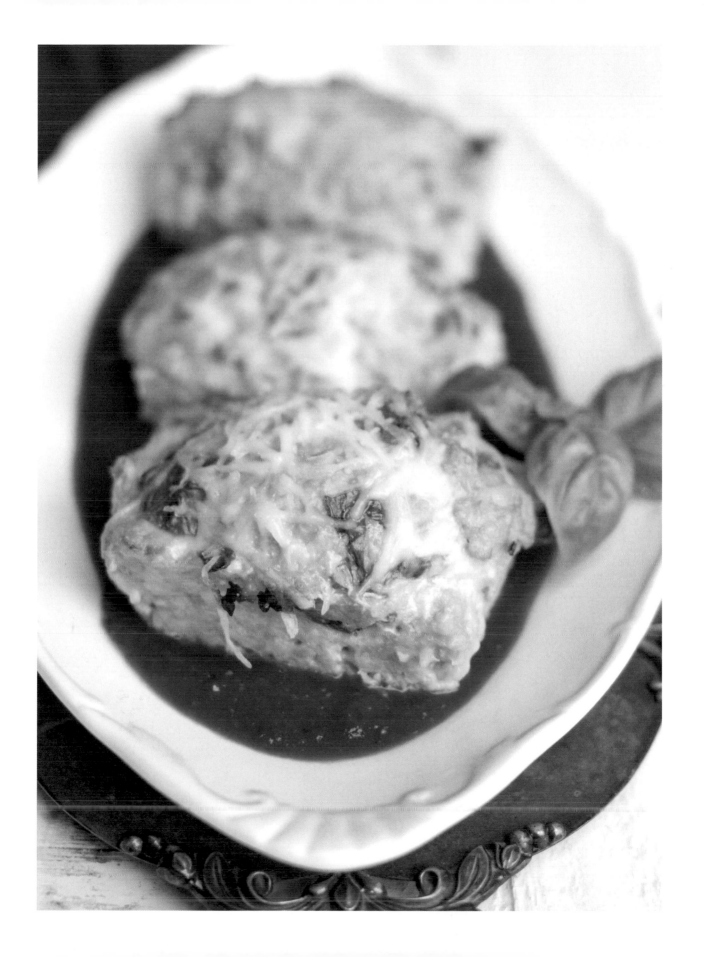

Ham 'n' Cheese Cones

L M H
KETO

filling

3 cups finely diced fully cooked ham

1 cup mayonnaise, homemade (page 359) or store-bought

1 tablespoon prepared yellow mustard

Fine sea salt and ground black pepper

cones

1 cup grated hard cheese, such as Parmesan, Asiago, or aged Gouda

for garnish

8 cherry tomatoes

1. In a large bowl, combine the ham, mayonnaise, and mustard. Stir to coat the ham well. Season to taste with salt and pepper. Refrigerate the filling until serving time.

2. To make the cones, preheat the oven to 375°F. Have on hand a cone-shaped object (I made a cone out of sheet metal; you can use a small funnel). Place a piece of parchment paper on a rimmed baking sheet and grease the paper with coconut oil spray. Place 2 tablespoons of cheese on one side of the paper and form it into a circle, about 4 inches in diameter. Repeat to make another 4-inch cheese circle, leaving at least 2 inches of space between them. Bake for 4 to 5 minutes, until golden brown.

3. Once you remove the baking sheet from the oven, you will need to move quickly. Using a spatula or knife, transfer one of the rounds of cheese to the cone-shaped object and form it around the mold. Allow to cool on the form for 10 minutes. Repeat with the second cheese circle. If the second round becomes too cool and brittle to mold, place it back in the hot oven for 30 seconds so it becomes flexible again.

4. Repeat with the rest of the cheese, making a total of 8 cones.

5. Once all of the cones are cool, fill them with the ham filling. Garnish each cone with a cherry tomato. Store extra filling and cones in separate airtight containers in the refrigerator for up to 4 days. Serve chilled.

nutritional info (per cone)				
calories	fat	protein	carbs	fiber
315	29g	12g	1g	0.2g

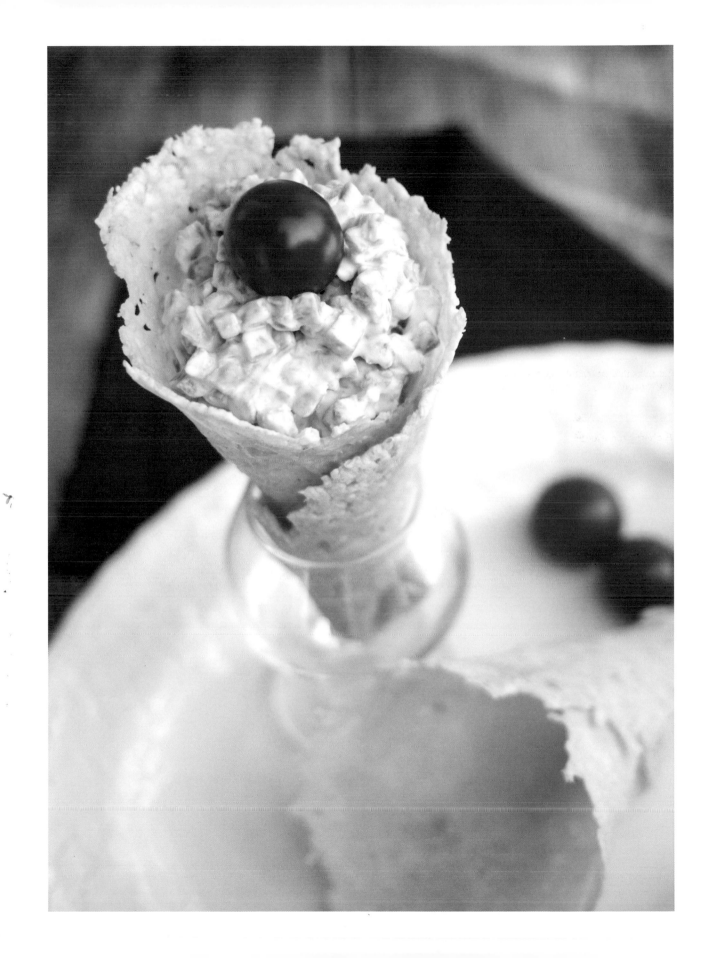

Chili Dogs

This is one of my boys' favorite meals. If your family enjoys this dish as much as we do, I suggest making a double batch of the chili to store in the fridge or freezer. I also keep keto hot dog buns in the freezer for easy meals. All you have to do is heat up a hot dog and heat up the chili and ta-da—dinner is ready in an instant! Plus, the chili tastes even better left over.

KETO OPTION

prep time: 10 minutes (not including time to make buns)
cook time: 40 minutes *yield:* 6 servings

1 pound ground beef

¼ cup chopped onions

1 cup tomato sauce

1 large tomato, diced, with juices

1 green chile pepper, chopped

½ cup beef bone broth, homemade (page 356) or store-bought

1 clove garlic, minced

1 tablespoon chili powder

1 teaspoon dried ground oregano

½ teaspoon ground cumin

½ teaspoon paprika

½ teaspoon fine sea salt

½ teaspoon ground black pepper

¼ teaspoon cayenne pepper

6 hot dogs

1 batch oblong Keto Buns (page 362)

additional toppings (optional)

Shredded sharp cheddar cheese (omit for dairy-free)

Sour cream (omit for dairy-free)

Sliced green onions

1. In a stockpot over medium heat, cook the ground beef with the onions, stirring often to break up the meat, until evenly browned, about 7 minutes. Pour in the tomato sauce. Add the diced tomato (with juices), chile pepper, and beef broth and stir to combine.

2. Season the meat mixture with the garlic, chili powder, oregano, cumin, paprika, salt, black pepper, and cayenne. Stir to blend, then cover and bring to a simmer over medium heat. Once at a simmer, reduce the heat to low and continue to simmer, covered, for at least 30 minutes, stirring occasionally. The longer the chili simmers, the better it will taste. After 30 minutes, taste and add more salt, pepper, and chili powder, if desired. Remove from the heat.

3. While the chili is simmering, make the hot dogs: Bring a pot of water to a boil. Place the hot dogs in the boiling water and cook for 3 minutes or until heated through. Alternatively, you can grill the hot dogs for about 3 minutes.

4. To assemble the chili dogs, slice the buns in half. Place the buns on a hot greased skillet over medium-high heat and fry until golden brown, about 1½ minutes. Place a hot dog in each fried bun. Top with ¼ to ½ cup of chili, then garnish with additional toppings, if desired.

5. The chili dogs are best served fresh, but any extra chili can be stored in an airtight container in the refrigerator for up to 5 days or frozen for up to 2 months. Reheat the chili in a pot on the stovetop over medium heat. Reheat the buns and hot dogs in a preheated 350°F oven for 3 minutes or until warm, then assemble the chili dogs as directed above.

nutritional info (per chili dog)				
calories	*fat*	*protein*	*carbs*	*fiber*
367	26g	25g	6g	1g

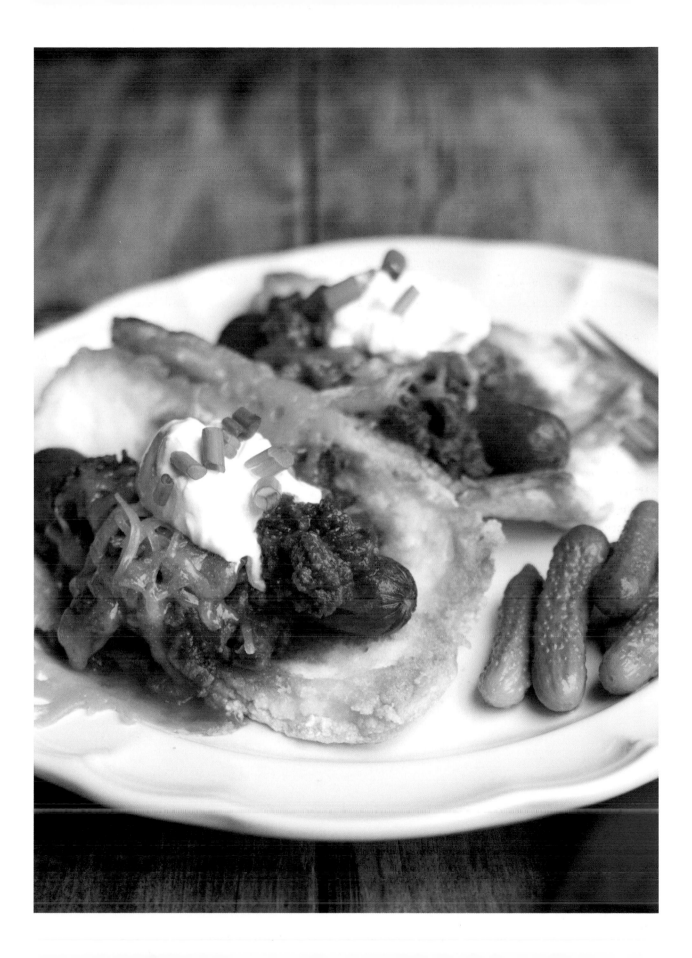

Deconstructed Bacon Cheeseburger Pizza

Bacon cheeseburgers and pizza, together at last! Even though you probably won't find this dish on any restaurant menus around town, it sounds like a fast-food match made in heaven. It marries two of America's fast-food favorites!

L M H
KETO

prep time: 15 minutes   *cook time:* 35 minutes   *yield:* 6 servings

14 slices thick-cut bacon

¼ pound ground beef

¼ teaspoon fine sea salt

¼ teaspoon ground black pepper

⅔ cup tomato sauce

2 tablespoons Swerve confectioners'-style sweetener or equivalent amount of liquid or powdered sweetener (see page 24)

2 tablespoons prepared yellow mustard

½ cup shredded mozzarella cheese

½ cup shredded sharp cheddar cheese

¼ cup chopped onions

for garnish

¼ large dill pickle, sliced into ¼-inch-thick rounds

¼ cup roughly chopped or torn lettuce

1 tomato, roughly chopped

1. Preheat the oven to 400°F.

2. On a rimmed baking sheet, weave the bacon strips together by overlapping each strip over and under the others, making a grid. Bake the bacon "crust" for 20 to 25 minutes, until crisp.

3. Meanwhile, heat a cast-iron skillet over medium heat. Place the ground beef, salt, and pepper in the skillet and cook, stirring often, until the meat is browned and crumbly, about 5 minutes. Set the skillet aside.

4. In a bowl, mix together the tomato sauce, sweetener, and mustard; spread this mixture over the bacon crust. Sprinkle the cheeses over the tomato sauce mixture and top with the beef and onions.

5. Bake the pizza until the cheese is melted, about 10 minutes. Remove from the oven and serve garnished with pickle slices, chopped lettuce, and chopped tomato.

6. This pizza is best served fresh, but any extras can be stored in an airtight container in the refrigerator for up to 3 days. Reheat on a rimmed baking sheet in a preheated 400°F oven for 4 minutes or until warmed through.

nutritional info (per serving)				
calories	fat	protein	carbs	fiber
283	23g	17g	3g	1g

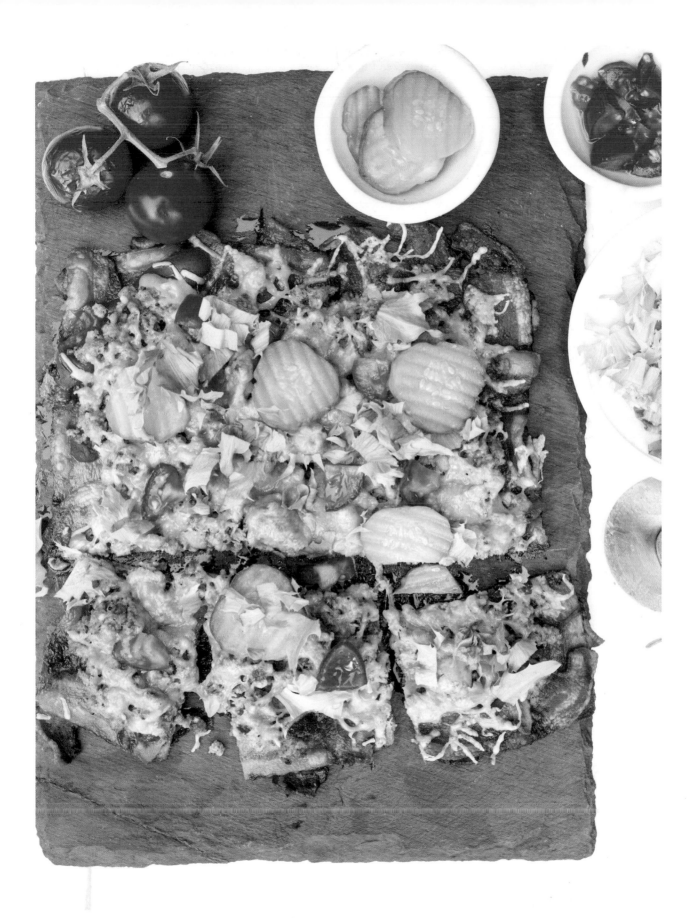

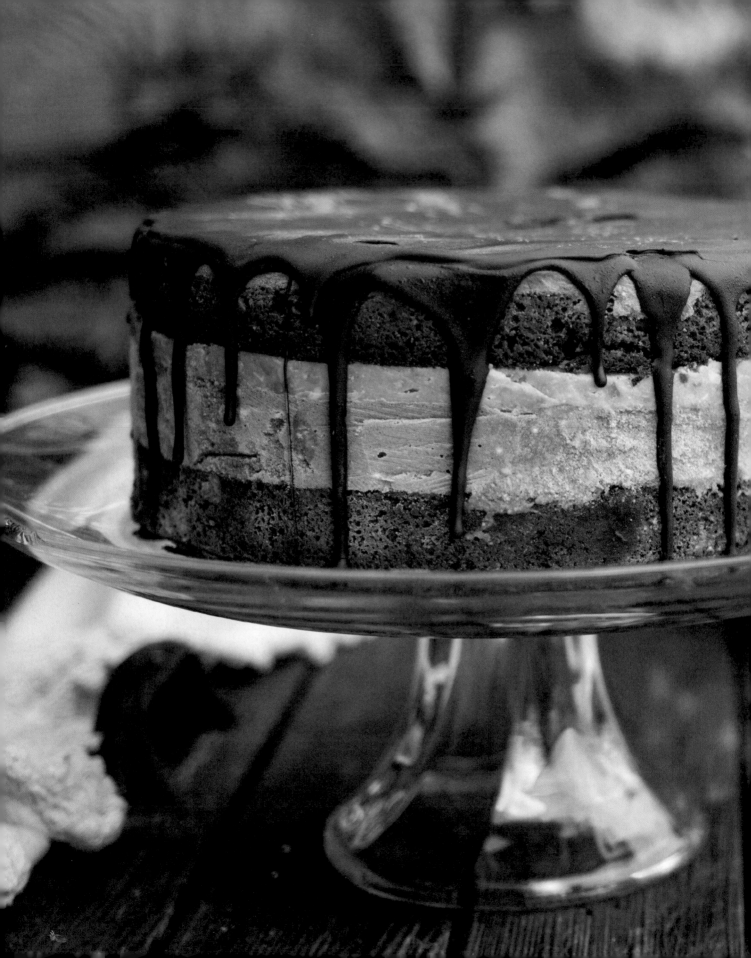

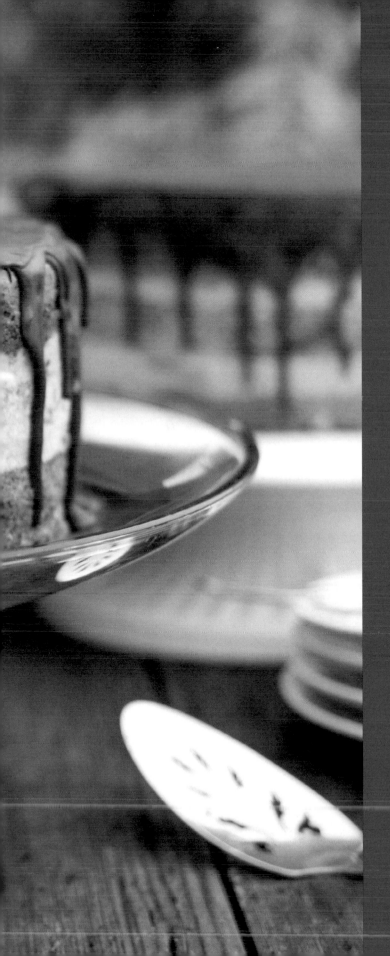

Sweet
Endings

Italian Cream Soda

Working at a coffee shop in high school was my favorite job (besides this job of writing cookbooks!). I adored getting up early; making muffins, scones, and lattes; and listening to good music while busy customers ran in before work. I always wanted to open my own keto bakery and coffee shop, and if I ever do, this Italian Cream Soda will certainly be on my menu!

Note: If you are looking to lose weight, I do not recommend drinking your calories, but ketosis is about more than just weight loss. If you are in "maintenance mode" or are trying to gain weight and muscle, this drink would be a great treat!

KETO   OPTION

Large ice cubes

1 cup sparkling mineral water or club soda

2 tablespoons Swerve confectioners'-style sweetener or equivalent amount of liquid or powdered sweetener (see page 24), or ¼ teaspoon flavored liquid stevia of choice

1 teaspoon strawberry extract or other extract of choice, or a few drops of strawberry oil

1 tablespoon heavy cream (or full-fat coconut milk if dairy-free)

2 tablespoons sweetened whipped cream, for garnish (see tip; omit for dairy-free)

prep time: 2 minutes (not including time to whip cream)   *yield:* 1 serving

1. Place the ice cubes in a tall glass. Pour in the sparkling mineral water. Stir in the sweetener and extract and adjust the sweetness to your liking.

2. Pour the heavy cream into the glass. Do not stir so you can watch the legs of the cream seep down into the drink. Top with the sweetened whipped cream and enjoy. This drink is best served fresh; it will lose its fizz if left overnight.

busy family tip:

I keep heavy cream in a whipped cream canister in my fridge at all times for easy additions to treats like this. I put 2 cups of cream and 2 tablespoons of powdered sweetener or ¼ teaspoon of liquid stevia in the canister and shake well to combine. Then it's presweetened and ready to go whenever I need it!

note: *To give this cream soda a pretty pink color, I added a few drops of natural red food dye. I also used Stur Strawberry Melon–flavored liquid water enhancer, which not only enhances the strawberry flavor but also gives the drink a pretty shade of pink.*

nutritional info				
calories	fat	protein	carbs	fiber
148	18g	0g	0g	0g

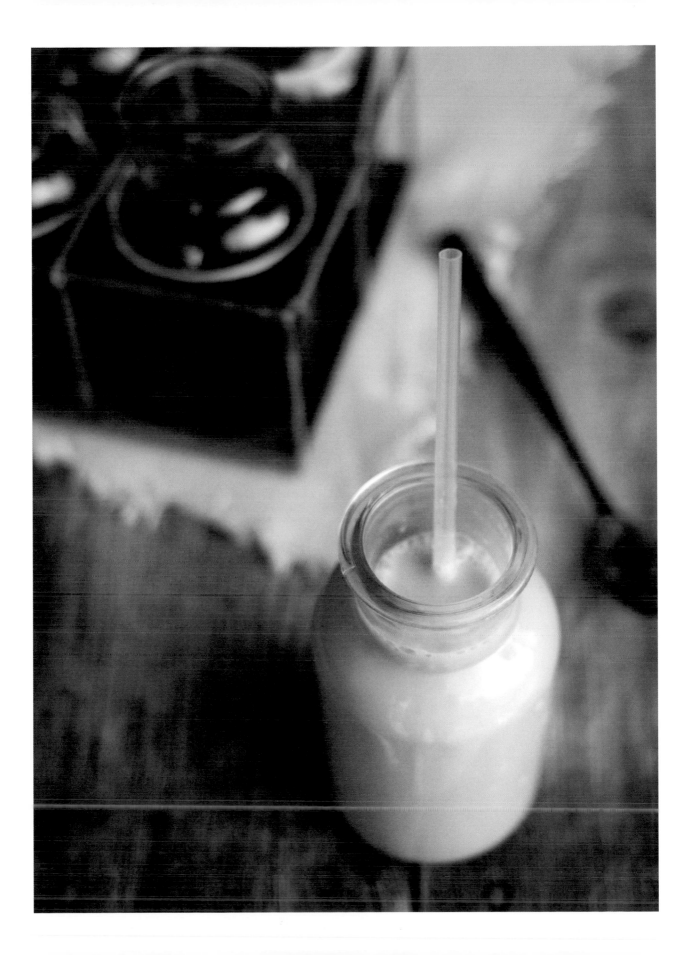

Persian Hot Chocolate

L M H
KETO OPTION OPTION

2 ounces unsweetened chocolate, chopped

⅓ cup Swerve confectioners'-style sweetener or equivalent amount of liquid or powdered sweetener (see page 24)

3 cups unsweetened cashew milk (or heavy cream or full-fat coconut milk for a richer drink)

1 teaspoon vanilla or chocolate extract

⅛ teaspoon toffee extract (optional)

⅛ teaspoon ground cinnamon, plus extra for garnish (optional)

Sweetened whipped cream, for garnish (see tip, page 298)

Melted ghee or unsalted butter, for garnish (omit for dairy-free)

prep time: 5 minutes (not including time to whip cream)
cook time: 2 minutes   *yield:* 2 servings

1. Place the chopped chocolate, sweetener, and cashew milk in a double boiler over medium-low heat. Stir often until everything is melted and well combined, about 2 minutes.

2. Stir in the extracts and cinnamon. Remove from the heat and serve in cute cups, garnished with whipped cream and a drizzle of melted ghee.

3. Store extras in an airtight container in the refrigerator for up to 4 days. To reheat, place in a saucepan over low heat and stir for 1 minute or until warmed through.

nutritional info (per serving)				
calories	fat	protein	carbs	fiber
134	10g	4g	6g	3g

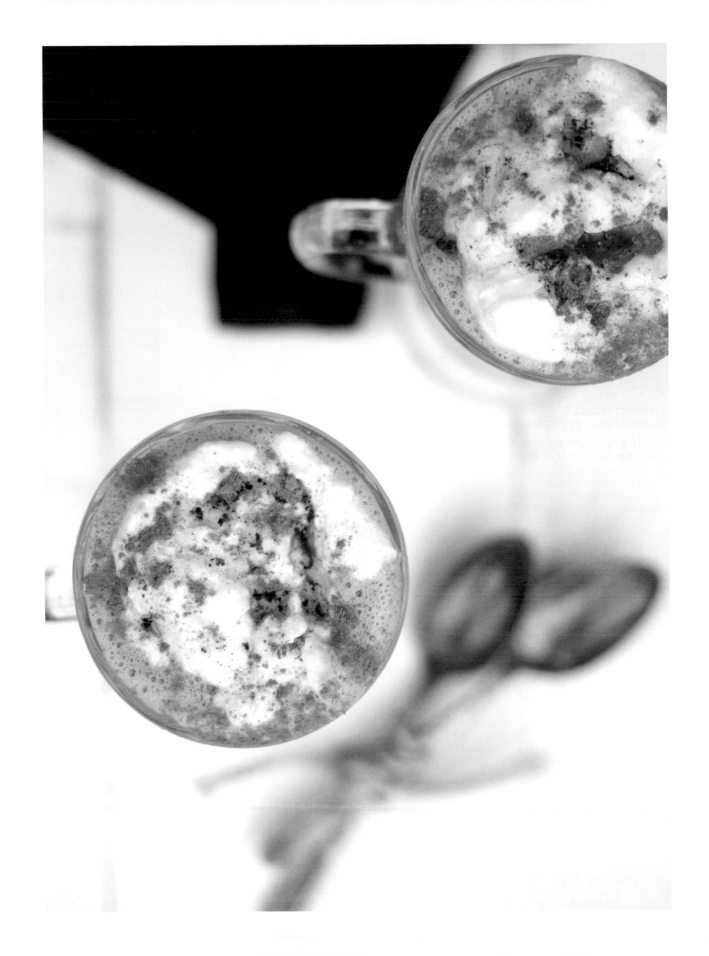

Pumpkin Dip
with Pie Fries

L M H ✕
KETO OPTION

dip

1 (8-ounce) package mascarpone or cream cheese (Kite Hill brand cream cheese style spread if dairy-free), softened

½ cup Swerve confectioners'-style sweetener or equivalent amount of liquid or powdered sweetener (see page 24)

¾ cup fresh or canned pumpkin puree

⅓ cup sour cream (or Kite Hill brand cream cheese style spread if dairy-free)

1 tablespoon vanilla extract

2½ teaspoons pumpkin pie spice

1 teaspoon ground cinnamon

pie fries

¾ cup blanched almond flour

¼ cup coconut flour

½ cup (1 stick) unsalted butter (or coconut oil if dairy-free), softened

½ cup Swerve confectioners'-style sweetener or equivalent amount of liquid or powdered sweetener (see page 24)

1 teaspoon fine sea salt

¼ cup Swerve granular-style sweetener

2 tablespoons ground cinnamon

1 large egg yolk, beaten

prep time: 10 minutes, plus 3 hours to chill dip   *cook time:* 15 minutes
yield: 10 servings

1. To make the dip, place the softened mascarpone cheese and sweetener in a medium-sized bowl and mix with a hand mixer until smooth. Add the pumpkin, sour cream, vanilla, pumpkin pie spice, and cinnamon and beat until combined. Cover and refrigerate for 3 hours.

2. When you're ready to make the pie fries, preheat the oven to 350°F. Line a baking sheet with parchment paper.

3. Place the almond flour, coconut flour, softened butter, ½ cup of confectioners'-style sweetener, and salt in a medium-sized bowl and mix well to combine. Place the dough between 2 pieces of parchment paper greased well with coconut oil spray. Roll out the dough into a ¼-inch-thick rectangle. Remove the top piece of parchment. Using a sharp knife or pizza wheel, cut the dough into strips that are ½ inch wide and 3 inches long.

4. Place the granular sweetener and cinnamon in a small dish and mix to combine. Set aside.

5. Brush the strips of dough with the beaten egg yolk, then sprinkle with the sweetened cinnamon mixture. Place the "fries" on the lined baking sheet, about 1 inch apart.

6. Bake the pie fries for 12 minutes or until golden brown. Allow to cool completely before removing from the baking sheet. Place on a serving platter and serve with the dip.

7. Store extra fries and dip in separate airtight containers in the refrigerator for up to 3 days. The fries can be frozen for up to 1 month.

busy family tip:
The dip can be made up to 2 days ahead.

nutritional info (per serving)				
calories	fat	protein	carbs	fiber
282	25g	5g	8g	3g

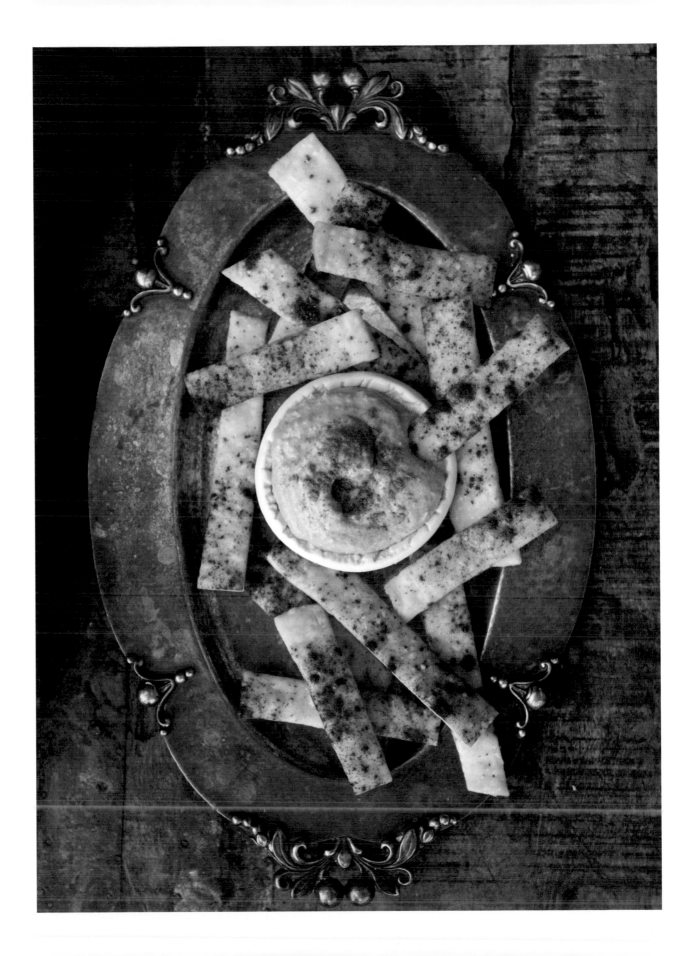

Malted Milk Ball Bûche de Noël

I adore this recipe because it is such an elegant-looking dessert; even though I am not an artist, the special bûche mold makes it look so fancy. But don't do what I did: early in the morning after assembling the dessert, I was excited to see how it looked. In the dark, I removed the mold from the freezer and started to push the dessert out of the mold onto a beautiful white serving dish. To my horror, the dish slid off the counter and shattered on the floor in a million pieces. So here's my tip: turn on some lights so you can see what you're doing!

prep time: 35 minutes, plus 5 hours to chill *cook time:* 3 minutes
yield: 12 servings

vanilla malted milk layer

¾ cup unsweetened cashew milk

1 tablespoon plus 1 teaspoon unflavored gelatin

4 (8-ounce) packages cream cheese (Kite Hill brand cream cheese style spread if dairy-free), softened

2 cups heavy cream (or full-fat coconut milk if dairy-free)

1½ cups Swerve confectioners'-style sweetener or equivalent amount of liquid or powdered sweetener (see page 24)

¼ cup plus 2 tablespoons maca powder, or more to taste

Seeds scraped from 2 vanilla beans (about 8 inches long), or 2 teaspoons vanilla extract

chocolate malted milk layer

½ batch Vanilla Malted Milk Layer (reserved from above)

3 tablespoons unsweetened cocoa powder, or more to taste

ganache

¾ cup heavy cream (or full-fat coconut milk if dairy-free)

⅓ cup Swerve confectioners'-style sweetener or equivalent amount of liquid or powdered sweetener (see page 24)

3 ounces unsweetened chocolate, finely chopped

Seeds scraped from 1 vanilla bean (about 8 inches long), or 1 teaspoon vanilla extract

⅛ teaspoon fine sea salt

for garnish (optional)
1 cup toasted crushed almonds

special equipment (optional)
Silicone bûche mold, about 10 by 3½ inches

1. Have on hand a silicone bûche mold or a 9 by 5-inch loaf pan. If using a loaf pan, line it with parchment paper, leaving some paper overhanging.

2. To make the vanilla malted milk layer, place the cashew milk and gelatin in a saucepan over medium-high heat and whisk until the gelatin melts. Remove from the heat and pour into a large bowl. Add the cream cheese, heavy cream, sweetener, and maca powder to the bowl and mix well with a hand mixer. Add the vanilla and beat until smooth. Taste and add more maca powder (for the malted milk flavor) and/or sweetener, if desired.

3. Pour half of the batter into the bûche mold or lined loaf pan. Gently place the mold in the freezer and allow the first layer to set, about 2 hours.

4. To make the chocolate malted milk layer, add the cocoa powder to the remaining half of the batter and mix with the hand mixer to combine. Taste and add more cocoa powder, if desired. Once the first layer in the freezer is set, gently spoon the chocolate layer over the vanilla layer. Place back in the freezer to set completely, about 3 hours.

5. Just before serving, make the ganache. Bring the cream and sweetener to a simmer in a saucepan over medium heat. Remove from the heat and stir in the chopped chocolate, vanilla, and salt. Allow to sit for 3 minutes, then stir again until completely smooth.

6. To serve, unmold the bûche onto a serving platter. Gently peel away the sides of the mold, pressing the top of the mold gently with your hand until the bûche releases. If you used a loaf pan, allow the bûche to thaw slightly, then use the overhanging paper to lift the bûche out of the pan and invert it onto a serving platter. Drizzle the top with the ganache and sprinkle with crushed almonds, if desired.

7. Store extras in an airtight container in the refrigerator for up to 3 days or in the freezer for up to a month. Allow to thaw before slicing and serving.

nutritional info (per serving)				
calories	fat	protein	carbs	fiber
587	55g	10g	12g	5g

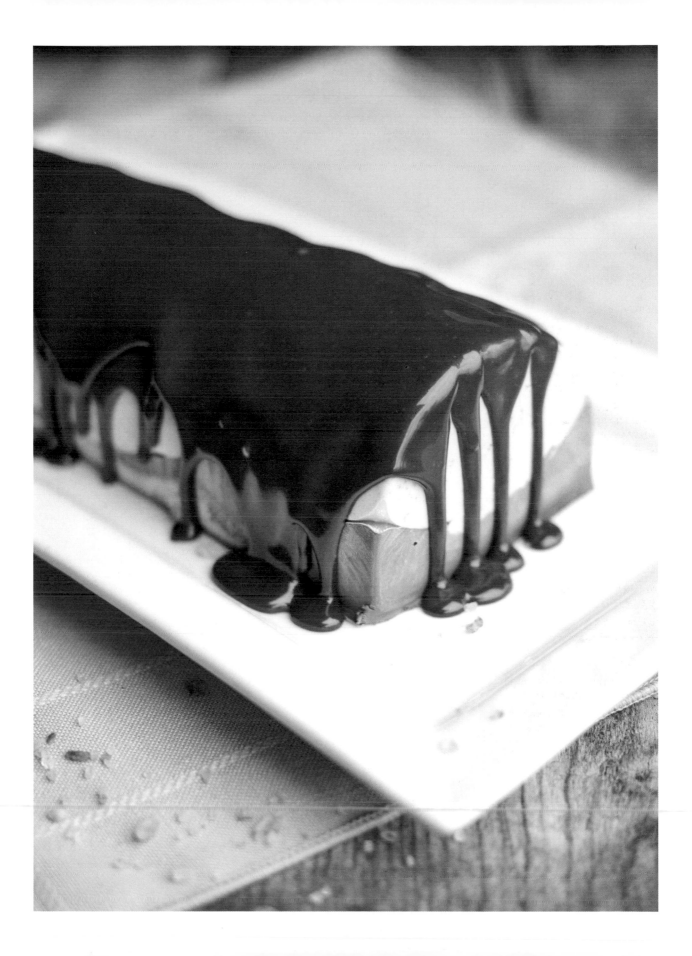

Gâteau au Chocolat

L M H
KETO OPTION

filling (omit for dairy-free)

¾ cup (1½ sticks) unsalted butter

6 ounces cream cheese or mascarpone cheese (¾ cup) (Kite Hill brand cream cheese style spread if dairy-free), softened

¾ cup Swerve confectioners'-style sweetener or equivalent amount of liquid or powdered sweetener (see page 24)

3 tablespoons unsweetened cocoa powder

3 tablespoons brewed decaf espresso or other strong brewed decaf coffee

Seeds scraped from 1 vanilla bean (about 8 inches long), or 1 teaspoon vanilla extract

cake

¾ cup (1½ sticks) unsalted butter (or coconut oil if dairy-free), plus extra for the pans

6 ounces unsweetened chocolate, finely chopped

1¼ cups Swerve confectioners'-style sweetener or equivalent amount of liquid or powdered sweetener (see page 24)

6 large eggs

1 tablespoon coconut flour

Seeds scraped from 1 vanilla bean (about 8 inches long), or 1 teaspoon vanilla extract

ganache

¾ cup heavy cream (or full-fat coconut milk if dairy-free)

⅓ cup Swerve confectioners'-style sweetener or equivalent amount of liquid or powdered sweetener (see page 24)

3 ounces unsweetened chocolate, finely chopped

Seeds scraped from 1 vanilla bean (about 8 inches long), or 1 teaspoon vanilla extract

⅛ teaspoon fine sea salt

If you are looking for a dairy-free cake, feel free to make this cake without the filling. The cake is like a fudgy brownie. You don't even need the filling!

prep time: 10 minutes, plus time to chill filling overnight

cook time: 20 minutes *yield:* one 8-inch two-layer cake (16 servings)

1. To make the filling, place the butter in a saucepan over medium-high heat. Stirring often, heat until the butter foams up and brown (but not black!) flecks appear. Remove from the heat and allow to cool a bit. Transfer the browned butter to a medium-sized bowl, add the cream cheese and sweetener, and cream with a hand mixer. Add the espresso to thin it out a little. Stir in the vanilla. Place the filling in the refrigerator to thicken overnight.

2. To make the cake, preheat the oven to 325°F. Grease two 8-inch cake pans, then line them with parchment paper and grease the paper. If desired, brown the butter as described in Step 1 (this makes the cake taste way better!). Otherwise, simply melt the butter (or coconut oil), then remove from the heat. Add the chopped chocolate and sweetener and stir well to combine. Add the eggs and mix well. Stir in the coconut flour and vanilla.

3. Pour the batter into the prepared pans and bake for 18 to 20 minutes, until a toothpick inserted in the center of a cake comes out clean. Remove from the oven and allow to cool completely in the pans.

4. To make the ganache, bring the cream and sweetener to a simmer in a saucepan over medium heat. Remove from the heat and stir in the chopped chocolate, vanilla, and salt. Allow to sit for 3 minutes, then stir again until completely smooth.

5. To assemble, place one cooled cake layer on a cake plate. Top with the filling, spreading it not quite to the edge of the cake. Place the second cake layer on top of the bottom layer. Pour the warm ganache over the cake, allowing it to drip down the sides, then smooth out the top with a knife. Serve at room temperature.

6. Store extras in an airtight container in the refrigerator for up to 4 days or in the freezer for up to 1 month. Allow to thaw to room temperature before slicing and serving.

---

busy family tip:
The cake layers can be made up to 2 days ahead and stored in an airtight container in the refrigerator, or frozen for up to 1 month.

nutritional info (per serving)				
calories	fat	protein	carbs	fiber
361	35g	6g	6g	4g

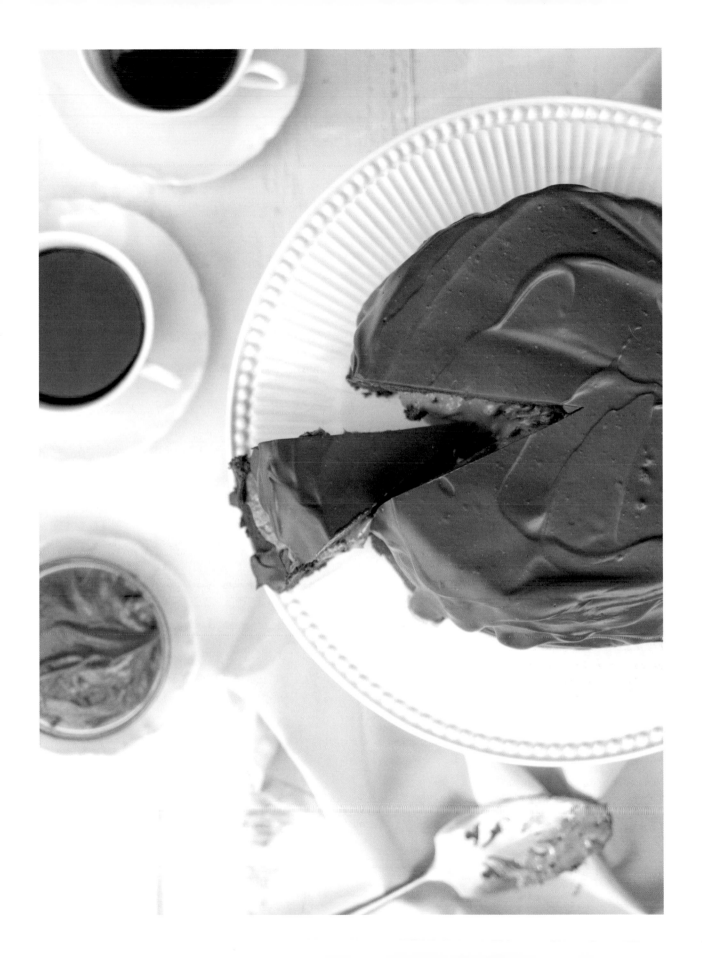

Pots de Crème

KETO OPTION OPTION

1¼ cups heavy cream (or full-fat coconut milk if dairy-free)

¾ cup unsweetened cashew milk (or hemp milk if nut-free)

6 ounces unsweetened chocolate, finely chopped

5 large egg yolks

⅔ cup Swerve confectioners'-style sweetener or equivalent amount of liquid or powdered sweetener (see page 24)

Seeds scraped from 1 vanilla bean (about 8 inches long), or 1 teaspoon vanilla extract

½ teaspoon fine sea salt

prep time: 5 minutes, plus at least 2 hours to chill *cook time:* 30 minutes
yield: 6 servings

1. Preheat the oven to 325°F.

2. Bring the cream and cashew milk to a simmer in a saucepan over medium-high heat. Once simmering, remove from the heat and immediately stir in the chopped chocolate. Let sit for 2 minutes, then stir until well combined.

3. Place the egg yolks, sweetener, vanilla, and salt in a small bowl. Stir well to combine. Slowly stream the egg mixture into the chocolate mixture while whisking so you do not scramble the eggs.

4. Evenly divide the mixture among six 4-ounce greased ramekins. Place the ramekins in an 11 by 9-inch baking dish. Pour hot water around the ramekins so that it comes two-thirds of the way up the sides of the ramekins. Bake for 30 minutes, until the custard is set (the center will jiggle ever so slightly when you shake the pan).

5. Remove the pan from the oven but leave the ramekins in the hot water for 5 minutes. After 5 minutes, remove them from the water and let cool completely. Cover and refrigerate for 2 hours or overnight.

6. These custards can be stored in the refrigerator, tightly covered, for up to 5 days. Do not freeze.

nutritional info (per serving)				
calories	*fat*	*protein*	*carbs*	*fiber*
396	38g	6g	9g	6g

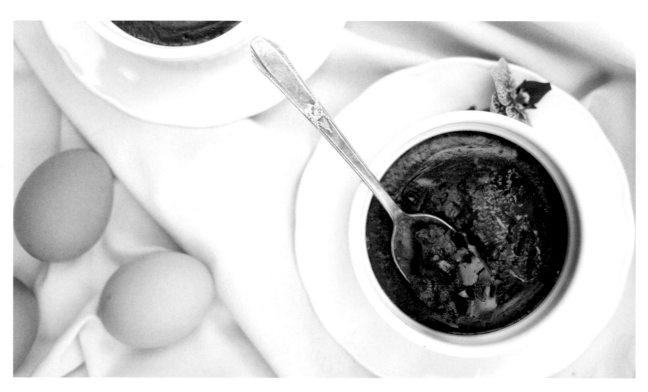

Deconstructed
Chocolate
Cannoli Cookies

I love to serve these tasty cookies alongside my Cannoli Mini Cheese Balls (page 328)!

L M H
KETO OPTION

prep time: 5 minutes   *cook time:* 12 minutes
yield: 2 dozen cookies (1 per serving)

½ cup (1 stick) unsalted butter (or coconut oil if dairy-free), softened

4 ounces cream cheese (½ cup) (Kite Hill brand cream cheese style spread if dairy-free), softened

¾ cup Swerve confectioners'-style sweetener or equivalent amount of liquid or powdered sweetener (see page 24)

1 large egg

1 teaspoon almond extract or other extract of choice, such as orange, lemon, or vanilla

½ teaspoon fine sea salt

2 cups blanched almond flour

¼ cup coconut flour

¼ cup unsweetened cocoa powder

¼ teaspoon baking powder

Pinch of fine sea salt

1. Preheat the oven to 300°F. Line a baking sheet with parchment paper and grease the parchment.

2. In a large bowl, cream the softened butter and cream cheese with a hand mixer for 1 minute. Add the sweetener and continue mixing until creamy. Add the egg, extract, and salt and mix again. Add the flours, cocoa powder, baking powder, and pinch of salt and mix well to combine.

3. Scoop up a heaping tablespoon of the dough and roll it into a ball between your hands, then place it on the greased parchment. Repeat with the rest of the dough, placing the balls about 2 inches apart. Bake for 12 to 15 minutes, until fine cracks form on the tops of the cookies. Let the cookies cool completely on the pan.

4. Store extras in an airtight container in the refrigerator for up to 3 days, or freeze for up to 1 month.

nutritional info (per cookie)				
calories	fat	protein	carbs	fiber
115	10g	3g	3g	2g

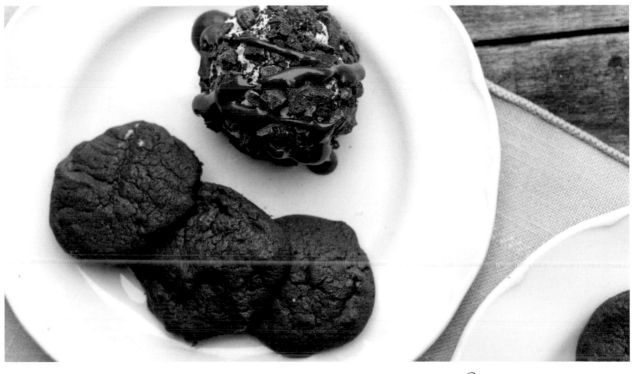

Death by Chocolate Cheesecake

M
L ⌐H   ✂   ✂
KETO   OPTION OPTION

crust

3½ tablespoons unsalted butter (or coconut oil if dairy-free), plus extra for the pan

1½ ounces unsweetened chocolate, finely chopped

⅓ cup Swerve confectioners'-style sweetener or equivalent amount of liquid or powdered sweetener (see page 24)

1 teaspoon stevia glycerite

1 large egg, beaten

2 teaspoons ground cinnamon

Seeds scraped from 1 vanilla bean (about 8 inches long), or 1 teaspoon vanilla extract

¼ teaspoon fine sea salt

filling

6 ounces unsweetened chocolate, finely chopped

1 tablespoon unsalted butter (or coconut oil if dairy-free)

4 (8-ounce) packages cream cheese (Kite Hill brand cream cheese style spread if dairy-free), softened

1 cup Swerve confectioners'-style sweetener or equivalent amount of liquid or powdered sweetener (see page 24)

⅓ cup unsweetened cashew milk (or heavy cream if nut-free)

Seeds scraped from 1 vanilla bean (about 8 inches long), or 1 teaspoon vanilla extract

½ teaspoon fine sea salt

3 large eggs

¼ cup unsweetened cocoa powder

special equipment

8-inch springform pan

prep time: 15 minutes, plus at least 4 hours to chill
cook time: about 1 hour *yield:* one 8-inch cake (12 servings)

1. Preheat the oven to 325°F. Grease an 8-inch springform pan, then line it with parchment paper and grease the paper.

2. To make the crust: If using butter, I suggest that you brown it (it tastes way better!). To brown the butter, heat the butter in a saucepan over high heat, stirring often. Once the butter foams and brown (but not black!) flecks start to appear, remove from the heat and allow to cool for 10 minutes, until it's warm but not hot. If you do not wish to brown the butter or are using coconut oil, melt the butter or oil in a saucepan over medium-low heat. Slowly add the chopped chocolate to the warm butter or oil, stirring constantly (don't let the chocolate burn). When the chocolate is melted, add the sweeteners. Let cool in the refrigerator. Once cool, add the beaten egg, cinnamon, vanilla, and salt. Pour the crust batter into the greased springform pan, spreading it with your hands to cover the bottom completely.

3. To make the filling, place the chopped chocolate and 1 tablespoon of butter in a medium-sized saucepan over low heat. Stir well to combine. When melted, remove from the heat and set aside.

4. In a large bowl or the bowl of a stand mixer, beat the cream cheese, sweetener, cashew milk, vanilla, and salt until well blended. Add the eggs, one at a time, mixing on low speed after each addition just until blended. Add the cocoa powder and reserved melted chocolate mixture. Combine until very smooth. Pour the batter over the crust in the pan.

5. Set up a water bath: Wrap aluminum foil entirely around the bottom and halfway up the sides of the springform pan to prevent water from leaking into the removable bottom of the pan. Place the cheesecake in a roasting pan (or any baking dish with sides) and place the pan in the oven. Pour hot water into the roasting pan so that it comes halfway up the sides of the springform pan. (*Note:* A water bath helps cook the cheesecake evenly; however, the cheesecake can be baked without it. See the note below if you choose not to use a water bath.) Bake for 55 minutes or until the center is almost set. Let the cheesecake cool completely in the pan before removing the outer ring. Refrigerate for 4 hours or overnight before serving.

note: *If you are not using a water bath, place the cheesecake on a lined rimmed baking sheet to catch any overflow or leaks. When done baking, turn the oven off and let the cake cool in the oven with the door closed for 5 to 6 hours; this keeps the top from cracking.*

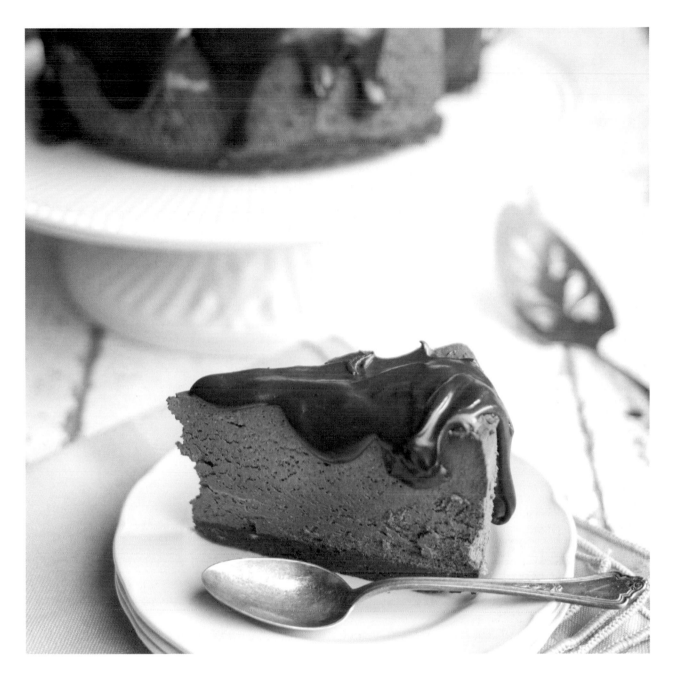

chocolate sauce

1 cup heavy cream (or full-fat coconut milk if dairy-free)

⅓ cup Swerve confectioners'-style sweetener or equivalent amount of liquid or powdered sweetener (see page 24)

2 ounces unsweetened chocolate, finely chopped

Seeds scraped from 1 vanilla bean (about 8 inches long), or 1 teaspoon vanilla extract

6. To make the chocolate sauce, place the cream, sweetener, and chopped chocolate in a double boiler or in a heat-safe bowl set over a pan of simmering water. Heat on low, stirring often, just until the chocolate melts. Remove from the heat. Stir in the vanilla. Pour the chocolate sauce over the chilled cheesecake.

7. Store extras in an airtight container in the refrigerator for up to 4 days or in the freezer for up to 1 month. Allow to thaw to room temperature before slicing and serving.

nutritional info (per serving)				
calories	fat	protein	carbs	fiber
552	50g	11g	11g	6g

French Silk Ice Cream

A woman mentioned to me that she didn't want to be a "stick in the mud" mom for not taking her kids to those frozen yogurt shops that are popping up on every corner. When I was a teenager, I mistakenly ate fat-free frozen yogurt for dessert thinking that it was a safe "diet" food. Nope, it isn't! At one of the top frozen yogurt chains, the ingredients for vanilla yogurt powder are pure crystalline fructose, dextrose, maltodextrin, non-fat milk, yogurt powder, and micro-encapsulated probiotic (Lactobacillus sporogenes).

And have you seen the prices at those places?! I often get questions about the cost of the ingredients I recommend. I calculated the price of my ice cream recipe with top-notch ingredients like organic coconut oil and farm-fresh organic eggs. The result: $3.13 per pint. Not bad considering that Ben & Jerry's costs about $4.00 a pint and Cold Stone Creamery's costs $7.50 a pint—and it has 2 grams of trans fat!

You can buy most of the ingredients used in my recipes in bulk and store them in a chest freezer to lower the cost even more. And ice cream tastes so much better when you make it fresh at home!

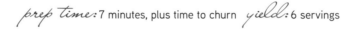

prep time: 7 minutes, plus time to churn   *yield:* 6 servings

1. Combine all the ingredients in a blender and blend until very smooth. Taste and add more sweetener, if desired.

2. Pour the mixture into an ice cream maker and churn according to the manufacturer's directions, and watch the magic happen! Serve immediately or store the ice cream in an airtight container in the freezer for up to 1 month.

---

tips: If you prefer a dark chocolate ice cream, you can add another ¼ cup of unsweetened cocoa powder.

To make this ice cream even more decadent, drizzle it with the chocolate sauce from my Death by Chocolate Cheesecake (see page 311).

Ingredients

¾ cup plus 2 tablespoons coconut oil (or unsalted butter if not dairy-sensitive), softened

½ cup unsweetened cashew milk (or water if nut-free)

¼ cup MCT oil

4 large eggs

4 large egg yolks

Seeds scraped from 1 vanilla bean (about 8 inches long), or 1 teaspoon vanilla extract

¼ cup Swerve confectioners'-style sweetener or equivalent amount of liquid or powdered sweetener (see page 24)

¼ cup unsweetened cocoa powder

½ teaspoon fine sea salt

special equipment

Ice cream maker

nutritional info (per serving)				
calories	fat	protein	carbs	fiber
460	49g	7g	2g	1g

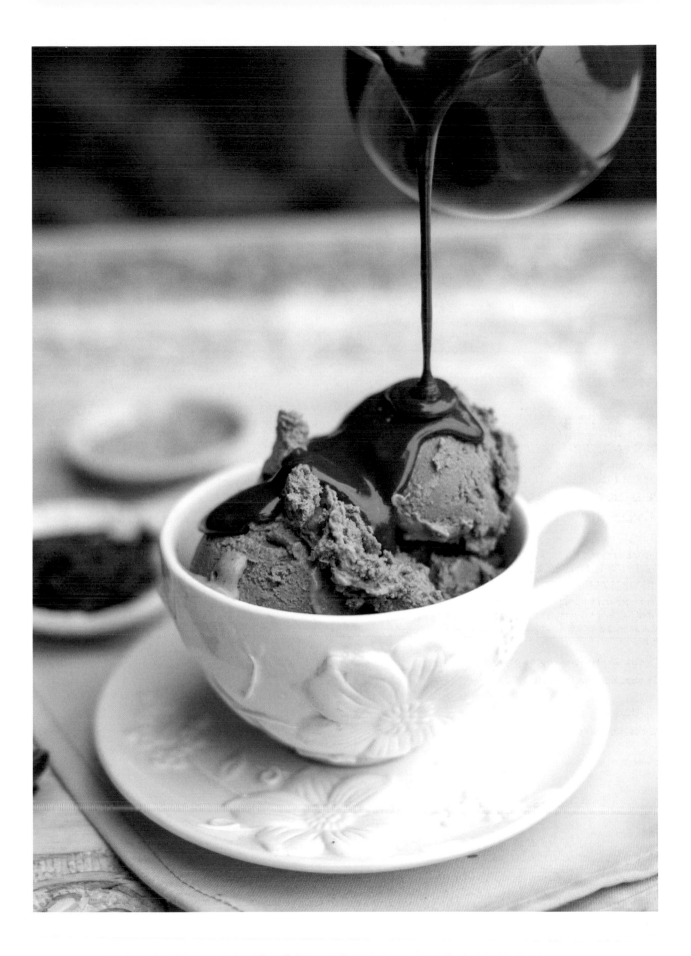

"Keto Debbie" Chocolate Cupcakes

L M H KETO OPTION

prep time: 15 minutes   *cook time:* 20 minutes   *yield:* 6 servings

cupcakes

3 large eggs, separated

¼ cup Swerve confectioners'-style sweetener or equivalent amount of liquid or powdered sweetener (see page 24)

¼ cup (½ stick) unsalted butter (or coconut oil if dairy-free), melted but not hot

1 teaspoon vanilla extract

½ cup blanched almond flour

2 tablespoons unsweetened cocoa powder

¼ teaspoon fine sea salt

¼ teaspoon baking soda

filling and decoration

1 (8-ounce) package cream cheese (Kite Hill brand cream cheese style spread if dairy-free), softened

½ cup Swerve confectioners'-style sweetener or equivalent amount of liquid or powdered sweetener (see page 24)

2 tablespoons unsweetened cashew milk or heavy cream

ganache

2 tablespoons unsalted butter (or coconut oil if dairy-free)

1 ounce unsweetened chocolate, chopped

¼ cup plus 1 tablespoon heavy cream (or full-fat coconut milk if dairy-free)

¼ cup Swerve confectioners'-style sweetener or equivalent amount of liquid or powdered sweetener (see page 24)

Seeds scraped from 1 vanilla bean (about 8 inches long), or 1 teaspoon vanilla extract

1. Preheat the oven to 350°F. Grease a 6-well jumbo muffin pan.

2. To make the cupcakes, place the egg whites in a bowl and whip until stiff peaks form. In a second bowl, combine the egg yolks, sweetener, butter, and vanilla and whisk until well blended. In a third bowl, whisk together the dry ingredients until fully combined. Gently fold the egg yolk mixture into the whipped whites, then slowly fold in the dry mixture. Fill the greased pan with the batter, filling each well about three-quarters full. Bake for 15 to 18 minutes, until a toothpick inserted in the center of a cupcake comes out clean. Let cool completely in the pan before removing.

3. While the cupcakes are cooling, make the filling: Place the softened cream cheese and sweetener in a small bowl. Using a hand mixer, combine until smooth. Slowly add the cashew milk to thin the filling. Transfer the filling to a piping bag. Fill the cupcakes by poking a hole in the bottom of each cupcake and piping in the filling. Reserve a few tablespoons of the filling for the white swirl on the top. (Leave the reserved filling on the counter; if it sets in the refrigerator, it will become too hard to pipe.)

4. To make the ganache, place the butter and chopped chocolate in a double boiler or in a heat-safe bowl set over a pan of simmering water. Heat on low, stirring often, until just melted (don't let the chocolate burn!), then add the cream, sweetener, and vanilla. Stir until smooth and thick.

5. Dunk the top of each cupcake into the ganache. Set the cupcakes upright on a serving platter. Place in the refrigerator for 5 minutes to set the ganache. Remove from the fridge and, using the reserved filling, pipe little swirls on the top of each cupcake, moving from one end to the other.

6. Store extras in an airtight container in the refrigerator for up to 4 days or in the freezer for up to 1 month. Allow to thaw to room temperature before serving.

nutritional info (per cupcake)				
calories	fat	protein	carbs	fiber
407	38g	9g	6g	2g

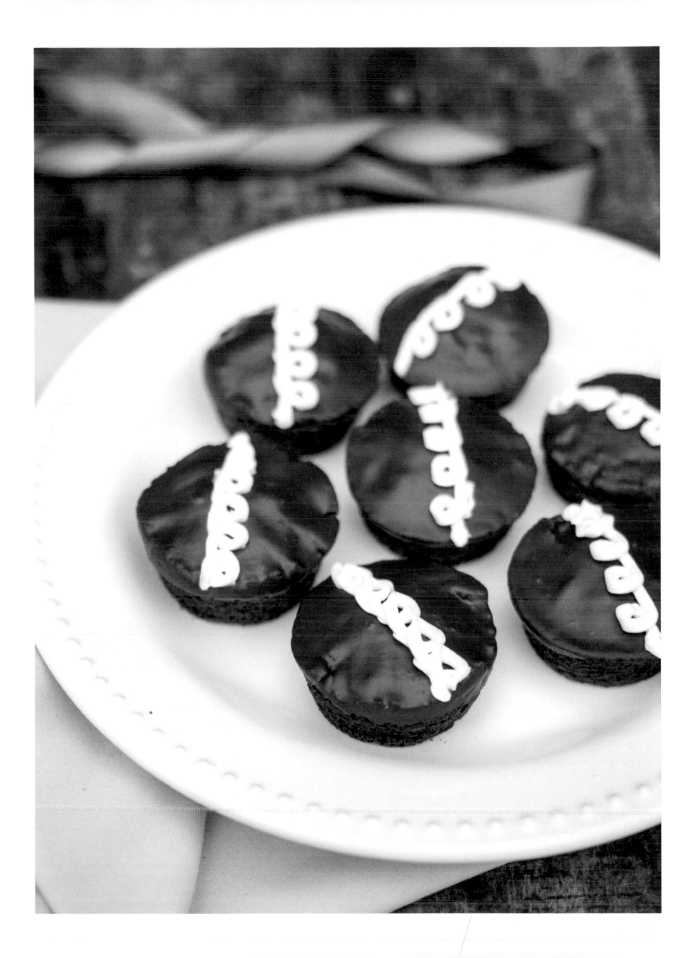

Penuche (Italian Fudge)

prep time: 10 minutes, plus time to chill overnight   *cook time:* 4 minutes
yield: 24 servings

1 cup (2 sticks) unsalted butter

¼ cup Swerve confectioners'-style sweetener or equivalent amount of liquid or powdered sweetener (see page 24)

1 teaspoon maple extract or a few drops of maple oil

1 (8-ounce) package mascarpone or cream cheese

¼ teaspoon ginger powder (optional)

1 cup chopped raw pecans or walnuts (optional)

for garnish (optional)

24 raw pecan or walnut halves

1. In a small saucepan, melt the butter over medium-high heat until brown (but not black!) flecks appear. Add the sweetener and stir to combine.

2. Add the extract and mascarpone cheese and stir until the cheese is melted. Pour the mixture into a blender and add the ginger, if using. Blend until smooth.

3. Stir in the nuts, if using.

4. Place a piece of parchment paper in an 8-inch square baking pan. Pour the fudge mixture into the lined pan. Refrigerate overnight; the fudge will thicken a lot. Remove it from the pan, peel away the parchment, and cut the fudge into 24 pieces. Garnish the top of each piece with a pecan or walnut half, if desired.

5. Store extras in an airtight container in the refrigerator for up to 4 days or in the freezer for up to 1 month. Allow to thaw before serving.

nutritional info (per serving)				
calories	fat	protein	carbs	fiber
157	16g	1g	1g	1g

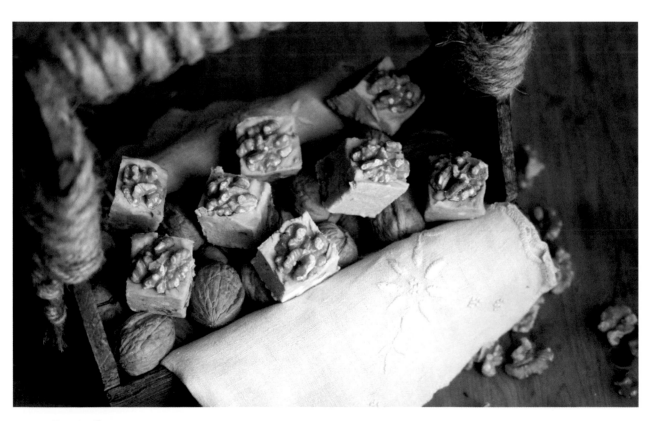

Peaches and Cream Sorbet

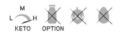

prep time: 10 minutes, plus time to churn *yield:* 4 servings

1½ cups heavy cream (or full-fat coconut milk if dairy-free)

½ cup strong brewed peach tea or Bai Panama Peach, chilled

1 teaspoon peach extract

1 teaspoon peach-flavored liquid stevia

3 tablespoons Swerve confectioners'-style sweetener or equivalent amount of liquid or powdered sweetener (see page 24)

½ teaspoon fine sea salt

special equipment

Ice cream maker

Place all the ingredients in a blender and blend until smooth. Pour into an ice cream maker and churn according to the manufacturer's directions. Serve immediately or store the sorbet in an airtight container in the freezer for up to 1 month.

nutritional info (per serving)				
calories	fat	protein	carbs	fiber
300	36g	0g	0g	0g

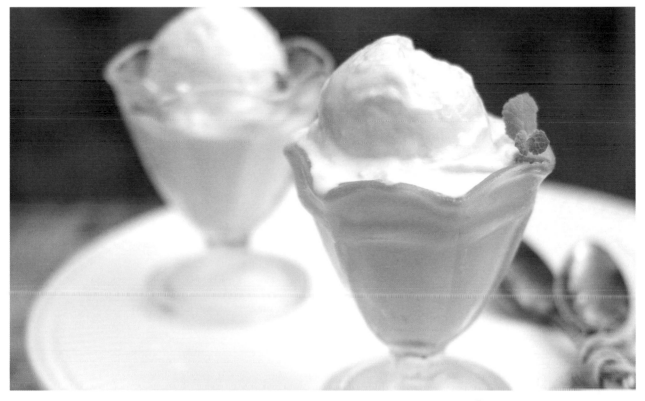

Chocolate Ice Cream Cake
with Almond Butter Swirl

L M H
KETO OPTION OPTION

prep time: 15 minutes, plus time to churn ice cream and freeze cake overnight
cook time: 35 minutes yield: one 8-inch four-layer cake (18 servings)

cake

3 cups blanched almond flour (or 1 cup coconut flour if nut-free)

¾ cup unsweetened cocoa powder

1 teaspoon ground cinnamon (optional)

1 teaspoon baking soda

½ teaspoon fine sea salt

6 large eggs (12 eggs if using coconut flour)

1 cup Swerve confectioners'-style sweetener or equivalent amount of liquid or powdered sweetener (see page 24)

1 tablespoon unsalted butter (or coconut oil if dairy-free), melted but not hot

3 tablespoons unsweetened cashew milk (or full-fat coconut milk if nut-free) (½ cup milk if using coconut flour)

1 teaspoon vanilla extract or other extract of choice, such as raspberry

1½ cups grated zucchini

ice cream

¾ cup (1½ sticks) plus 2 tablespoons unsalted butter (or coconut oil if dairy-free), softened

4 large eggs

4 large egg yolks

½ cup unsweetened cashew milk (or water if nut-free)

¼ cup MCT oil (creates a smooth ice cream)

Seeds scraped from 2 vanilla beans (about 8 inches long), or 2 teaspoons vanilla extract

¼ cup Swerve confectioners'-style sweetener or equivalent amount of powdered stevia or erythritol (see page 24)

¼ cup unsweetened cocoa powder

½ teaspoon fine sea salt (keeps the ice cream soft)

1. Preheat the oven to 350°F. Spray two 8-inch round cake pans with coconut oil spray.

2. To make the cake, in a large mixing bowl, whisk together the flour, cocoa powder, cinnamon (if using), baking soda, and salt until blended.

3. In a separate bowl, using a hand mixer, beat the eggs and sweetener for 2 to 3 minutes, until frothy and lightened in color. Add the melted butter, cashew milk, and extract to the egg mixture and mix to combine.

4. Squeeze the water out of the grated zucchini if it seems wet, then add the zucchini to the egg mixture and stir to combine. Add the wet ingredients to the dry, stirring only enough to combine.

5. Pour the batter evenly into the pans and bake for 20 to 30 minutes, until a toothpick inserted in the center comes out clean. Allow the cake layers to cool completely in the pans.

6. Meanwhile, make the ice cream layer: In a blender, combine the butter, whole eggs, egg yolks, cashew milk, MCT oil, vanilla, sweetener, cocoa powder, and salt. Blend until very smooth. Place in an ice cream maker and churn according to the manufacturer's directions.

7. While the ice cream is churning, make the almond butter swirl, if using: Combine the almond butter, melted butter, and sweetener in a small bowl and beat until smooth with the hand mixer. Place in the refrigerator to chill until the ice cream is almost done. In the last 30 seconds of churning, add the swirl to the ice cream maker.

8. When the cake layers are fully cool, run a knife around the edge of each pan to loosen the cake, then tip the pan over and pop out the cake. With a large sharp knife, cut each cake layer in half horizontally to create 4 thin layers. At this point, the cake layers can be frozen, or you can assemble the ice cream cake immediately and then freeze it.

9. To assemble, take one sliced layer of cake and set it in a parchment paper–lined springform pan (the walls of the springform pan will help support the cake as you build it). Then scoop some ice cream on top of it and spread it in an even layer. Once the ice cream layer is level, place a second cake layer on top, then add another layer of ice cream. Repeat with the remaining layers of cake and ice cream so you have 4 even layers. Freeze overnight.

10. Once frozen, make the chocolate glaze: Place the butter and chopped chocolate in a double boiler or in a heat-safe bowl set over a pot of simmering water. Heat on medium, stirring often, until the chocolate

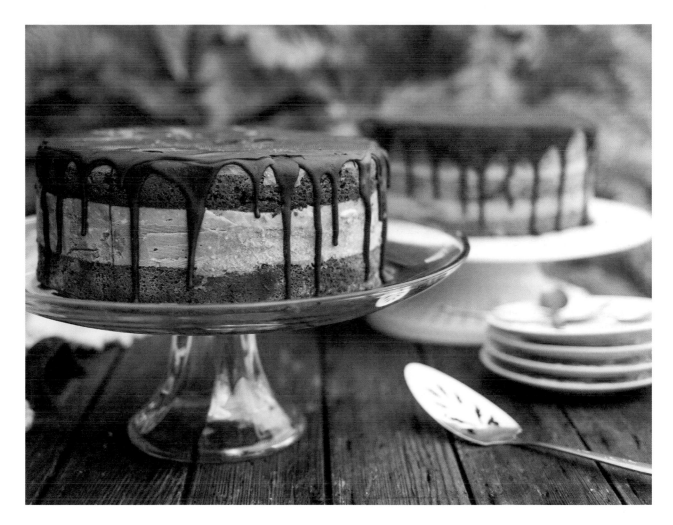

almond butter swirl (omit for nut-free)

½ cup almond butter, at room temperature

¼ cup (½ stick) unsalted butter (or coconut oil if dairy-free), melted

¼ cup Swerve confectioners'-style sweetener or equivalent amount of liquid or powdered sweetener (see page 24)

chocolate glaze

2 tablespoons unsalted butter (or coconut oil if dairy-free)

1 ounce unsweetened chocolate, chopped

8 tablespoons heavy cream (or full-fat coconut milk if dairy-free)

¼ cup Swerve confectioners'-style sweetener or equivalent amount of powdered stevia or erythritol (see page 24)

1 teaspoon vanilla extract

is just melted (don't let it burn!), then add the cream, sweetener, and vanilla. Stir until smooth and thick. Remove from the heat and place in the refrigerator to cool for a few minutes before using.

11. Remove the frozen ice cream cake from the freezer. Drizzle the glaze on top of the cake and put it back in the freezer to set. Allow to thaw a bit before slicing and serving. Store extras in an airtight container in the freezer for up to 1 month.

note: *This is just one option for layering this cake. You could also put one unsliced cake layer in the bottom of the pan, add all the ice cream to form the middle layer, and then add the second cake layer and the glaze on top, as shown in the photo. For the cake pictured, I also used the almond butter swirl mixture to make a separate layer on top of the ice cream instead of adding it to the ice cream to create a swirl. However you layer it, it will be delicious!*

special equipment

Ice cream maker

nutritional info (per serving)				
calories	fat	protein	carbs	fiber
385	35g	11g	8g	4g

Deconstructed
Chocolate Waffle Cones

prep time: 10 minutes (not including time to make ice cream)
cook time: 20 minutes   *yield:* 6 servings

hot fudge sauce

¾ cup heavy cream (or full-fat coconut milk if dairy-free)

⅓ cup Swerve confectioners'-style sweetener or equivalent amount of liquid or powdered sweetener (see page 24)

2 ounces unsweetened chocolate, finely chopped

Seeds scraped from 1 vanilla bean (about 8 inches long), or 1 teaspoon vanilla extract

chocolate waffles

4 large eggs

4 hard-boiled eggs

¼ cup Swerve confectioners'-style sweetener or equivalent amount of liquid or powdered sweetener (see page 24)

¼ cup unsweetened cocoa powder

2 tablespoons egg white protein powder

¾ teaspoon baking powder

¼ teaspoon fine sea salt

¼ cup coconut oil, plus extra for the waffle iron

2 teaspoons vanilla extract (option: substitute almond extract for 1 teaspoon if not allergic to almonds)

1 batch French Silk Ice Cream (page 312)

1. To make the hot fudge sauce, place the heavy cream, sweetener, and chopped chocolate in a double boiler or in a heat-safe bowl over a pot of simmering water. Heat on low, while stirring, just until the chocolate melts, then slide the pot off the heat. Stir in the vanilla. Keep the top part of the double boiler (or the bowl) over the warm water to keep the sauce hot while you make the waffles.

2. To make the waffles, heat a waffle iron to high. Place the raw eggs, hard-boiled eggs, sweetener, cocoa powder, protein powder, baking powder, and salt in a blender or food processor and combine until smooth and thick. Add the coconut oil and extract and pulse until well combined. Grease the hot waffle iron with coconut oil. Place 3 tablespoons of the batter in the center of the iron and close. Cook for 3 to 4 minutes, until the waffle is golden brown and crisp. Repeat with the remaining batter, making a total of 6 waffles.

3. Serve the waffles topped with a scoop of French Silk Ice Cream and the hot fudge sauce.

4. Store extra waffles in an airtight container in the refrigerator for up to 3 days or in the freezer for up to 1 month. Reheat the waffles in a preheated 375°F oven or toaster oven for 3 minutes or until warmed through. Store the hot fudge in an airtight container in the refrigerator for up to 4 days or in the freezer for up to 2 months. Reheat the hot fudge in a double boiler or heavy-bottomed saucepan over low heat, stirring often, for about 1 minute. Heat gently or the chocolate will break.

busy family tip:

Save time by having the ice cream made ahead. You can even make the hot fudge and waffles in advance and reheat them just before serving.

nutritional info (per serving)				
calories	fat	protein	carbs	fiber
810	82g	19g	7g	4g

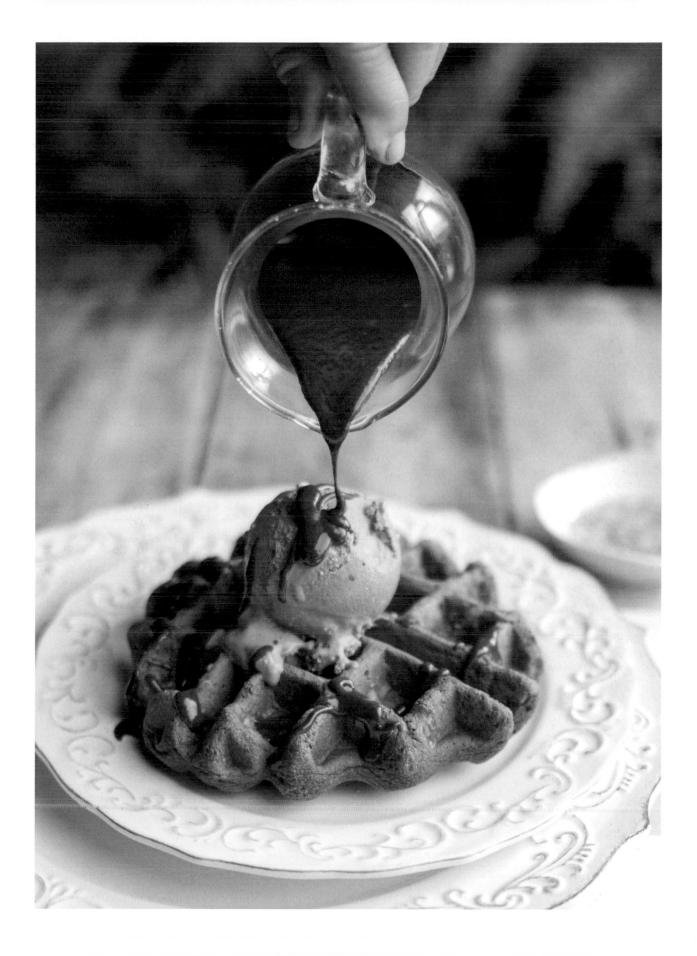

Maple Bacon Ice Cream
in Bacon Cones

Oh my word! This ice cream is amazing! If you adore ice cream like I do, you must try this recipe. If you don't have maple extract, you can substitute the seeds scraped from 1 vanilla bean (about 8 inches long), or 1 teaspoon vanilla extract. Vanilla and bacon isn't quite as delicious as maple and bacon, but it's not too shabby!

12 strips bacon

¾ cup (1½ sticks) plus 2 tablespoons unsalted butter (or coconut oil if dairy-sensitive)

½ cup unsweetened cashew milk, almond milk, or water

¼ cup MCT oil (creates a smooth ice cream)

4 large eggs

4 large egg yolks

¼ cup Swerve confectioners'-style sweetener or equivalent amount of liquid or powdered sweetener (see page 24)

2 teaspoons maple extract

¼ teaspoon fine sea salt (keeps the ice cream soft)

special equipment
Ice cream maker

prep time: 10 minutes, plus time to churn ice cream *cook time:* 20 minutes
yield: 6 servings

1. Preheat the oven to 400°F.

2. Line a rimmed baking sheet with parchment paper. Have on hand 6 cone-shaped metal objects (I made my own with sheet metal; you can use a funnel). Take a strip of bacon and wrap it tightly around the form, overlapping the edges so the bacon totally covers the form. Place the cone on the baking sheet, on its side, with the bacon ends seam side down. Repeat with another 5 strips of bacon and the remaining forms to make 6 cones. Bake for 15 to 20 minutes, until the bacon is crisp. Allow to cool completely on the forms before removing the cones.

3. While the bacon cones are baking, dice the remaining 6 strips of bacon and cook in a skillet over medium heat until crispy. Set the cooked bacon aside for use as a garnish; reserve the rendered bacon fat for another purpose.

4. If browning the butter, place the butter in a saucepan over medium-high heat. Using a whisk, stir occasionally while the butter heats, foams up, and forms brown (but not black!) specks. Do not allow the butter to burn. Once browned, remove the pan from the heat and allow the butter to cool. If not browning the butter, or if using coconut oil, simply heat the butter or oil until melted, then set aside to cool.

5. In a blender, combine the cooled browned butter, cashew milk, MCT oil, whole eggs, egg yolks, sweetener, extract, and salt. Blend until very smooth. Place in an ice cream maker and churn according to the manufacturer's directions.

6. To serve, scoop some ice cream into a cooled bacon cone and sprinkle the cooked diced bacon on top.

7. Store the ice cream in an airtight container in the freezer for up to 1 month.

nutritional info (per serving)				
calories	fat	protein	carbs	fiber
514	50g	14g	1g	0g

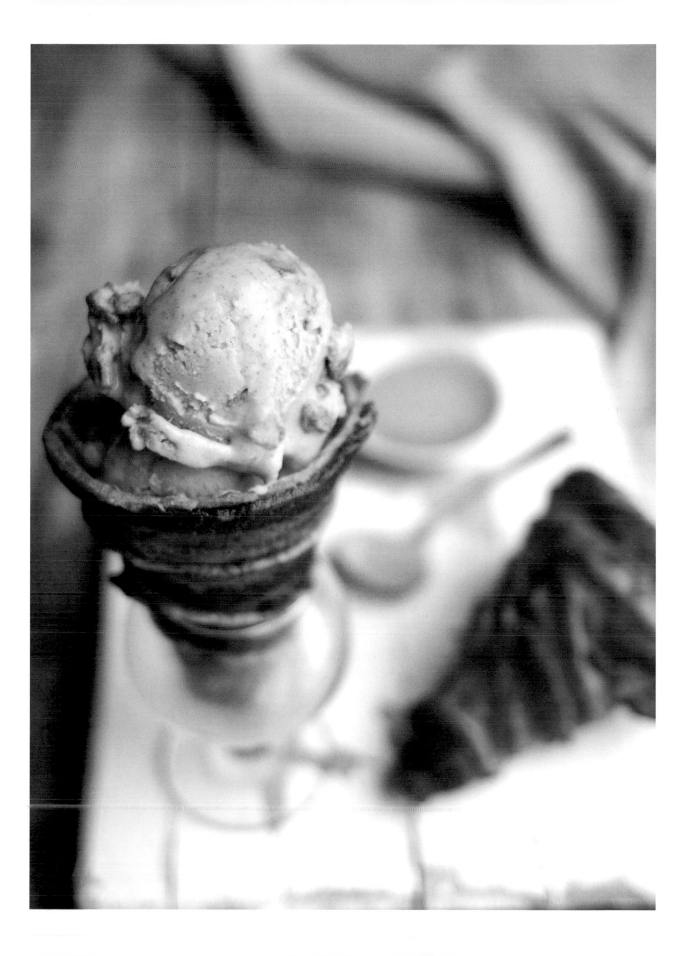

Strawberries and Cream Snowballs

I like to call these snowballs because I first made them on a cold, wintry day after making a snow fort with my little boys. We came in with icicles hanging from our eyelashes and warmed up by baking these beautiful little cakes.

^M
L ↑ H
KETO

prep time: 10 minutes, plus at least 1 hour to chill   *cook time:* 12 minutes
yield: 12 snowballs (1 per serving)

cakes

2¾ cups blanched almond flour or 1 cup coconut flour

2 teaspoons baking powder

1 teaspoon baking soda

¾ teaspoon fine sea salt

¾ cup (1½ sticks) unsalted butter, softened

1½ cups Swerve confectioners'-style sweetener or equivalent amount of liquid or powdered sweetener (see page 24)

3 large eggs (8 eggs if using coconut flour)

2 teaspoons strawberry extract

1½ cups sour cream

frosting

1½ cups (3 sticks) unsalted butter, softened

1½ (8-ounce) packages cream cheese or mascarpone cheese, softened

1½ cups Swerve confectioners'-style sweetener or equivalent amount of liquid or powdered sweetener (see page 24)

2 tablespoons unsweetened cashew milk or almond milk

½ teaspoon strawberry extract

Natural red or pink food coloring (optional)

Unsweetened shredded coconut, for garnish

special equipment

2 (6-cavity) silicone round-bottomed (sphere- or ball-shaped) cupcake pans

1. Preheat the oven to 350°F. Grease two 6-cavity round-bottomed cupcake pans.

2. In a small bowl, sift together the almond flour, baking powder, baking soda, and salt. In a large bowl, beat together the butter and sweetener with a hand mixer on medium-high speed until pale and fluffy, 3 to 5 minutes. Beat in the eggs one at a time, beating well after each addition, then beat in the extract. Reduce the speed to low, then add the flour mixture and sour cream alternately in batches, beginning and ending with the flour mixture and mixing until the batter is just smooth.

3. Spoon the batter evenly into the pans, filling the cavities about two-thirds full. Smooth the tops, then rap the pans on the counter once or twice to expel any air bubbles. Bake until the cakes are pale golden and a toothpick inserted in the center comes out clean, about 12 minutes. Remove from the oven and let cool completely in the pan. (*Tip:* Once you've removed the cakes from the pan, place them in the freezer until frozen for easier frosting.)

4. To make the frosting, combine the butter, cream cheese, sweetener, cashew milk, and extract in small bowl. Beat on medium speed until smooth; if the frosting is too thick, gradually add more milk until it reaches the desired spreading consistency. Add natural food coloring, if desired.

5. To assemble the snowballs, cut ¼ inch off the bottom (the rounded side) of half of the cakes and eat or set aside. This will help keep the balls from rolling over as you work. Set the cakes with the bottoms cut off on a baking sheet or serving platter with the broad, flat side facing up. Frost the flat top part of each cake. Top with an uncut cake to make a ball. Spread the frosting over the whole ball and sprinkle with shredded coconut. Cover loosely and place in the refrigerator for at least 1 hour to allow the frosting to harden before serving.

6. Store extras in an airtight container in the refrigerator for up to 4 days.

nutritional info (per snowball)				
calories	*fat*	*protein*	*carbs*	*fiber*
591	58g	9g	7g	3g

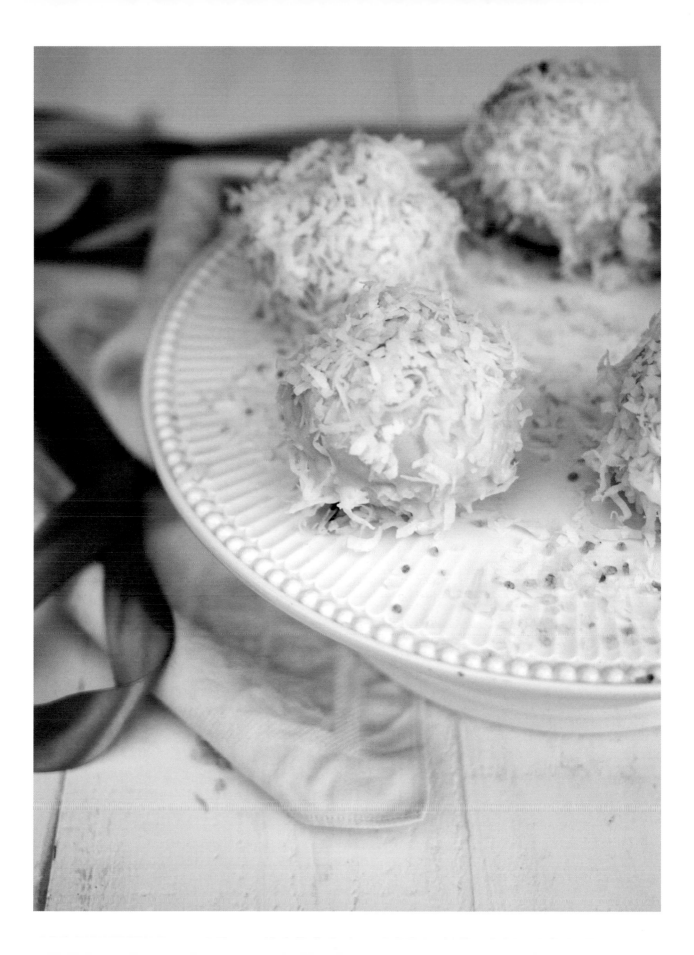

Malted Milk Ball Cheesecake

There's something special about the flavor of malted milk. When I was in high school, I worked at the front desk of a hotel, and across the parking lot was the Medford Café. I would get dinner from the café and always ordered their classic malt. I always wondered what was in malted milk, and when I finally looked it up, I was horrified by the ingredients!

Malt powder is made from grains, typically barley, which are not part of a keto diet. It was tricky to recreate that malted milk flavor without barley. After experimenting for a few years (yes, *years*), I finally found the perfect malted milk flavor! It is a superfood called maca powder.

L M H
KETO   OPTION

prep time: 10 minutes, plus time to chill overnight   *cook time:* 1 hour

yield: one 8-inch cake (16 servings)

crust

3½ tablespoons unsalted butter (or coconut oil if dairy-free), plus extra for the pan

1½ ounces unsweetened chocolate, finely chopped

⅓ cup Swerve confectioners'-style sweetener or equivalent amount of liquid or powdered sweetener (see page 24)

1 teaspoon stevia glycerite

1 large egg, beaten

2 teaspoons ground cinnamon

Seeds scraped from 1 vanilla bean (about 8 inches long), or 1 teaspoon vanilla extract

¼ teaspoon fine sea salt

filling

6 (8-ounce) packages cream cheese (Kite Hill brand cream cheese style spread if dairy-free)

¾ cup Swerve confectioners'-style sweetener or equivalent amount of liquid or powdered sweetener (see page 24)

½ cup maca powder

Seeds scraped from 1 vanilla bean (about 8 inches long), or 1 teaspoon vanilla extract

3 large eggs

ganache

1 cup heavy cream (or full-fat coconut milk if dairy-free)

⅓ cup Swerve confectioners'-style sweetener or equivalent amount of liquid or powdered sweetener (see page 24)

2 ounces unsweetened chocolate, finely chopped

Seeds scraped from 1 vanilla bean (about 8 inches long), or 1 teaspoon vanilla extract

⅛ teaspoon fine sea salt

special equipment

8-inch springform pan

1. Preheat the oven to 350°F. Grease an 8-inch springform pan, then line it with parchment paper and grease the paper.

2. Mix together the crust ingredients, then press the crust mixture into the prepared pan.

3. Combine the cream cheese, sweetener, maca powder, and vanilla with a hand mixer until blended. Add the eggs one at a time, mixing on low after each addition, just until blended. Pour the batter on top of the crust in the springform pan.

4. Set up a water bath: Wrap aluminum foil entirely around the bottom and halfway up the sides of the springform pan to prevent water from leaking into the removable bottom of the pan. Place the wrapped pan inside a roasting pan (or any baking dish with sides) and place the pans in the oven. Pour hot water into the roasting pan so that it comes halfway up the sides of the springform pan. (*Note:* A water bath helps cook the cheesecake evenly; however, the cheesecake can be baked without it. See the note on page 310 if you choose not to use a water bath.) Bake for 1 hour or until the center of the cheesecake is almost set. Let the cake cool completely in the pan before removing the outer ring. Refrigerate the cheesecake overnight.

5. Just before serving, make the ganache: Bring the cream and sweetener to a simmer in a saucepan over medium heat. Remove from the heat and add the chopped chocolate, vanilla, and salt. Stir, then allow to sit for 3 minutes. Stir again until completely smooth. Pour the ganache over the chilled cheesecake, then place the cake in the refrigerator to set for 10 minutes before serving.

6. Store extras in an airtight container in the refrigerator for up to 4 days.

nutritional info (per serving)				
calories	fat	protein	carbs	fiber
358	31g	8g	9g	3g

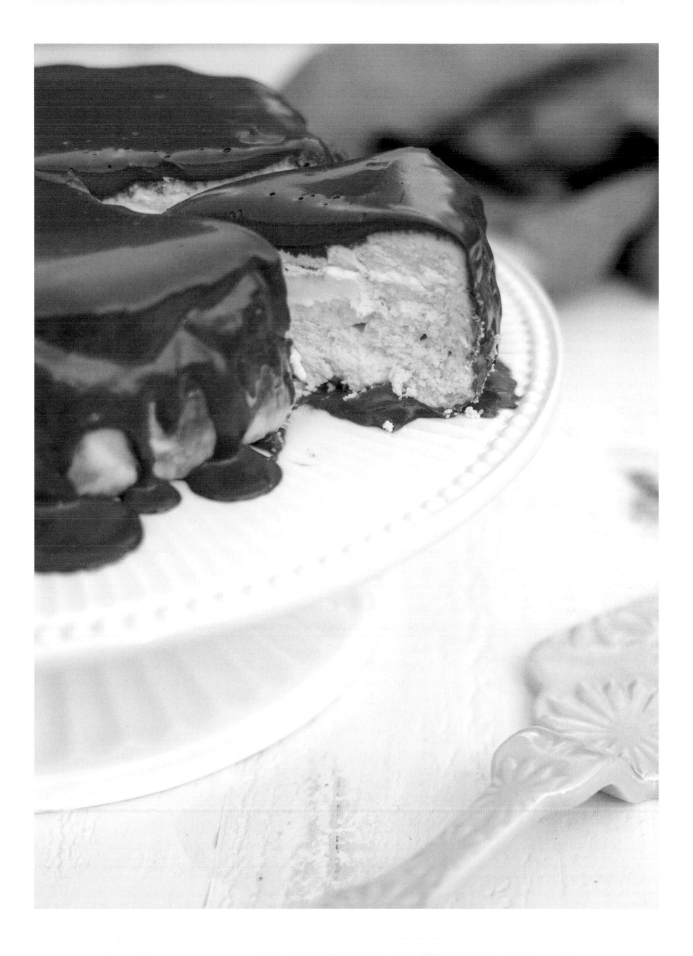

Cannoli Mini Cheese Balls

These amazingly tasty cannoli cheese balls are yummy on their own, but if you prefer to serve them like a chip and dip, pair them with Deconstructed Chocolate Cannoli Cookies (page 309), as pictured.

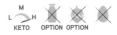

L M H KETO OPTION OPTION

prep time: 10 minutes, plus 30 minutes to chill   *yield:* 8 balls (1 per serving)

cannoli balls

1 (8-ounce) package cream cheese or mascarpone cheese (Kite Hill brand cream cheese style spread if dairy-free), softened

½ cup ricotta cheese (or Kite Hill brand cream cheese style spread, softened, if dairy-free)

½ cup Swerve confectioners'-style sweetener or equivalent amount of liquid or powdered sweetener (see page 24)

1 teaspoon ground cinnamon

chocolate chunks

1 cup (2 sticks) unsalted butter (or coconut oil if dairy-free), melted

1 cup unsweetened cocoa powder

¾ cup Swerve confectioners'-style sweetener or equivalent amount of liquid or powdered sweetener (see page 24)

1 teaspoon almond extract (omit for nut-free)

1 teaspoon vanilla extract

¼ teaspoon fine sea salt

chocolate drizzle

¼ cup heavy cream (or full-fat coconut milk if dairy-free)

1 ounce unsweetened chocolate, finely chopped

2 tablespoons Swerve confectioners'-style sweetener or equivalent amount of liquid or powdered sweetener (see page 24)

Seeds scraped from 1 vanilla bean (about 8 inches long), or 1 teaspoon vanilla extract

1. To make the cannoli balls, place the cream cheese, ricotta, sweetener, and cinnamon in a medium-sized bowl. Mix well with a hand mixer. Using your hands, form the mixture into eight 2-inch balls and place on a rimmed baking sheet or tray. Cover and refrigerate for at least 30 minutes, until firm.

2. To make the chocolate chunks, place a piece of parchment paper in a 9-inch pie pan. Place all the ingredients for the chunks in a blender and pulse until smooth. Taste and adjust the sweetness to your liking. Pour the mixture onto the parchment and place the pie pan in the refrigerator or freezer to set, about 20 minutes in the fridge or 10 minutes in the freezer. Once hard, chop the chocolate into small pieces and place them in a shallow bowl.

3. To make the drizzle, place the cream, chopped chocolate, and sweetener in a double boiler or in a heat-safe bowl set over a pan of simmering water. Heat on low, stirring, just until the chocolate melts. Remove from the heat and stir in the vanilla. Place in the refrigerator to cool for 8 minutes or until thickened, but still a bit warm; if the chocolate hardens too much, return it to the double boiler and reheat gently.

4. Remove the cream cheese balls from the fridge and roll them in the chocolate pieces. Drizzle the chocolate-coated balls with the chocolate drizzle.

5. Store extras in an airtight container in the refrigerator for up to 4 days.

tip: *The chocolate chunks can be made ahead and stored in an airtight container in the refrigerator for up to 1 week or in the freezer for up to 1 month.*

nutritional info (per ball)				
calories	fat	protein	carbs	fiber
417	40g	6g	7g	3g

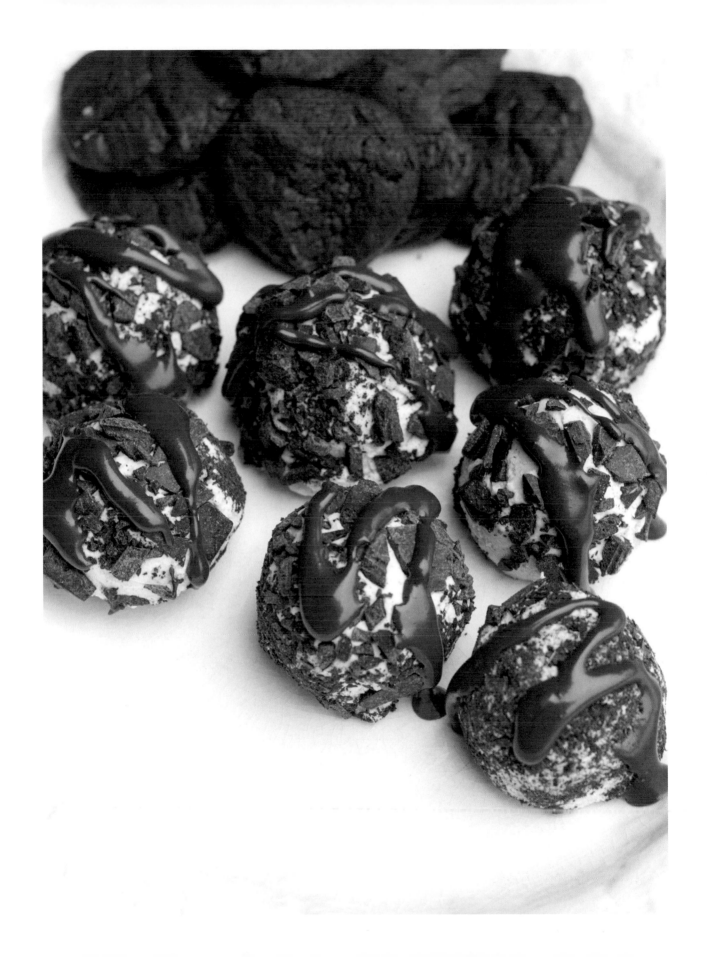

Mini Mocha Bundt Cakes

If you love mocha, then use decaf espresso in the glaze for a double dose of mocha flavor; if you like just a little bit of mocha flavor, like me, use hot water in the glaze for more of a vanilla flavor.

L M H
KETO OPTION

prep time: 10 minutes   *cook time:* 15 minutes   *yield:* 12 servings

cakes

3 cups blanched almond flour, or 1 cup coconut flour

¾ cup unsweetened cocoa powder

1 teaspoon baking soda

½ teaspoon fine sea salt

6 large eggs (12 eggs if using coconut flour)

1 cup Swerve confectioners'-style sweetener or equivalent amount of liquid or powdered sweetener (see page 24)

3 tablespoons ghee or unsalted butter (or coconut oil if dairy-free), melted but not hot

3 tablespoons brewed decaf espresso or other strong brewed decaf coffee (½ cup if using coconut flour)

1 teaspoon vanilla extract

1½ cups grated zucchini

glaze

1½ cups Swerve confectioners'-style sweetener or equivalent amount of powdered stevia or erythritol (see page 24)

¼ cup melted ghee or unsalted butter (or coconut oil if dairy-free)

2 tablespoons hot water (for vanilla-flavored glaze) or hot brewed decaf espresso or other strong brewed decaf coffee (for mocha-flavored glaze)

½ teaspoon vanilla extract

½ cup chopped walnuts or pecans, for garnish (optional)

special equipment

2 (6-well) mini Bundt cake pans (see note)

1. Preheat the oven to 350°F. Spray 2 mini Bundt pans with coconut oil spray.

2. To make the cakes, place the flour, cocoa powder, baking soda, and salt in a medium-sized bowl and whisk until blended. In a large bowl, beat the eggs and sweetener with a hand mixer for 2 to 3 minutes, until light and fluffy. Add the melted ghee, espresso, and vanilla to the egg mixture.

3. Squeeze the water out of the zucchini if it seems wet, then add it to the egg mixture and stir to combine. Add the wet ingredients to the dry ingredients and stir just to combine.

4. Pour the cake batter into the prepared pans, filling each well two-thirds full, and bake for about 15 minutes, until a toothpick inserted into the center of a cake comes out clean. Allow the cakes to cool completely in the pans before removing them.

5. To make the glaze, combine the sweetener with the melted ghee. Stir in the hot water or espresso and vanilla; it should be fairly thick, but thin enough to be stirred with ease. Add more water or espresso if the glaze is too thick; if it's too thin, add more sweetener.

6. Gently spoon the glaze over the cakes, covering the tops. If desired, garnish the cakes with chopped nuts.

7. Store extras in an airtight container in the refrigerator for up to 4 days or in the freezer for up to 1 month.

note: If you have only one 6-well mini Bundt pan, simply bake the cakes in two batches.

nutritional info (per cake)				
calories	fat	protein	carbs	fiber
328	29g	11g	9g	4g

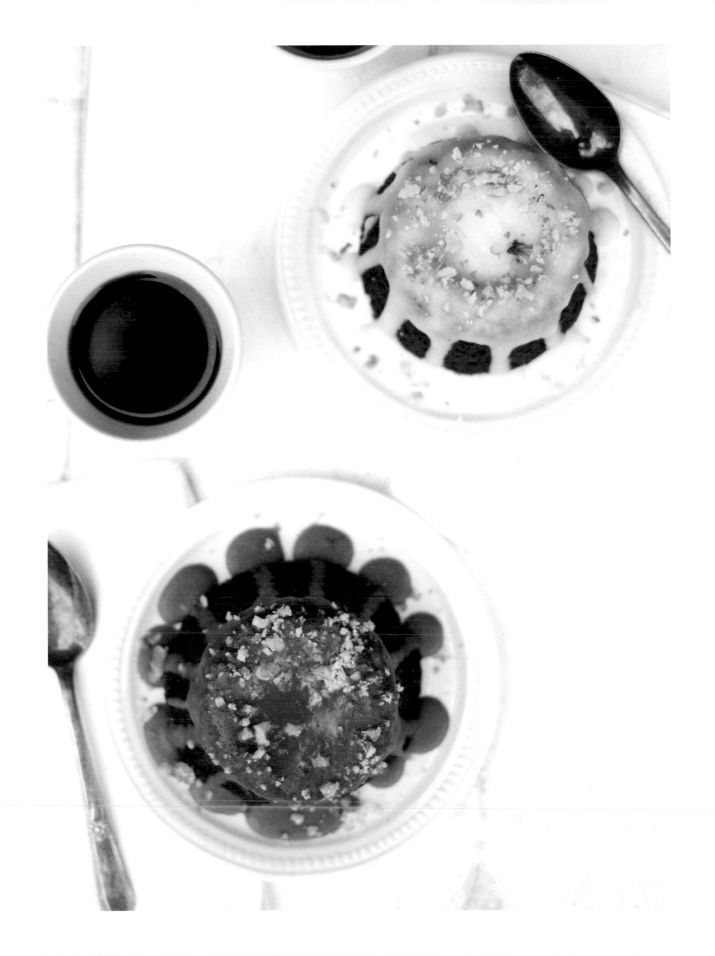

Mint Chocolate Whoopie Pies

1¼ cups blanched almond flour, or ½ cup coconut flour

¼ cup unsweetened cocoa powder

½ teaspoon baking soda

¼ teaspoon fine sea salt

¼ cup (½ stick) unsalted butter or coconut oil, softened, plus extra for the pans

⅓ cup Swerve confectioners'-style sweetener or equivalent amount of liquid or powdered sweetener (see page 24)

3 large eggs (6 eggs and ¼ cup unsweetened almond milk if using coconut flour)

1 teaspoon mint extract

filling

¾ cup (1½ sticks) unsalted butter, softened

6 ounces cream cheese or mascarpone cheese (¾ cup), softened

¾ cup Swerve confectioners'-style sweetener or equivalent amount of liquid or powdered sweetener (see page 24)

1 tablespoon heavy cream

1 teaspoon mint extract

chocolate drizzle

¼ cup heavy cream

2 tablespoons Swerve confectioners'-style sweetener or equivalent amount of liquid or powdered sweetener (see page 24)

½ ounce unsweetened chocolate, finely chopped

½ teaspoon vanilla extract

Fresh mint leaves, for garnish (optional)

special equipment

12-well whoopie pie pan or muffin top pan

prep time: 10 minutes   *cook time:* 12 minutes
yield: 6 pies (1 per serving)

1. Preheat the oven to 325°F. Grease a 12-well whoopie pie pan (or muffin top pan).

2. In a mixing bowl, whisk together the flour, cocoa powder, baking soda, and salt until blended. In a separate bowl, beat the butter, sweetener, eggs, and extract with a hand mixer until smooth. Stir the wet ingredients into the flour mixture. Spoon the batter into the prepared pan, filling each well about two-thirds full. Bake for 12 minutes or until a toothpick inserted into the center of a pie comes out clean. Allow to cool in the pan.

3. Meanwhile, make the filling: Using the hand mixer, cream the butter, cream cheese, and sweetener in a medium-sized bowl. Add the heavy cream to thin it out a little, then add the mint extract and mix to combine. Set the filling aside.

4. To make the chocolate drizzle, place the cream, sweetener, and chopped chocolate in a double boiler or in a heat-safe bowl set over a pan of simmering water. Heat on low, stirring, just until the chocolate is melted. Remove from the heat and stir in the vanilla. Taste and add more sweetener, if desired.

5. To assemble the whoopie pies, place one pie flat side up on a plate. Place 2 tablespoons of filling on the pie, then top with another pie. Repeat with the rest of the pies and filling. Drizzle the chocolate over each whoopie pie. Serve garnished with mint leaves, if desired.

6. Store extras in an airtight container in the refrigerator for up to 4 days.

nutritional info (per pie)				
calories	*fat*	*protein*	*carbs*	*fiber*
609	59g	11g	8g	4g

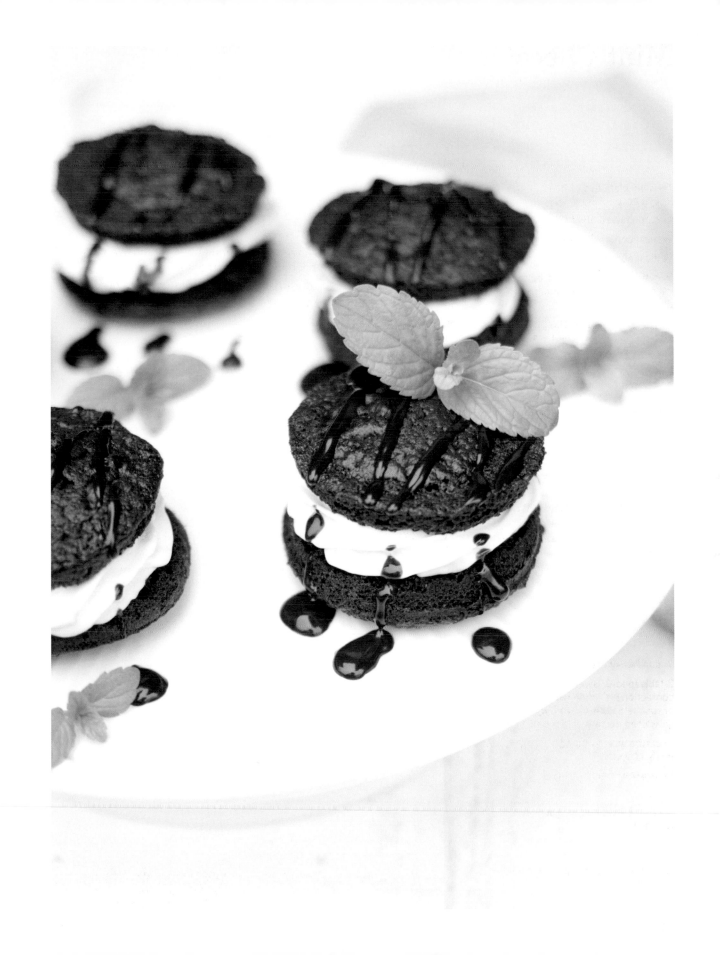

Mint Chocolate Cheesecake Bûche de Noël

Like its malted milk ball cousin on page 304, this is an elegant-looking dessert. If you don't have a bûche mold, you can make it in a loaf pan instead.

prep time: 1 hour, plus at least 3 hours to chill *cook time:* 2 minutes *yield:* 12 servings

mint cheesecake layer

½ cup unsweetened cashew milk

1 teaspoon unflavored gelatin

1 (8-ounce) package cream cheese, softened

1 cup heavy cream

¾ cup Swerve confectioners'-style sweetener or equivalent amount of liquid or powdered sweetener (see page 24)

2 teaspoons peppermint extract

Natural green food coloring (optional)

chocolate mousse layer

¼ cup unsweetened almond milk

1 teaspoon unflavored gelatin

3 large egg yolks

½ cup Swerve confectioners'-style sweetener or equivalent amount of liquid or powdered sweetener (see page 24)

3 ounces unsweetened chocolate, finely chopped

1 cup heavy cream

chocolate glaze

¾ cup heavy cream

⅓ cup Swerve confectioners'-style sweetener or equivalent amount of powdered stevia or erythritol (see page 24)

2 ounces unsweetened chocolate, finely chopped

Seeds scraped from 1 vanilla bean (about 8 inches long), or 1 teaspoon vanilla extract

Fresh mint leaves, for garnish

1. Have on hand a silicone bûche mold or a 9 by 5-inch loaf pan. If using a loaf pan, line it with parchment paper, leaving some paper overhanging.

2. To make the cheesecake layer, heat the cashew milk and gelatin in a large saucepan over low heat until the gelatin melts, about 2 minutes (or in the microwave for 10 seconds or until liquefied). Add the cream cheese, heavy cream, and sweetener and mix well with a hand mixer. Add the extract and food coloring, if using, and beat until smooth. Pour the batter into the bûche mold or lined loaf pan. Gently set the mold in the freezer while you make the chocolate mousse layer.

3. To make the mousse layer, heat the almond milk in the microwave or in a saucepan over low heat until hot, then set aside. Place 1 tablespoon of water in a small saucepan and whisk in the gelatin; let soften for 1 minute. Whisk in the egg yolks and sweetener, then stir in the hot almond milk. Cook over medium heat, stirring constantly, for 5 minutes or until the mixture thickens and coats a spoon. Add the 3 ounces of chopped chocolate and stir until the chocolate is totally melted, about 3 more minutes. Transfer the chocolate custard to a mixing bowl and place it in the refrigerator to cool slightly.

4. When the custard is just slightly warm, whip the cream until stiff peaks form. Gradually fold the whipped cream into the custard, then smooth the mousse over the cheesecake layer in the bûche pan and smooth the top. Cover and freeze for at least 3 hours or overnight, until firm.

5. To unmold, gently peel the sides of the silicone mold away from the bûche, pressing the top of the mold gently with your hand until the bûche releases. If you used a loaf pan, allow the bûche to thaw slightly, then use the overhanging paper to lift the bûche out of the pan. Place the bûche on a serving platter and set it in the freezer while you prepare the glaze.

6. To make the chocolate glaze, place the cream, sweetener, and chopped chocolate in a double boiler or in a heat-safe bowl set over a pan of simmering water. Heat on low, stirring, just until the chocolate is melted. Remove from the heat and stir in the vanilla. Pour the chocolate glaze over the cooled bûche. Cut into slices and garnish with mint leaves. Cover and refrigerate until ready to serve.

7. Store extras in an airtight container in the refrigerator for up to 4 days or in the freezer for up to 1 month.

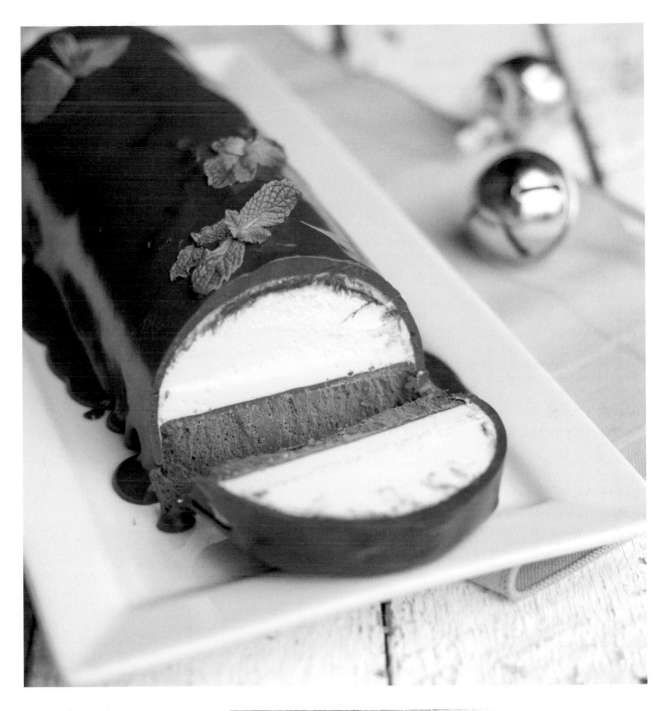

special equipment (optional)

Silicone bûche mold, about 10 by 3½ inches

serving tip :

The bûche is easier to cut into pretty slices when it's semi-frozen. I like to slice it before dinner (when slightly frozen) and then allow the slices to warm at room temperature until soft but still chilled.

health tip :

After fructo-oligosaccharides, the highest short-chain fatty acid–yielding prebiotic is collagen. That's right. Collagen (like the Great Lakes gelatin collagen hydrolysate) is a great prebiotic. So adding gelatin can be a great prebiotic without adding carbs.

nutritional info (per serving)				
calories	fat	protein	carbs	fiber
343	35g	4g	4g	3g

Decadent Black Forest Dessert
for Two

L M H — KETO — X OPTION

I adore my toaster oven! I often use it to make simple desserts like this.

simple vanilla ice cream

½ cup heavy cream (or coconut cream if dairy-free)

½ cup unsweetened cashew milk

3 tablespoons Swerve confectioners'-style sweetener or equivalent amount of liquid or powdered sweetener (see page 24), or more as desired

Seeds scraped from 1 vanilla bean (about 8 inches long), or 1 teaspoon vanilla extract

Pinch of fine sea salt

cake

¼ cup blanched almond flour

2 tablespoons Swerve confectioners'-style sweetener or equivalent amount of liquid or powdered sweetener (see page 24)

1 tablespoon unsweetened cocoa powder

½ teaspoon baking powder

Pinch of fine sea salt

2 tablespoons melted (but not hot) ghee or unsalted butter (or butter-flavored coconut oil if dairy-free), plus extra for greasing the pans

1 large egg

½ teaspoon cherry extract

cherry glaze

3 tablespoons unsalted butter (or butter-flavored coconut oil if dairy-free)

1½ tablespoons Swerve confectioners'-style sweetener or equivalent amount of powdered stevia or erythritol (see page 24)

1 to 2 teaspoons cherry extract

special equipment

Ice cream maker

prep time: 10 minutes, plus time to churn ice cream   *cook time:* 12 minutes
yield: 2 servings

1. To make the ice cream, place all the ingredients for the ice cream in a blender and puree for 1 minute or until frothy. Place in an ice cream maker and churn according to the manufacturer's directions. Transfer the ice cream to an airtight container and place in the freezer while you make the cake and glaze. (*Note:* The ice cream can be made ahead and stored in the freezer for up to 1 month.)

2. To make the cakes, preheat the oven or toaster oven to 325°F. Grease 2 wells of a standard-size muffin pan or two 4-ounce ramekins.

3. Place the almond flour, powdered sweetener (if using powdered), cocoa powder, baking powder, and salt in a medium-sized bowl and stir to combine well. Add the melted ghee, egg, cherry extract, and liquid sweetener (if using liquid) and stir until well combined. Pour into the prepared pan and bake for 10 to 13 minutes, until a toothpick inserted in the middle of a cake comes out clean. Let cool in the pan.

4. While the cake is baking, make the cherry glaze: Place the butter in a saucepan over medium-high heat. Stirring often, heat until the butter foams up and brown (but not black!) flecks appear. Remove from the heat and allow to cool a bit. (If using coconut oil, simply heat the oil until melted.) Add the sweetener and 1 teaspoon of cherry extract to the browned butter (or coconut oil). Taste and add more sweetener or extract, if desired.

5. To assemble the dessert, remove the ice cream from the freezer. (If you made the ice cream ahead of time and it's frozen solid, allow it to soften for 15 to 25 minutes.) Slice a cake into 4 wedges and arrange them in a serving bowl. Scoop half of the ice cream into the bowl, then drizzle half of the cherry glaze over the ice cream. Repeat with the other cake and remaining ice cream and glaze.

nutritional info (per serving)				
calories	fat	protein	carbs	fiber
613	65g	7g	4g	2g

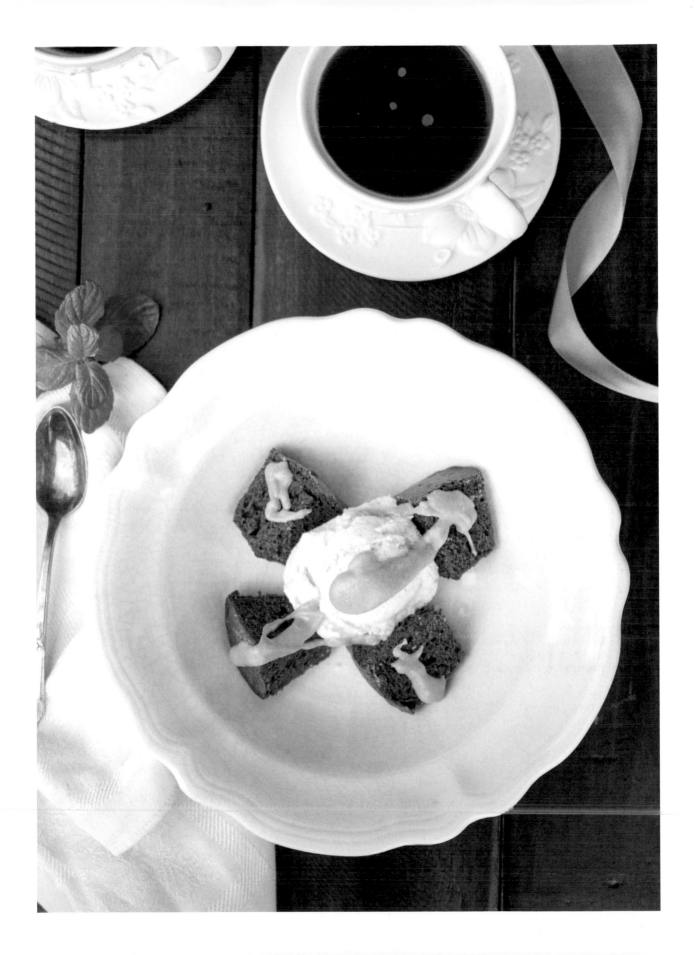

"Rice" Pudding

prep time: 5 minutes   *cook time:* 5 minutes   *yield:* 4 servings

6 large egg yolks

½ cup unsweetened cashew milk (or hemp milk if nut-free, or heavy cream if not dairy-sensitive)

¼ cup Swerve confectioners'-style sweetener or equivalent amount of liquid or powdered sweetener (see page 24)

1 teaspoon vanilla extract or other extract of choice, such as cherry

¼ cup coconut oil, melted (or melted unsalted butter if not dairy-sensitive)

1 (8-ounce) package Miracle Rice

Ground cinnamon

Melted unsalted butter or ghee, for drizzling (omit for dairy-free)

1. In a medium-sized bowl, combine the egg yolks, cashew milk, sweetener, and extract. Slowly mix in the melted coconut oil so the eggs don't cook unevenly. Set the bowl over a saucepan of simmering water.

2. Whisk the mixture constantly and vigorously until it is thick enough to coat the back of a spoon and an instant-read thermometer inserted into the mixture registers 140°F, 3 to 5 minutes.

3. Remove the mixture from the water and stir in the Miracle Rice. Add cinnamon to taste. Serve warm or chilled, garnished with a dusting of extra cinnamon and a drizzle of melted butter, if desired.

4. Store extra pudding in an airtight container in the refrigerator for up to 4 days.

tip : *If you're serving the pudding chilled, it can be prepared up to 4 days ahead and stored in the refrigerator. Whisk before serving.*

nutritional info (per serving)				
calories	fat	protein	carbs	fiber
206	21g	4g	1g	0.1g

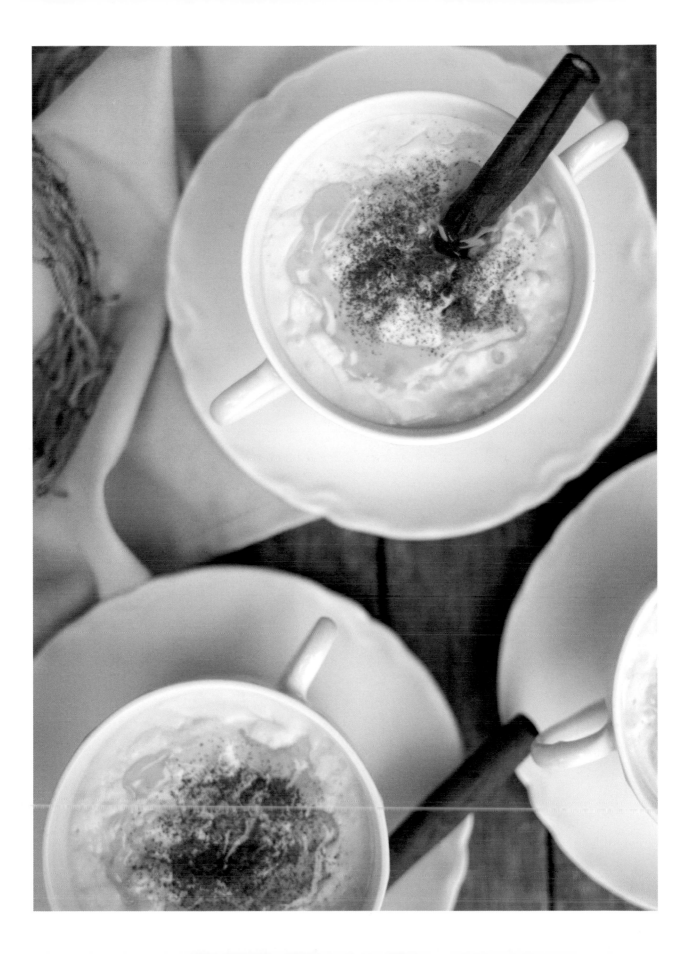

Creamy Chocolate Mint Truffles

L M H   KETO   OPTION   OPTION

5 ounces cream cheese (½ cup plus 2 tablespoons) (Kite Hill brand cream cheese style spread if dairy-free), softened

¼ cup Swerve confectioners'-style sweetener or equivalent amount of liquid or powdered sweetener (see page 24)

1 teaspoon unsweetened cashew milk (or hemp milk if nut-free)

1 teaspoon mint extract

chocolate drizzle

¼ cup heavy cream (or full-fat coconut milk if dairy-free)

2 tablespoons Swerve confectioners'-style sweetener or equivalent amount of liquid or powdered sweetener (see page 24)

1 ounce unsweetened chocolate, finely chopped

1 teaspoon mint extract

Fresh mint leaves, for garnish

1. Place the cream cheese, sweetener, cashew milk, and extract in a bowl and mix with a hand mixer until smooth. Taste and adjust the sweetness to your liking, adding more sweetener or extract, if desired. Cover and refrigerate for at least 3 hours or overnight.

2. Using a mini ice cream scooper or spoon, scoop out 1-inch balls of the mixture. Place the balls on a serving platter. Place the platter in the refrigerator while you make the chocolate drizzle.

3. To make the drizzle, place the cream, sweetener, and chopped chocolate in a double boiler or in a heat-safe bowl set over a pan of simmering water. Heat on low, stirring, just until the chocolate is melted. Remove from the heat and stir in the extract. Allow the drizzle to cool in the refrigerator for 8 minutes or until thickened, but still a bit warm; if it hardens too much, return the drizzle to the double boiler and reheat gently.

4. Remove the truffles from the fridge and use a spoon to drizzle the chocolate over each truffle. Serve chilled, garnished with mint leaves.

5. Store extras in an airtight container in the refrigerator for up to 4 days. Freezing is not recommended.

nutritional info (per truffle)				
calories	fat	protein	carbs	fiber
111	10g	2g	2g	1g

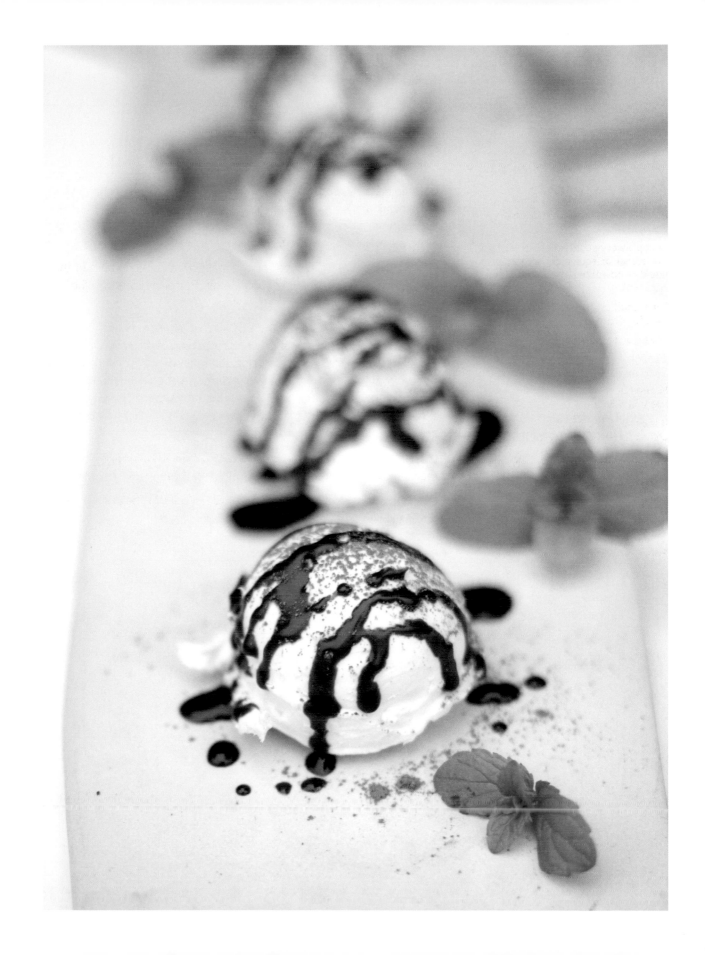

Malted Milk Ball Truffles

5 ounces cream cheese (½ cup plus 2 tablespoons) (Kite Hill brand cream cheese style spread if dairy-free), softened

¼ cup Swerve confectioners'-style sweetener or equivalent amount of liquid or powdered sweetener (see page 24)

2 tablespoons maca powder

1 teaspoon unsweetened cashew milk (or hemp milk if nut-free)

Seeds scraped from 1 vanilla bean (about 8 inches long), or 1 teaspoon vanilla extract

chocolate drizzle

¼ cup heavy cream (or full-fat coconut milk if dairy-free)

2 tablespoons Swerve confectioners'-style sweetener or equivalent amount of liquid or powdered sweetener (see page 24)

1 ounce unsweetened chocolate, finely chopped

Seeds scraped from 1 vanilla bean (about 8 inches long), or 1 teaspoon vanilla extract

1. Place the cream cheese, sweetener, maca powder, cashew milk, and vanilla in a bowl and mix with a hand mixer until smooth. Taste and adjust the sweetness to your liking, adding more sweetener or maca powder, if desired. Cover and refrigerate for at least 3 hours or overnight.

2. Using a mini ice cream scooper or spoon, scoop out 1-inch balls of the mixture. Place the balls on a serving platter. Place the platter in the refrigerator while you make the chocolate drizzle.

3. To make the drizzle, place the cream, sweetener, and chopped chocolate in a double boiler or in a heat-safe bowl set over a pan of simmering water. Heat on low, stirring, just until the chocolate is melted. Remove from the heat and stir in the vanilla. Allow the drizzle to cool in the refrigerator for 8 minutes or until thickened, but still a bit warm; if it hardens too much, return the drizzle to the double boiler and reheat gently.

4. Remove the truffles from the fridge and use a spoon to drizzle the chocolate over each truffle. Serve chilled.

5. Store extras in an airtight container in the refrigerator for up to 4 days. Freezing is not recommended.

nutritional info (per truffle)				
calories	fat	protein	carbs	fiber
123	10g	2g	4g	2g

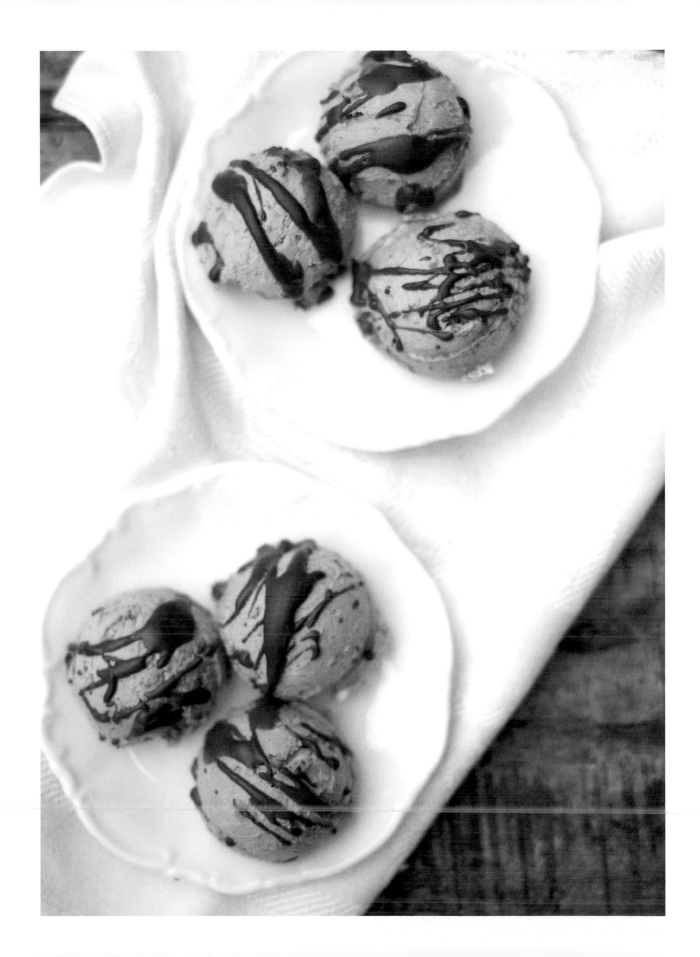

Pecan Pie Truffles

KETO

1 cup (2 sticks) unsalted butter

¼ cup Swerve confectioners'-style sweetener or equivalent amount of liquid or powdered sweetener (see page 24)

¼ cup raw pecans, finely chopped

Seeds scraped from 1 vanilla bean (about 8 inches long), or 1 teaspoon vanilla extract

¼ teaspoon fine sea salt

chocolate drizzle

¼ cup heavy cream

2 tablespoons Swerve confectioners'-style sweetener or equivalent amount of liquid or powdered sweetener (see page 24)

1 ounce unsweetened chocolate, finely chopped

Seeds scraped from 1 vanilla bean (about 8 inches long), or 1 teaspoon vanilla extract

Crushed raw pecans, for garnish

prep time: 10 minutes *cook time:* 5 minutes
yield: 2 dozen truffles (2 per serving)

1. Melt the butter in a small saucepan over medium-high heat until it foams up and brown (but not black!) flecks appear. Remove from the heat and place in the refrigerator to cool for 10 minutes.

2. Add the sweetener, pecans, vanilla, and salt to the browned butter and stir well to combine.

3. When the mixture is at room temperature and has returned to a solid consistency, use a mini ice cream scooper or spoon to scoop out 1-inch balls of the mixture. Place the balls on a serving platter and set the platter in the refrigerator while you make the chocolate drizzle.

4. To make the drizzle, combine the cream, sweetener, and chopped chocolate in a double boiler or in a heat-safe bowl set over a pan of simmering water. Heat on low, stirring, just until the chocolate is melted. Remove from the heat and stir in the vanilla. Allow to cool in the refrigerator for 8 minutes or until thickened, but still a bit warm; if it hardens too much, return the drizzle to the double boiler and reheat gently.

5. Remove the truffles from the fridge and use a spoon to drizzle the chocolate over each truffle. Garnish each truffle with crushed pecans. Serve at room temperature.

6. Store extras in an airtight container in the refrigerator for up to 4 days or in the freezer for up to 1 month.

nutritional info (per serving)				
calories	fat	protein	carbs	fiber
182	19g	1g	1g	1g

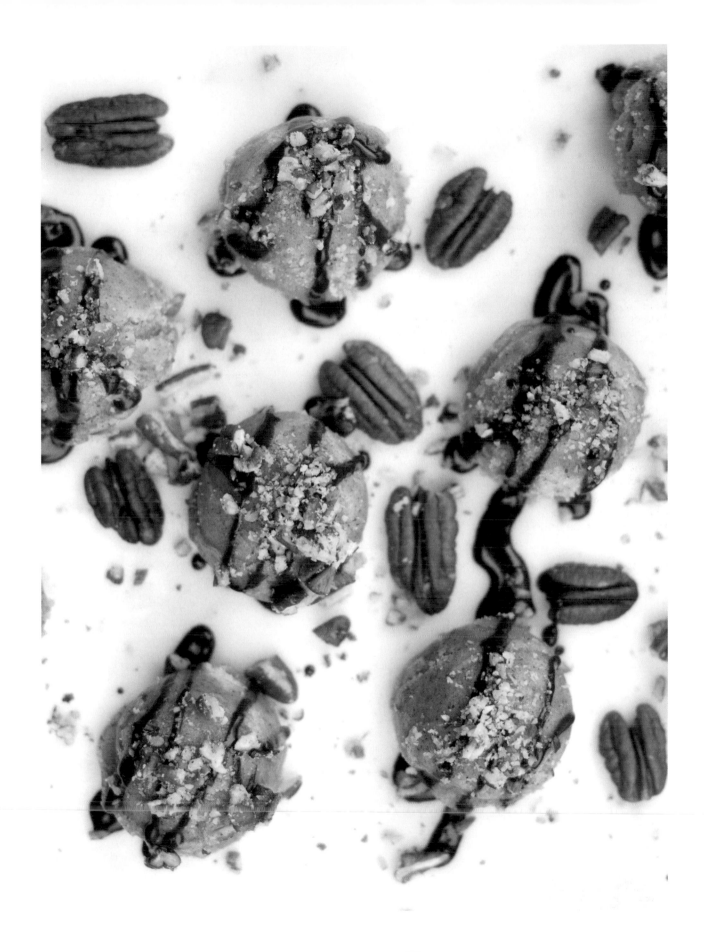

Dark Chocolate Raspberry Truffles

L M H KETO · OPTION · OPTION · ✕

prep time: 10 minutes, plus at least 3 hours to chill · *cook time:* 2 minutes · *yield:* 8 truffles (1 per serving)

5 ounces cream cheese (½ cup plus 2 tablespoons) (Kite Hill brand cheese style spread if dairy-free), softened

¼ cup Swerve confectioners'-style sweetener or equivalent amount of liquid or powdered sweetener (see page 24)

1 to 2 teaspoons unsweetened cashew milk (or hemp milk if nut-free), warmed

2 tablespoons unsweetened cocoa powder, or more if you prefer darker chocolate, plus extra for garnish

1 teaspoon raspberry extract

chocolate drizzle

¼ cup heavy cream (or full-fat coconut milk if dairy-free)

2 tablespoons Swerve confectioners'-style sweetener or equivalent amount of liquid or powdered sweetener (see page 24)

1 ounce unsweetened chocolate, finely chopped

1 teaspoon raspberry extract

1. Place the cream cheese and sweetener in a bowl and mix with a hand mixer until smooth. Remove 2 tablespoons of the sweetened cream cheese and place it in a small bowl for the topping. Add a teaspoon of warm cashew milk to thin the topping and mix until smooth. If it's still too thick, add another teaspoon of milk. Transfer the topping to a small resealable plastic bag or piping bag and set in the refrigerator.

2. Add the cocoa powder and extract to the bowl with the remaining sweetened cream cheese and beat with the hand mixer on high speed until combined. Taste and add more sweetener, cocoa powder, or extract, if desired. Cover and refrigerate for at least 3 hours or overnight.

3. Using a mini ice cream scooper or spoon, scoop out 1-inch balls of the chocolate mixture. Place the balls on a serving platter. Cut a tiny hole in the corner of the plastic bag with the topping and drizzle each truffle with a little bit of the topping. Return the truffles to the refrigerator while you make the chocolate drizzle.

4. To make the drizzle, place the cream, sweetener, and chopped chocolate in a double boiler or in a heat-safe bowl set over a pan of simmering water. Heat on low, stirring, just until the chocolate is melted. Remove from the heat and stir in the extract. Allow to cool in the refrigerator for 8 minutes or until thickened, but still a bit warm; if it hardens too much, return it to the double boiler and reheat gently.

5. Remove the truffles from the fridge and use a spoon to drizzle the chocolate over each truffle. Dust each truffle with cocoa powder. Serve chilled.

6. Store extras in an airtight container in the refrigerator for up to 4 days. Freezing is not recommended.

nutritional info (per truffle)				
calories	fat	protein	carbs	fiber
116	11g	2g	2g	1g

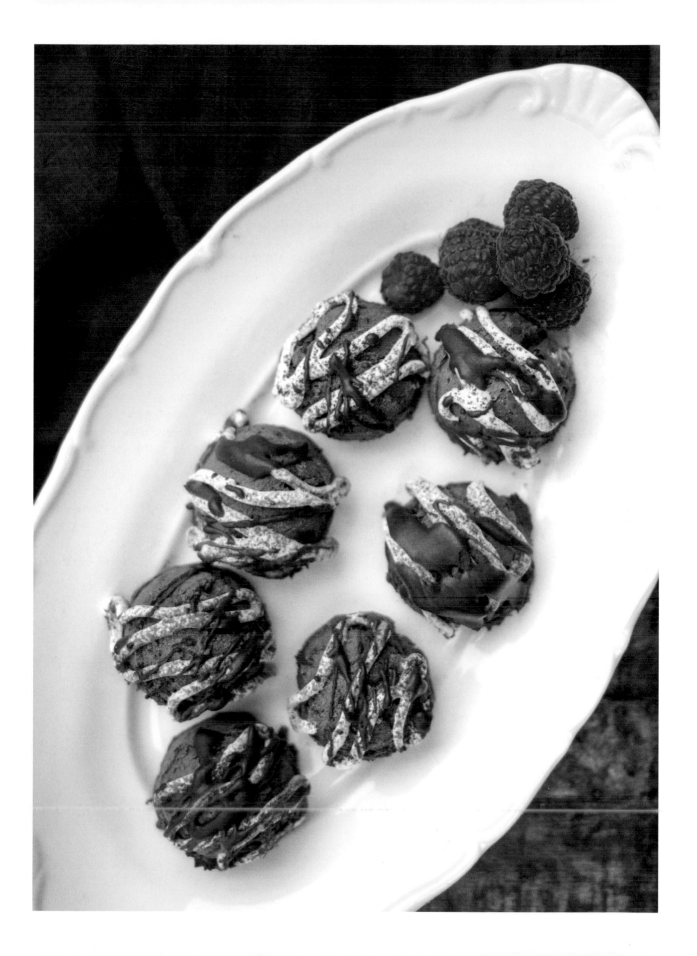

Pumpkin Cheesecake Truffles

L →H · M
KETO   OPTION

prep time: 5 minutes, plus at least 3 hours to chill
yield: 8 truffles (1 per serving)

5 ounces cream cheese (½ cup plus 2 tablespoons) (Kite Hill brand cream cheese style spread if dairy-free), softened

¼ cup Swerve confectioners'-style sweetener or equivalent amount of liquid or powdered sweetener (see page 24)

1 to 2 teaspoons unsweetened cashew milk or hemp milk, warmed

¼ cup pecan meal or almond meal

2 tablespoons fresh or canned pumpkin puree

¾ teaspoon pumpkin pie spice

½ teaspoon ground cinnamon

3 tablespoons crushed walnuts or pili nuts, for garnish (optional)

Pinch of ground nutmeg, for garnish

1. Place the cream cheese and sweetener in a bowl and mix with a hand mixer until smooth. Remove 2 tablespoons of the sweetened cream cheese and place it in a small bowl for the topping. Add a teaspoon of warm cashew milk to thin the topping and mix until smooth. If it's still too thick, add another teaspoon of milk. Transfer the topping to a small resealable plastic bag or piping bag and set in the refrigerator.

2. Add the pecan meal, pumpkin puree, pumpkin pie spice, and cinnamon to the bowl with the remaining sweetened cream cheese and beat with the hand mixer on high speed until combined. Cover and refrigerate for at least 3 hours or overnight.

3. Using a mini ice cream scooper or spoon, scoop out 1-inch balls of the pumpkin cheesecake mixture. Place the balls on a serving platter. Cut a tiny hole in the corner of the plastic bag with the topping and drizzle each truffle with a little bit of the topping. Sprinkle with crushed walnuts, if desired, and a touch of nutmeg. Serve chilled.

4. Store extras in an airtight container in the refrigerator for up to 4 days. Freezing is not recommended.

tip : I used leftover pumpkin puree that I had in my freezer, which had a bit of liquid in the container. If you use frozen puree, make sure to drain the excess liquid or the truffles will be too soft.

nutritional info (per truffle)				
calories	fat	protein	carbs	fiber
137	12g	2g	2g	1g

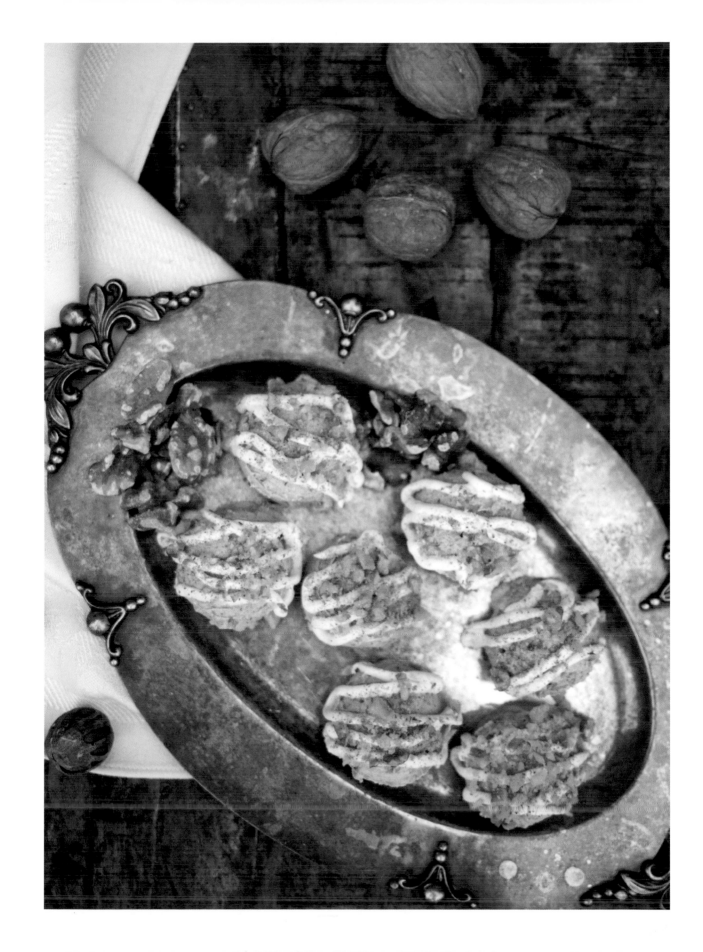

Bananas Foster
for Two

L M H KETO   OPTION

My first taste of Bananas Foster was at a four-star restaurant on Maui called Nick's. It was the most amazing meal I've ever had. Whenever I make this dessert, I am immediately transported back to that meal.

A toaster oven is perfect for making simple desserts like this.

prep time: 10 minutes, plus time to churn ice cream (not including time to make sweetened whipped cream) *cook time:* 12 minutes *yield:* 2 servings

simple vanilla ice cream

½ cup heavy cream (or coconut cream if dairy-free)

½ cup unsweetened cashew milk

3 tablespoons Swerve confectioners'-style sweetener or equivalent amount of liquid or powdered sweetener (see page 24), or more as desired

Seeds scraped from 1 vanilla bean (about 8 inches long), or 1 teaspoon vanilla extract

Pinch of fine sea salt

cake

¼ cup blanched almond flour

2 tablespoons Swerve confectioners'-style sweetener or equivalent amount of liquid or powdered sweetener (see page 24)

½ teaspoon baking powder

Pinch of fine sea salt

2 tablespoons melted (but not hot) ghee or unsalted butter (or butter-flavored coconut oil if dairy-free)

1 large egg

1 teaspoon banana extract

caramel glaze

3 tablespoons unsalted butter (or butter-flavored coconut oil if dairy-free)

1½ tablespoons Swerve confectioners'-style sweetener or equivalent amount of powdered stevia or erythritol (see page 24)

1 to 2 teaspoons rum or banana extract

1. To make the ice cream, place all the ingredients for the ice cream in a blender and puree for 1 minute or until frothy. Pour into an ice cream maker and churn according to the manufacturer's directions. Transfer the ice cream to an airtight container and place in the freezer while you make the cake and glaze. (*Note:* The ice cream can be made ahead and stored in the freezer for up to 1 month.)

2. To make the cake, preheat the oven or toaster oven to 325°F. Grease 2 wells of a standard-size muffin pan or two 4-ounce ramekins.

3. Place the almond flour, powdered sweetener (if using powdered), baking powder, and salt in a medium-sized bowl and stir to combine well. Add the melted ghee, egg, extract, and liquid sweetener (if using liquid) and stir until well combined. Pour the batter into the prepared pan and bake for 10 to 13 minutes, until a toothpick inserted in the middle of a cake comes out clean. Let cool in the pan.

4. While the cakes are cooling, make the glaze: Place the butter in a small saucepan over medium-high heat. Stirring often, heat until the butter foams up and brown (but not black!) flecks appear. Remove from the heat and allow to cool a bit. (If using coconut oil, simply heat the oil until melted.) Add the sweetener and 1 teaspoon of the extract to the browned butter (or coconut oil), then taste and add more sweetener or extract, if desired.

5. To assemble the dessert, remove the ice cream from the freezer. (If you made the ice cream ahead of time and it's frozen solid, allow it to soften for 15 to 25 minutes.) Slice a cake into 4 pieces and arrange the pieces in a serving bowl. Scoop half of the ice cream into the bowl, then drizzle half of the glaze over the ice cream. Repeat with the other cake and remaining ice cream and glaze. Garnish with whipped cream and walnuts, if desired.

for garnish (optional)

Sweetened whipped cream (see tip, page 298; omit for dairy-free)

Chopped walnuts

special equipment

Ice cream maker

nutritional info (per serving)				
calories	*fat*	*protein*	*carbs*	*fiber*
650	69g	7g	4g	2g

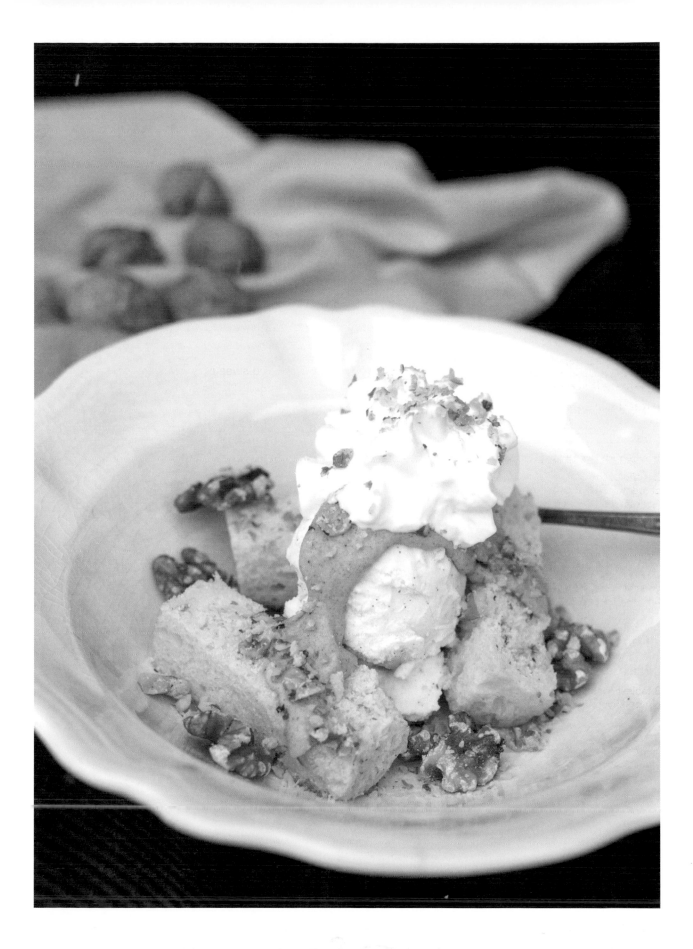

Banana Cream Pie

L M H — KETO OPTION

prep time: 10 minutes (not including time to make sweetened whipped cream)
cook time: 15 minutes *yield:* one 8-inch pie (12 servings)

crust

¾ cup blanched almond flour

¼ cup coconut flour

½ cup Swerve confectioners'-style sweetener or equivalent amount of liquid or powdered sweetener (see page 24)

½ cup (1 stick) unsalted butter (or coconut oil if dairy-free)

1 teaspoon fine sea salt

filling

6 large egg yolks

½ cup unsweetened almond milk

¼ cup Swerve confectioners'-style sweetener or equivalent amount of liquid or powdered sweetener (see page 24)

¼ cup (½ stick) unsalted butter (or coconut oil if dairy-free), melted

1 teaspoon banana extract or a few drops of banana oil

optional topping

Sweetened whipped cream (see tip, page 298; omit for dairy-free)

1. Preheat the oven to 325°F. Grease an 8-inch pie pan.

2. To make the crust, mix together the crust ingredients in a medium-sized bowl. Press the mixture into the bottom of the greased pie pan. Par-bake the crust for 15 minutes or until lightly golden brown. Set aside to cool.

3. While the crust is in the oven, make the filling: Place the egg yolks, almond milk, and sweetener in a medium-sized heat-safe bowl and whisk to blend. Slowly whisk the melted butter into the egg mixture (be sure to go slowly so the eggs don't cook). Set the bowl over a saucepan of simmering water. Whisk the filling mixture constantly and vigorously until it is thick enough to coat the back of a spoon and an instant-read thermometer inserted into the mixture registers 140°F, about 5 minutes. Stir in the extract, then remove the filling from the heat. Place the bowl of filling in an ice bath, stirring often, until completely chilled. (Or let it cool to room temperature, then place the filling in the refrigerator until completely chilled.)

4. Pour the chilled filling into the cooled crust and top the pie with sweetened whipped cream, if desired.

busy family tip:
The filling can be made 1 to 3 days ahead and refrigerated.

nutritional info (per serving)				
calories	fat	protein	carbs	fiber
212	21g	3g	3g	2g

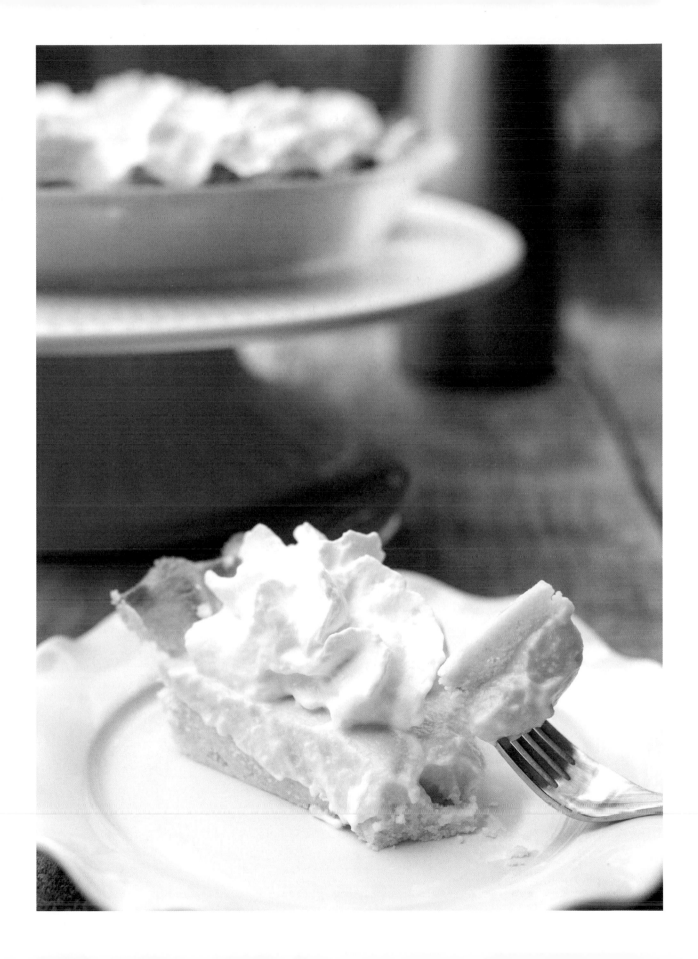

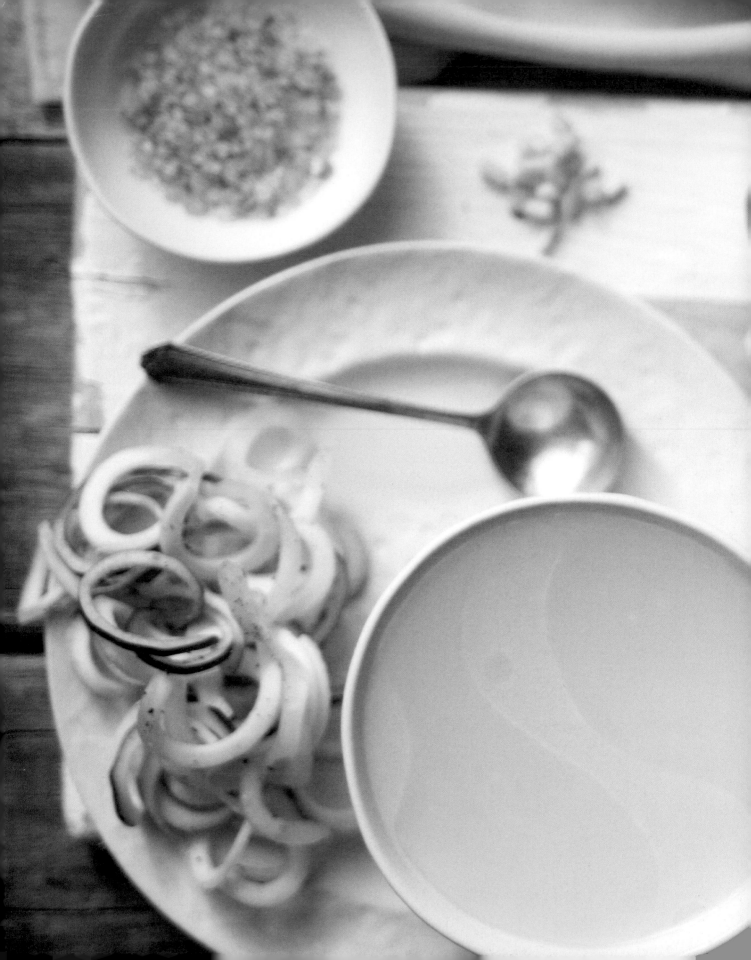

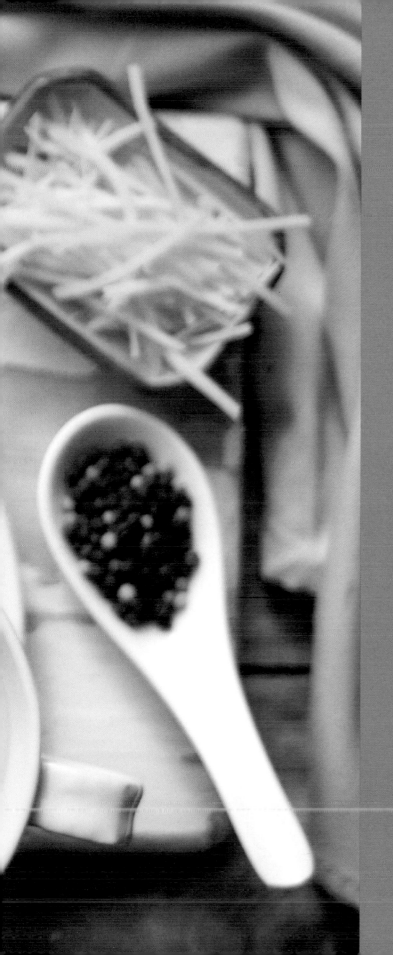

Basics

This chapter is home to the some of my favorite ketogenic sauces and other recipe components. Many of them are building blocks in a ketogenic kitchen that you will find yourself turning to again and again. If you have already started on your ketogenic journey, you may have some of these basics, like bone broth and mayonnaise, under your belt. If you're new to ketogenic cooking, I've collected the basics here for easy access.

Bone Broth:
Beef, Chicken, or Fish

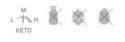

KETO

4 quarts cold water (filtered or reverse-osmosis water is best)

4 large beef bones (about 4 pounds), or leftover bones and skin from 1 pastured chicken (ideally with the feet), or 4 pounds fish bones and head

1 medium onion, chopped

2 stalks celery, sliced ¼ inch thick

2 tablespoons coconut vinegar or apple cider vinegar

2 tablespoons fresh rosemary or other herb of choice

2 teaspoons finely chopped garlic

2 teaspoons fine sea salt

1 teaspoon fresh or dried thyme leaves

Nothing could be easier to make than this broth. Once you get all the ingredients in the slow cooker, it does all the work for you. The longer you cook the broth, the thicker and more nutritious it will get. If you roast the beef bones before making the broth, they will create a darker, more flavorful broth (see note below). You can use this broth to make soups and sauces or drink it as a nourishing beverage.

prep time: 10 minutes   *cook time:* 1 to 3 days

yield: 4 quarts (1 cup per serving)

1. Place all the ingredients in a 6-quart slow cooker. Set the slow cooker to high, then, after 1 hour, turn it down to low. Simmer for a minimum of 1 day and up to 3 days. The longer the broth cooks, the more nutrients and minerals will be extracted from the bones!

2. When the broth is done, pour it through a strainer and discard the solids, but do not skim the fat off the top. The fat makes this broth even more keto-friendly.

3. The broth will keep in the refrigerator for about 5 days or in the freezer for several months.

note: For a richer, more deeply flavored beef broth, roast large beef bones on a rimmed baking sheet at 375°F for 50 to 60 minutes and smaller bones for 30 to 40 minutes.

busy family tip:
Make a double batch in two slow cookers and freeze the broth in freezer-safe mason jars to have on hand as needed.

nutritional info (per serving)				
calories	fat	protein	carbs	fiber
10	2g	0.7g	0.8g	0g

Béarnaise Sauce

I am a sauce lover. That is almost an understatement. In my former life, I would dredge my steaks in ketchup or steak sauce, but there is a ton of sugar in those common staples. I still need my sauces, though, so now I just make my own. For my béarnaise sauce, I wanted that amazing browned butter flavor. Browning the butter is not a prerequisite for this tasty sauce, but like my friend Julie says, anything with browned butter is a game-changer!

KETO

¼ cup (½ stick) unsalted butter

2 tablespoons chopped fresh tarragon leaves

1 shallot, minced

2 tablespoons coconut vinegar or white wine vinegar

6 large egg yolks

Fine sea salt

prep time: 5 minutes   *cook time:* 15 minutes
yield: 1 cup (3 tablespoons per serving)

1. Place the butter in a medium-sized saucepan over high heat. Once the butter is melted, you may skip ahead to Step 2 if you don't want to use browned butter to make the béarnaise. To make browned butter, continue heating the butter until it starts to sizzle. (It will foam up and then fall down.) Watch closely for small brown flecks. As soon as you see these flecks, remove the saucepan from the heat and whisk the butter vigorously. You don't want the specks to turn black—that means it's turned into black butter (which is common in French cuisine, but it just tastes burnt to me).

2. Add the tarragon, shallot, and vinegar to the browned butter and place over medium heat. Simmer for 15 minutes. Remove the pan from the heat and allow the sauce to cool a bit.

3. Place the egg yolks in a blender and turn it to low speed. Slowly pour in the warm (not hot) browned butter mixture in a very slow, steady stream while the blender is running. If you do it too fast, the sauce will break. Taste the sauce and add salt to your liking. Set aside at the back of the stove or other warm spot to keep warm until ready to serve.

4. Store extras in an airtight container in the refrigerator for up to 3 days. Reheat in a double boiler, heating it gently so the sauce doesn't separate.

nutritional info (per serving)				
calories	fat	protein	carbs	fiber
152	14g	4g	2g	0.1

Hollandaise

This is a dairy-free hollandaise, and it's one of my basic sauces that I've used for years. If you have some of my other cookbooks or follow my site, MariaMindBodyHealth.com, you are likely familiar with this recipe. To make a vegetarian version, use avocado oil as the fat. If you're not sensitive to dairy, feel free to use unsalted butter as the fat to create a traditional hollandaise.

1 cup bacon fat, beef tallow, duck fat, or lard (or unsalted butter or ghee if not dairy-sensitive)

4 large egg yolks

½ cup lemon juice

½ teaspoon fine sea salt (more if not using bacon fat)

¼ teaspoon ground black pepper

prep time: 5 minutes   *cook time:* 5 minutes
yield: 1½ cups (about 2 tablespoons per serving)

1. Heat the fat in a small saucepan over high heat (or in the microwave) until very hot and melted. Set aside.

2. Combine the egg yolks and lemon juice in a blender and puree until very smooth. With the blender running on low speed, drizzle in the hot melted fat until a thick, creamy mixture forms. Add the salt and pepper and pulse to combine; adjust the seasoning to taste.

3. Use immediately or keep warm for up to 1 hour in a heat-safe bowl set over a pot of warm water. Store in a covered jar in the fridge for up to 5 days. Reheat in a double boiler or a heat-safe bowl set over a pot of simmering water, whisking often, until it is warm and thick.

variation:

Easy Basil Hollandaise. In Step 2, add 1 cup (1 ounce) loosely packed fresh basil leaves to the blender with the egg yolks and lemon juice. Continue with the recipe as written.

nutritional info (per serving)				
calories	fat	protein	carbs	fiber
175	19g	1g	1g	0.1g

Pizza Sauce

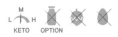

1 cup tomato sauce

3 tablespoons grated Parmesan cheese (or nutritional yeast if dairy-free)

2 tablespoons Swerve confectioners'-style sweetener or equivalent amount of liquid or powdered sweetener (see page 24) (optional)

2 teaspoons Italian seasoning

1 teaspoon garlic powder

¾ teaspoon onion powder

¼ teaspoon ground black pepper

prep time: 7 minutes   *yield:* 1¼ cups (¼ cup per serving)

Place all the ingredients in a small bowl and combine until smooth. Cover and refrigerate until ready to use. Store the sauce in a jar in the refrigerator for up to 5 days.

nutritional info (per serving)				
calories	fat	protein	carbs	fiber
52	3g	4g	3g	1g

Mayonnaise

2 large egg yolks

2 teaspoons lemon juice

1 cup MCT oil or other neutral-flavored oil, such as macadamia nut oil or avocado oil

1 tablespoon Dijon mustard

½ teaspoon fine sea salt

special equipment

Immersion blender

Homemade mayonnaise is so much tastier and healthier than store-bought mayo! You can personalize this basic mayo to your taste by adding garlic paste, roasted garlic, or your favorite herb.

prep time: 5 minutes   *yield:* 1½ cups (about 1 tablespoon per serving)

1. Place the ingredients in the order listed in a wide-mouth, pint-sized mason jar. Place an immersion blender at the bottom of the jar. Turn the blender on and very slowly move it to the top of the jar. Be patient! It should take you about a minute to reach the top. Moving the blender slowly is the key to getting the mayonnaise to emulsify.

2. Store the mayo in a jar in the refrigerator for up to 5 days.

note: To make this mayo nut-free, don't use a nut-based oil.

nutritional info (per serving)				
calories	fat	protein	carbs	fiber
91	10g	0.2g	0.1g	0g

Ranch Dressing

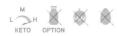

1 (8-ounce) package cream cheese (Kite Hill brand cream cheese style spread if dairy-free), softened

½ cup chicken or beef bone broth, homemade (page 356) or store-bought

½ teaspoon dried chives

½ teaspoon dried dill weed

½ teaspoon dried parsley

¼ teaspoon garlic powder

¼ teaspoon onion powder

⅛ teaspoon fine sea salt

⅛ teaspoon ground black pepper

prep time: 5 minutes, plus 2 hours to chill

yield: 1½ cups (2 tablespoons per serving)

1. In a blender or food processor, mix together all the ingredients until smooth. Cover and refrigerate for 2 hours before serving. (It will thicken up as it rests.)

2. Store the dressing in a jar in the refrigerator for up to 1 week.

nutritional info (per serving)				
calories	fat	protein	carbs	fiber
71	6g	2g	1g	0g

Cilantro Lime Ranch Dressing

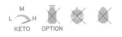

prep time: 5 minutes, plus 2 hours to chill
yield: 2 cups (2 tablespoons per serving)

1 (8-ounce) package cream cheese (Kite Hill brand cream cheese style spread if dairy-free), softened

¾ cup chicken or beef bone broth, homemade (page 356) or store-bought, or more if needed

½ cup fresh cilantro leaves and stems

¼ cup lime juice

½ teaspoon dried chives

½ teaspoon dried parsley

½ teaspoon dried dill weed

¼ teaspoon garlic powder

¼ teaspoon onion powder

⅛ teaspoon fine sea salt

⅛ teaspoon ground black pepper

1. Place all the ingredients in a blender or food processor and puree until smooth. Cover and refrigerate for 2 hours before serving (it will thicken up as it rests). Add more broth if the dressing is too thick.

2. Store the dressing in a jar in the refrigerator for up to 1 week.

nutritional info (per serving)				
calories	fat	protein	carbs	fiber
56	5g	1g	1g	0.1g

The Best Blue Cheese Dressing

prep time: 5 minutes   yield: 2 cups (2 tablespoons per serving)

8 ounces crumbled blue cheese, plus extra if desired for a chunky texture

¼ cup sour cream

¼ cup beef bone broth, homemade (page 356) or store-bought

¼ cup red wine vinegar or coconut vinegar

1½ tablespoons Swerve confectioners'-style sweetener or equivalent amount of liquid or powdered sweetener (see page 24)

1 tablespoon MCT oil

1 clove garlic

1. Place all the ingredients in a food processor and blend until smooth. Transfer to a jar. Stir in extra chunks of blue cheese, if desired.

2. Store the dressing in a jar in the refrigerator for up to 5 days.

nutritional info (per serving)				
calories	fat	protein	carbs	fiber
66	5g	4g	0.2g	0g

Greek Feta Dressing

3 ounces feta cheese

¼ to ½ cup beef or chicken bone broth, homemade (page 356) or store-bought

¼ cup avocado oil, MCT oil, or extra-virgin olive oil

2 tablespoons coconut vinegar

¼ teaspoon minced raw garlic or cloves squeezed from ½ head roasted garlic

1 teaspoon dried oregano leaves

½ teaspoon fine sea salt

prep time: 5 minutes *yield:* ¾ cup (2 tablespoons per serving)

1. Place all the ingredients in a food processor and puree until smooth. If you prefer a thicker dressing, use only ¼ cup of broth. If you prefer a thinner dressing, add up to ¼ cup more broth. Taste and add more salt, if needed.

2. Store the dressing in a jar in the refrigerator for up to 2 weeks.

nutritional info (per serving)				
calories	fat	protein	carbs	fiber
158	16g	3g	1g	0g

Keto Grits

KETO

4 large eggs

¼ cup beef bone broth, homemade (page 356) or store-bought

½ teaspoon fine sea salt

¼ cup (½ stick) unsalted butter

¼ cup shredded sharp cheddar cheese

If you own some of my other cookbooks, you are likely already familiar with these indispensable keto grits. I find that they have a million uses and go with just about any flavor or type of cuisine.

prep time: 2 minutes *cook time:* 4 minutes
yield: 2 servings (¾ cup per serving)

1. To make the grits, whisk together the eggs, broth, and salt in a small bowl. In a medium-sized saucepan, melt the butter over medium heat. Add the egg mixture and cook until the mixture thickens and small curds form, scraping the bottom of the pan and stirring to keep large curds from forming. (A whisk works well for this task.)

2. Once curds have formed and the mixture has thickened, add the shredded cheese and stir until well combined. Remove from the heat and transfer to a serving bowl.

3. Store leftovers in an airtight container in the refrigerator for up to 3 days. Reheat in a sauté pan over medium heat, stirring often, for 3 minutes or until warmed through.

nutritional info (per serving)				
calories	fat	protein	carbs	fiber
405	37g	16g	1g	0g

Keto Buns

These light and fluffy buns are often described as having the texture of Wonder Bread. If you properly whip the whites until very stiff, you will end up with light and airy buns rather than eggy, soufflé-like bread.

It is best to use real eggs and separate the yolks from the whites yourself. Egg whites in a carton do not whip as well.

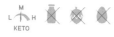

KETO

3 large eggs, separated

½ teaspoon cream of tartar

2 tablespoons unflavored egg white protein powder

prep time: 10 minutes   *cook time:* 15 minutes   *yield:* 6 buns

1. Preheat the oven to 325°F.

2. In a large bowl, whip the egg whites with the cream of tartar for a few minutes until very stiff. Very slowly add the protein powder. Fold the reserved yolks into the whipped whites.

3. Grease a baking sheet. Use a spatula to gently scoop up about ⅓ cup of the dough and place it on the prepared baking sheet. With the spatula, form the dough into either a round hamburger bun, about 3½ inches in diameter, or an oblong hot dog bun, about 6 inches long and 2 inches wide. Repeat with the rest of the dough to make a total of 6 buns.

4. Bake the buns for 15 to 20 minutes, until they are golden brown and cooked through. Let cool completely on the baking sheet before slicing and serving.

5. Store extras in an airtight container in the refrigerator for up to 5 days or in the freezer for up to 2 months.

nutritional info (per bun)				
calories	fat	protein	carbs	fiber
36	2g	4g	0.5g	0g

Cauliflower Rice

KETO

2 cups small cauliflower florets, about 1 inch in size

2 tablespoons coconut oil (or unsalted butter if not dairy-sensitive)

Fine sea salt

prep time: 5 minutes   *cook time:* 5 minutes
yield: 4 servings (½ cup per serving)

1. Place the cauliflower florets in a food processor. Pulse until you have small pieces of "rice." In a skillet, heat the oil. When hot, add the riced cauliflower and cook over medium-low heat for 4 minutes, stirring occasionally, or until the cauliflower is soft but not mushy. Season with salt to taste.

2. Store extras in an airtight container in the refrigerator for up to 3 days. Reheat in a lightly greased sauté pan over medium heat, stirring, for 2 minutes or until warmed through.

tip : You can also use the core of the cauliflower for rice, or you can slice the core into ¼-inch-thick sticks and make Steak Fries (page 131).

nutritional info (per serving)				
calories	fat	protein	carbs	fiber
70	7g	1g	2g	1g

Zoodles—
Two Ways

There's not much more comforting than a bowl of noodles topped with sauce. When made with zucchini or other low-carb vegetables, noodles absolutely can be part of a ketogenic lifestyle.

One of the tricks to making zucchini noodles is to use zucchini that aren't too large. The seeds in a large zucchini can make a mess of your spiral slicer. I look for zucchini that are no larger than 12 inches long and 2 inches wide.

The other trick is to remove some of the water from the zoodles so that your beautiful sauce doesn't become a watery mess when tossed with the zoodles. The two easiest ways to remove the excess water are to salt and drain the raw zoodles (salt draws out water) or to bake them in a low-temperature oven (so that you're essentially dehydrating them).

If you are a visual learner like me and would like to see how zoodles are made, check out the video on my site, MariaMindBodyHealth.com (type the word *video* in the search field).

To increase the ketogenic level to high, toss the zoodles with melted butter or a ketogenic sauce.

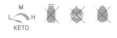

2 medium zucchini, not more than 12 inches long

1 tablespoon fine sea salt (if making salted and drained zoodles)

special equipment

Spiral slicer

prep time: 5 minutes (plus 5 minutes to drain if making salted, raw noodles)
cook time: 20 minutes (if making baked noodles)
yield: 4 servings (1 cup per serving)

1. If making baked zoodles, preheat the oven to 250°F. Place a paper towel on a rimmed baking sheet.

2. To prepare the zucchini for either method: Cut the ends off the zucchini to create nice, even edges. If you desire white noodles, peel the zucchini.

3. Using a spiral slicer, swirl the zucchini into long, thin, noodle-like shapes by gently pressing down on the handle while turning it clockwise.

4. To make baked zoodles: Spread out the zucchini noodles on the paper towel–lined baking sheet and bake for 20 minutes. Serve immediately.

   To make salted and drained noodles: Place the raw zucchini noodles in a colander over the sink and sprinkle with the salt. Allow to sit for 5 minutes, then press to ring out the excess water. Serve immediately.

5. Store leftover zoodles, unsauced, in an airtight container in the refrigerator for up to 5 days. Wait to sauce salted and drained or baked zoodles until ready to serve. (Once sauced, the noodles get a little soggy when stored.) Freezing is not recommended; frozen zoodles tend to get soggy.

busy family tip:
To enjoy zoodles throughout the week, prepare a double or triple batch of raw zoodles by completing Steps 2 and 3 above. Store the raw zoodles in an airtight container in the refrigerator for up to 5 days. Following Step 4 above, bake or salt and drain the amount of zoodles you need just before serving them.

nutritional info (per serving)				
calories	fat	protein	carbs	fiber
18	0.2g	1.4g	3.8g	1.2g

Umami Broth

LESS / KETO / MH

Wondering what you can do with those leftover Parmesan rinds? Here is a great way to use them and add flavor to your soups. Clean the rinds and store them in an airtight container in the freezer until you need them. I like to serve this broth with Zoodles (page 363).

2 or 3 rinds Parmesan cheese, about 3½ inches wide and ½ inch thick, rinsed

Veggies and herbs of choice:

1 pound sliced mushrooms

¼ cup diced onions

2 cloves garlic, minced

2 tablespoons fresh basil, thyme, or other herb of choice

Fine sea salt and ground black pepper

prep time: 5 minutes   *cook time:* 2 hours
yield: 2 quarts (1 cup per serving)

1. Place the Parmesan rinds in a large pot with 8 cups of water.

2. Add any veggies and/or herbs you like. I like to use mushrooms to give the broth more umami flavor.

3. Bring to a boil, then lower the heat to a simmer. Simmer for 2 hours. The longer the broth simmers, the more the flavors will open up. Add salt and pepper to taste. Strain the broth and use it in place of water or other types of broth in your favorite soups, stews, or cauliflower rice or risotto dishes.

4. Store extras in an airtight container in the refrigerator for 4 days or in the freezer for up to 1 month.

nutritional info (per serving)				
calories	fat	protein	carbs	fiber
30	1g	3g	3g	1g

quick reference

H L→M→H KETO   M L→M→H KETO   L L→M→H KETO   • omits this ingredient   O option

RECIPES	PAGE	M L→H KETO	DAIRY FREE	NUT FREE	EGG FREE
Browned Butter Mocha Latte	36	H	O	O	•
Lovers' Omelet	38	H		•	
Quiche Lorraine Dutch Baby	40	H	O	O	
Garlicky Cheddar Biscuits and Gravy	42	H	O		
Creamy Stuffed Blintzes	44	H	O	O	
Flappers	46	H			
Buttery Scones	48	M			
Cinnamon Roll Bread Pudding	50	H	O	O	
Cream Cheese Pumpkin Muffins	52	L	O		
Grandma Suzie's Kringle	54	H			
Sour Cream Coffee Cake with Browned Butter Glaze	56	M			
Tiramisu Muffins	58	H	O	O	
Amazing Breakfast Sausage Bake	60	H		•	•
Monte Cristo Crepes	62	H	O	O	
Chicken and Waffles with Hollandaise	64	H	O	•	
Glazed Chocolate Donuts	66	M	O	O	
Chocolate Donut Bread Pudding	68	H	O	O	
Red Velvet Pancakes with Cream Cheese Syrup	70	H	O	O	
Snickerdoodle Breakfast Pots de Crème	72	H	O	O	
BBQ Pulled Pork Hash with Eggs	74	H	O	•	O
Maple Bacon Waffle Breakfast Sundaes	76	H	O	•	
Croque Madame Waffles	78	H		•	
Sweet Breakfast Biscuits with Chocolate or Caramel Mocha Gravy	80	H			
Crab Cake Eggs Benedict	82	H	O	•	
BLT Party Cheese Ball	86	H		•	•
BLT Stuffed Mushrooms	87	H		•	•
Twice-Baked Mashed Fauxtato Bites	88	L		•	
Bacon Poppers	89	M	O	•	•
Buffalo Chicken Cannoli	90	H		•	•
Loaded Fries with Ranch	92	H		•	
Pizza Fat Bombs	94	H		•	•
Bacon-Wrapped Stuffed Portobellos	95	H		•	•
Loaded Chicken Nachos	96	H		•	•
The Best Browned Butter Cheese Fondue	98	H		•	•
Parmesan Chips	100	H		•	•
Buffalo Chicken Wings with The Best Blue Cheese Dressing	101	H	O	•	•
Baked Brie with Keto Cherry Jelly	102	H			
Spanakopita Flatbread	104	H			
Bacon-Wrapped Stuffed Meatballs	106	H	O	•	
Hush Puppies with Pimiento Mayo	108	H		•	
Seafood Bisque	112	H	O	•	•
Clam Chowder	114	M	O	•	•
Chicken "Wild Rice" Soup	116	H	O	•	•
Cream of Chicken Soup	118	H	O	•	•
Mushroom Truffle Bisque	119	H	O	•	•
Fauxtato Leek Soup	120	M	O	•	•
Beef Stew	122	M	•	•	•
Slow Cooker Chipotle Lime Steak Soup	123	M	O	•	•
Italian Sausage Soup	124	M	O	•	•
Philly Cheesesteak Soup	126	H	O	•	•
Warm Goat Cheese Salad with Bacon Vinaigrette	128	H		O	•
Mashed Fauxtatoes	129	L		•	•
Roasted Cauliflower with Béarnaise Sauce	130	L		•	
Steak Fries	131	H		•	
Brussels Sprouts with Soft-Boiled Eggs and Avocado	132	L	O	O	O
Yorkshire Pudding	134	H	•	O	
Roasted Asparagus with Poached Eggs and Hollandaise	136	M	O	•	

RECIPES	PAGE	KETO	DAIRY FREE	NUT FREE	EGG FREE
Zucchini and Bacon Gratin	138	M		•	•
"Cornbread" Muffins	139	H	O		
Stuffing Cupcakes	140	H	O	•	
Creamed Collards with Browned Butter and Bacon	142	L	O	•	•
Scalloped Fauxtatoes with Bacon, Leeks, and Gruyère	144	H		•	•
Pimiento Cheese Muffins	146	M			
Cordon Bleu Lasagna	150	H		•	•
Poulet Grand-Mère	152	H	O	•	•
Chicken and Gravy Cobbler	154	H	O		
Lemon Pepper Roast Turkey with Bacon Gravy	156	H		•	
Turkey Tetrazzini	158	H		•	
Skillet Enchilada Casserole	160	H		•	
Turkey Meatloaf Cupcakes	162	M		•	
Saucy Crispy Chicken	164	H		•	
Braised Turkey Legs with Creamy Gravy	166	M		•	
Chicken Club Hand Pies	168	H			
Fried Chicken with Cheesy Grits	170	H		•	
Chicken Divan	172	H		•	
Smothered Fried Cabin Chicken	174	H	O	•	
Shredded Amish Chicken and Gravy	176	L	O	O	O
BBQ Chicken Lasagna	178	M		•	•
Turkey Goulash Over Mashed Fauxtatoes	180	L		•	•
Red Curry Chicken Over Cauliflower Rice	182	L	O	•	•
Herb Roasted Chicken	184	H	•	•	•
Chicken Cordon Bleu	186	H		•	•
Slow Cooker Creamy Picante Chicken	188	L	O	•	•
Buffalo Chicken Casserole	190	M	O	•	•
Duck à l'Orange	192	H		•	•
Braised Duck Legs with Bacon and Mushrooms	194	H		•	•
Chicken Pot Pies	196	H			
Sunday Supper Pot Roast Over Mashed Fauxtatoes	200	H	O	•	•
Skillet Moussaka	202	M		•	
Philly Cheesesteak Cupcakes	204	H		•	
Gyro Loaf with Tzatziki Sauce	206	H		•	
Joe's Special	208	H	O	•	
Meatloaf Cordon Bleu	209	H		•	
Steak Frites with Béarnaise Sauce	210	H	O	•	O
Rib-Eye Steak with Asparagus Puree and Bacon Custard	212	H		•	
Filet Mignons Florentine	214	H	•		•
Meatballs with Brown Gravy	216	H	O	•	
Steak with Blue Cheese Whip	218	H		•	
Perfect Reverse-Sear Prime Rib with Tiger Sauce	220	H		•	
Greek Burgers with Feta Dressing	222	H		•	
Country-Fried Steak and Gravy	224	M	O	•	
Taco Pizza	226	M			
Pizza Supreme	228	M			
French Dip Sandwiches	230	H		•	
Garlic and Rosemary Rack of Lamb	232	H	O	•	•
Shrimp Thermidor	236	H		•	
Walleye Simmered in Basil Cream	238	H	O	•	
Cheesy Tuna Casserole	240	H	O	•	
Charleston Shrimp 'n' Gravy Over Grits	242	H		•	
Seafood Risotto	244	M		•	
Surf and Turf for Two	245	H	•	•	
Crawfish Étouffée	246	H	O	•	
Halibut Smothered in Creamy Lemon-Dill Sauce	248	H	O	•	•
Sole Meunière	250	H		•	•
Creole Catfish	252	L	O	•	•
Butter-Poached Lobster Tails Over Creamy Keto Risotto	254	H		•	
BBQ Pulled Pork Sandwiches with Wilted Bacon Slaw	258	H	O	•	
Saucy Stuffed Cabbage Rolls	260	L	O	•	
Schnitzel	262	H	O	•	

RECIPES	PAGE	KETO (L-M-H)	DAIRY FREE	NUT FREE	EGG FREE
Smothered Pork Chops in Mushroom and Onion Gravy	264	M	O	•	•
Ham 'n' Grits with Redeye Gravy	265	H		•	•
Pork and Cheddar Sausages	266	H		•	•
Bangers and Mash with Onion Gravy	268	L		•	•
Crispy Pork Belly Over Grits with Bacon Jam	270	H		•	
Creamy Cajun Pasta	272	H		•	•
Bomba Burgers	276	H			
Hot Beef Sundaes	278	H		•	•
Grilled Cheese Waffles and Tomato Gorgonzola Bisque	280	H		•	
Cheeseburger Soup	282	H		•	•
Chili Cheese Dog Casserole	284	M		•	•
Pizza Waffles	286	H		•	
Chicken Parmesan Mini Meatloaves	288	H	O	•	
Ham 'n' Cheese Cones	290	H		•	
Chili Dogs	292	H	O	•	•
Deconstructed Bacon Cheeseburger Pizza	294	H			•
Italian Cream Soda	298	H	O	•	•
Persian Hot Chocolate	300	M	O	O	•
Pumpkin Dip with Pie Fries	302	M		O	
Malted Milk Ball Bûche de Noël	304	L	O		•
Gâteau au Chocolat	306	H	O	•	
Pots de Crème	308	M	O	O	
Deconstructed Chocolate Cannoli Cookies	309	M	O		
Death by Chocolate Cheesecake	310	L	O	O	
French Silk Ice Cream	312	H	•	O	
"Keto Debbie" Chocolate Cupcakes	314	H	O		
Penuche (Italian Fudge)	316	H		O	•
Peaches and Cream Sorbet	317	H	O	•	•
Chocolate Ice Cream Cake with Almond Butter Swirl	318	M	O	O	
Deconstructed Chocolate Waffle Cones	320	H	O	O	
Maple Bacon Ice Cream in Bacon Cones	322	H	O	O	
Strawberries and Cream Snowballs	324	M			
Malted Milk Ball Cheesecake	326	M	O	•	
Cannoli Mini Cheese Balls	328	H	O	O	•
Mini Mocha Bundt Cakes	330	M	O		
Mint Chocolate Whoopie Pies	332	H			
Mint Chocolate Cheesecake Bûche de Noël	334	H			
Decadent Black Forest Dessert for Two	336	H	O		
"Rice" Pudding	338	H	O	O	
Creamy Chocolate Mint Truffles	340	H	O	O	•
Malted Milk Ball Truffles	342	M	O	O	•
Pecan Pie Truffles	344	H			•
Dark Chocolate Raspberry Truffles	346	H	O	O	•
Pumpkin Cheesecake Truffles	348	H	O		
Bananas Foster for Two	350	H	O		
Banana Cream Pie	352	H	O		
Bone Broth: Beef, Chicken, or Fish	356	M	•	•	•
Béarnaise Sauce	357	H		•	
Hollandaise	358	H	•	•	
Pizza Sauce	358	M	O	•	•
Mayonnaise	359	H	•	O	
Ranch Dressing	359	H	O	•	•
Cilantro Lime Ranch Dressing	360	H	O	•	•
The Best Blue Cheese Dressing	360	H		•	
Greek Feta Dressing	361	H		•	
Keto Grits	361	H		•	
Keto Buns	362	H	•	•	
Cauliflower Rice	362	M	•	•	•
Zoodles—Two Ways	363	L	•	•	•
Umami Broth	364	L		•	•

recipe index

Breakfast

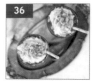
36
Browned Butter Mocha Latte

38
Lovers' Omelet

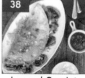
40
Quiche Lorraine Dutch Baby

42
Garlicky Cheddar Biscuits and Gravy

44
Creamy Stuffed Blintzes

46
Flappers

48
Buttery Scones

50
Cinnamon Roll Bread Pudding

52
Cream Cheese Pumpkin Muffins

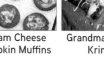
54
Grandma Suzie's Kringle

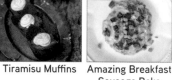
56
Sour Cream Coffee Cake with Browned Butter Glaze

58
Tiramisu Muffins

60
Amazing Breakfast Sausage Bake

62
Monte Cristo Crepes

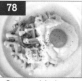
64
Chicken and Waffles with Hollandaise

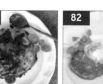
66
Glazed Chocolate Donuts

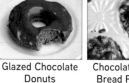
68
Chocolate Donut Bread Pudding

70
Red Velvet Pancakes with Cream Cheese Syrup

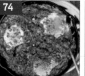
72
Snickerdoodle Breakfast Pots de Crème

74
BBQ Pulled Pork Hash with Eggs

76
Maple Bacon Waffle Breakfast Sundaes

78
Croque Madame Waffles

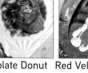
80
Sweet Breakfast Biscuits with Chocolate or Caramel Mocha Gravy

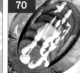
82
Crab Cake Eggs Benedict

Appetizers and Snacks

86
BLT Party Cheese Ball

87
BLT Stuffed Mushrooms

88
Twice-Baked Mashed Fauxtato Bites

89
Bacon Poppers

90
Buffalo Chicken Cannoli

92
Loaded Fries with Ranch

94
Pizza Fat Bombs

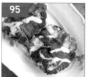
95
Bacon-Wrapped Stuffed Portobellos

96
Loaded Chicken Nachos

98
The Best Browned Butter Cheese Fondue

100
Parmesan Chips

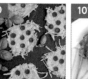
101
Buffalo Chicken Wings

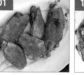
102
Baked Brie with Keto Cherry Jelly

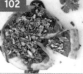
104
Spanakopita Flatbread

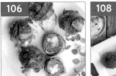
106

108

Bacon-Wrapped
Stuffed Meatballs

Hush Puppies
with Pimiento
Mayo

Soups, Salads, and Sides

112

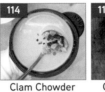
114

116

118

119

120

122

Seafood Bisque

Clam Chowder

Chicken "Wild
Rice" Soup

Cream of Chicken
Soup

Mushroom Truffle
Bisque

Fauxtato Leek
Soup

Beef Stew

123

124

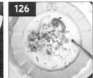
126

128

129

130

131

Slow Cooker
Chipotle Lime
Steak Soup

Italian Sausage
Soup

Philly Cheesesteak
Soup

Warm Goat
Cheese Salad with
Bacon Vinaigrette

Mashed
Fauxtatoes

Roasted
Cauliflower with
Béarnaise Sauce

Steak Fries

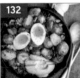
132

134

136

138

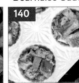
139

140

142

Brussels Sprouts
with Soft-Boiled
Eggs and Avocado

Yorkshire Pudding

Roasted Asparagus
with Poached Eggs
and Hollandaise

Zucchini and
Bacon Gratin

"Cornbread"
Muffins

Stuffing Cupcakes

Creamed Collards
with Browned
Butter and Bacon

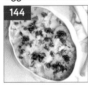
144

146

Scalloped
Fauxtatoes with
Bacon, Leeks, and
Gruyère

Pimiento Cheese
Muffins

Main Dishes: Poultry

150

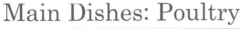
152

154

156

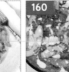
158

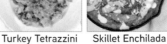
160

162

Cordon Bleu
Lasagna

Poulet Grand-Mère

Chicken and Gravy
Cobbler

Lemon Pepper
Roast Turkey with
Bacon Gravy

Turkey Tetrazzini

Skillet Enchilada
Casserole

Turkey Meatloaf
Cupcakes

Maria Emmerich 369

164
Saucy Crispy
Chicken

166
Braised Turkey
Legs with
Creamy Gravy

168
Chicken Club
Hand Pies

 170
Fried Chicken
with Cheesy Grits

172
Chicken Divan

 174
Smothered Fried
Cabin Chicken

176
Shredded Amish
Chicken and Gravy

 178
BBQ Chicken
Lasagna

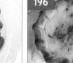 **180**
Turkey Goulash
Over Mashed
Fauxtatoes

182
Red Curry Chicken
Over Cauliflower
Rice

184
Herb Roasted
Chicken

186
Chicken Cordon
Bleu

188
Slow Cooker
Creamy Picante
Chicken

190
Buffalo Chicken
Casserole

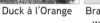 **192**
Duck à l'Orange

 194
Braised Duck Legs
with Bacon and
Mushrooms

196
Chicken Pot Pies

Main Dishes: Beef and Lamb

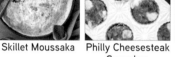 **200**
Sunday Supper
Pot Roast Over
Mashed Fauxtatoes

202
Skillet Moussaka

 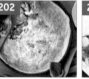 **204**
Philly Cheesesteak
Cupcakes

 206
Gyro Loaf with
Tzatziki Sauce

208
Joe's Special

209
Meatloaf
Cordon Bleu

210
Steak Frites with
Béarnaise Sauce

 212
Rib-Eye Steak with
Asparagus Puree and
Bacon Custard

 214
Filet Mignons
Florentine

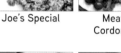 **216**
Meatballs with
Brown Gravy

 218
Steak with Blue
Cheese Whip

 220
Perfect Reverse-
Sear Prime Rib
with Tiger Sauce

222
Greek Burgers
with Feta Dressing

 224
Country-Fried
Steak and Gravy

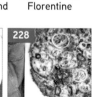 **226**
Taco Pizza

 228
Pizza Supreme

 230
French Dip
Sandwiches

232
Garlic and
Rosemary
Rack of Lamb

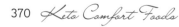

Main Dishes: Fish and Seafood

 236
Shrimp Thermidor

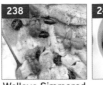 238
Walleye Simmered in Basil Cream

 240
Cheesy Tuna Casserole

 242
Charleston Shrimp 'n' Gravy Over Grits

 244
Seafood Risotto

 245
Surf and Turf for Two

246
Crawfish Étouffée

 248
Halibut Smothered in Creamy Lemon-Dill Sauce

 250
Sole Meunière

 252
Creole Catfish

 254
Butter-Poached Lobster Tails Over Creamy Keto Risotto

Main Dishes: Pork

 258
BBQ Pulled Pork Sandwiches with Wilted Bacon Slaw

 260
Saucy Stuffed Cabbage Rolls

262
Schnitzel

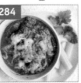 264
Smothered Pork Chops in Mushroom and Onion Gravy

 265
Ham 'n' Grits with Redeye Gravy

266
Pork and Cheddar Sausages

 268
Bangers and Mash with Onion Gravy

270
Crispy Pork Belly Over Grits with Bacon Jam

272
Creamy Cajun Pasta

Comfort Food Favorites for Grown-up Kids

 276
Bomba Burgers

278
Hot Beef Sundaes

280
Grilled Cheese Waffles and Tomato Gorgonzola Bisque

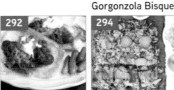 282
Cheeseburger Soup

284
Chili Cheese Dog Casserole

286
Pizza Waffles

288
Chicken Parmesan Mini Meatloaves

290
Ham 'n' Cheese Cones

 292
Chili Dogs

294
Deconstructed Bacon Cheeseburger Pizza

Sweet Endings

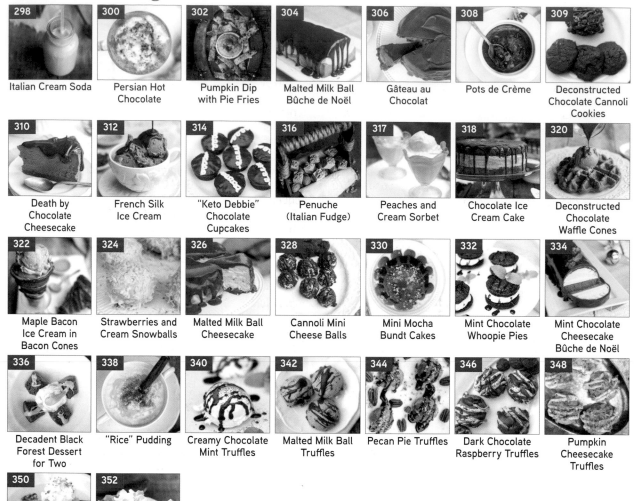

298 Italian Cream Soda

300 Persian Hot Chocolate

302 Pumpkin Dip with Pie Fries

304 Malted Milk Ball Bûche de Noël

306 Gâteau au Chocolat

308 Pots de Crème

309 Deconstructed Chocolate Cannoli Cookies

310 Death by Chocolate Cheesecake

312 French Silk Ice Cream

314 "Keto Debbie" Chocolate Cupcakes

316 Penuche (Italian Fudge)

317 Peaches and Cream Sorbet

318 Chocolate Ice Cream Cake

320 Deconstructed Chocolate Waffle Cones

322 Maple Bacon Ice Cream in Bacon Cones

324 Strawberries and Cream Snowballs

326 Malted Milk Ball Cheesecake

328 Cannoli Mini Cheese Balls

330 Mini Mocha Bundt Cakes

332 Mint Chocolate Whoopie Pies

334 Mint Chocolate Cheesecake Bûche de Noël

336 Decadent Black Forest Dessert for Two

338 "Rice" Pudding

340 Creamy Chocolate Mint Truffles

342 Malted Milk Ball Truffles

344 Pecan Pie Truffles

346 Dark Chocolate Raspberry Truffles

348 Pumpkin Cheesecake Truffles

350 Bananas Foster for Two

352 Banana Cream Pie

Other Books by Maria Emmerich

The Ketogenic Cookbook

Quick & Easy Ketogenic Cooking

The 30-Day Ketogenic Cleanse

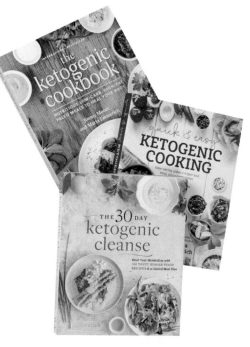

general index

gratitude

If you weren't aware already, I am a huge Green Bay Packers fan. You could call me a cheesehead. If you love football like I do, you know that it takes a whole team to create champions, even though the quarterback often gets most of the credit. I am honored to be the quarterback of this book; however, it took a whole team to create such a champion.

The quarterback often buys the offensive line special gifts to show his gratitude for a successful and safe season, and I would like to take a moment to thank my team for such an amazing book.

If I had to break down my team, I would have to thank our coach, Erich, who calls me even on Sunday afternoons just to check in and say, "Hi!" And offensive line coach, Lance, who always keeps me updated on the latest.

I want to thank my "center," marketing and sales, which is Susan and the sales team at Victory Belt.

The "guards" on my team were my amazingly talented editors, Holly and Pam, who have the most spectacular eyes for detail and make the recipes (our "plays") read smoothly.

My "tackles" would be Bill and Haley, who helped create such a beautiful cover for my book!

My "running backs" are my recipe testers, to whom I can "hand off" recipes to test with their families and make sure every recipe is extra-tasty. Thank you, Wendy and Kristie, for tackling the intense job of testing my recipes.

My "draft scout," Jimmy Moore, introduced me to Victory Belt years ago and is my coauthor on the international bestselling book *The Ketogenic Cookbook*.

And I couldn't forget to mention my fans in the stands. This means all of you who cheer me on through the thick of it. Without you filling the stadium and cheering for keto, I wouldn't be able to do what I do. I can't thank you all enough.

Lastly, I couldn't be more blessed to have such an amazing husband, Craig, who never complains about the messes I make in the kitchen, even an hour after he cleaned it, as well as my sons, Micah and Kai, who are brutally honest when it comes to taste-testing. I love you all so much!